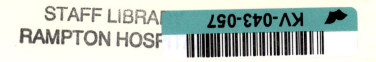
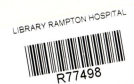

HOW THE BRITISH NATIONAL HEALTH SERVICE DEALS WITH DIVERSITY

HOW THE BRITISH NATIONAL HEALTH SERVICE DEALS WITH DIVERSITY

Professional Problems, Patient Problems

Nick Johns

The Edwin Mellen Press
Lewiston•Queenston•Lampeter

Library of Congress Cataloging-in-Publication Data

Johns, Nick (Nicolas)
    How the British national health service deals with diversity : professional problems,
patient problems / Nick Johns.
        p. cm.
    Includes bibliographical references and index.
    ISBN-13: 978-0-7734-5733-1
    ISBN-10: 0-7734-5733-X
    I. Title.

hors série.

A CIP catalog record for this book is available from the British Library.

The Edwin Mellen Press   The Edwin Mellen Press
        Box 450   Box 67
Lewiston, New York   Queenston, Ontario
    USA 14092-0450   CANADA L0S 1L0

The Edwin Mellen Press, Ltd.
Lampeter, Ceredigion, Wales
UNITED KINGDOM SA48 8LT

Printed in the United States of America

For Heather, Ben and the baby, my reasons for hoping for a better world

TABLE OF CONTENTS

Chapter 3 – Institutional racism in the NHS

Section Two – Improving service provision to minority ethnic communities

Chapter 4 - The internal market

Chapter 5 – Minding our language

LIST OF CHARTS AND TABLES

Charts

Tables

PREFACE

This book is a very timely contribution to the urgent debate taking place in the United Kingdom about equal opportunities, diversity and multiculturalism. It reveals the confusions and contradictions at the heart of employment and service delivery policies in the National Health Service (NHS), long seen as a pioneer in all these fields. Based on thorough scholarship and research, it offers a new way forward on pressing issues.

Since the New Labour government came to power in 1997, ministers have confidently pursued a programme to combine New Managerialism, choice for 'customers' and social inclusion in the public services. This assumes that the potential tensions between autonomous, mobile individuals in the mainstream seeking competitive advantage over health, education and social care, and policies for community cohesion in disadvantaged districts, can be reconciled. The research on which this book is based reveals worrying discrepancies between the perceptions of (predominantly white) managers and professionals in the NHS, and those of minority ethnic service-user representatives.

It was a founding assumption of the NHS that the interactions between staff of public agencies and service users would consolidate democratic and egalitarian citizenship. But the basis for that citizenship is itself now contested. Although the aspiration for diversity in staffing (including management) was shared by all respondents in this research, as was the belief that this would improve services to minorities, in practice it was neglected in favour of other priorities.

Nick Johns shows that the persistence of cultures of professional exclusion, blaming and stereotyping in the NHS is complex and multi-layered. Partly it is related to ideas about 'equal treatment' – that no group should be favoured over any other. Partly it reflects structural factors, where the ethos and location of hospitals and clinics effectively discriminate against recruitment from minorities. But most subtly, efficiency-driven criteria for service organisations do not allow the special contribution of staff from minority communities to be recognised and valued. Hence many of the needs of these groups of patients go unmet.

He reviews the theoretical literature on equal opportunities and diversity, and policy measures to implement the various principles, which are interestingly reflected in the research interviews. He concludes with an assessment of new initiatives associated with 'managing diversity'; these have particularly attracted human resources managers in the NHS.

I commend this book for its contribution to the debate about public services, as the context for citizenship and civic culture in the United Kingdom. But it is also of great value to the wider discussion of how diversity can be seen as a strength in our society, and how our institutions can encompass equality and difference.

Bill Jordan
Professor of Social Policy,
University of Huddersfield

ACKNOWLEDGEMENTS

I would like to acknowledge the overwhelming majority of NHS staff who do an incredibly difficult job in testing circumstances, and particularly those from minority ethnic backgrounds whose contributions have not always been recognised much less rewarded. From the perspective of the book I would like most of all to thank those who took part in the study in whatever capacity, but the respondents especially without whose time and effort nothing could have been achieved. I would also like to thank the University of Plymouth for its financial support during the development and fulfilment of this project.

On a personal and professional level I would like to thank a number of colleagues and friends. First, to Daniel Gilling for his advice and assistance at a critical phase in the research, it was much appreciated. Thanks are also due to Paul Iganski who got the ball rolling and showed me the way to proceed. For giving me a kick when I needed it I would like to thank Mike Sheppard – I needed to be told that it could be and indeed had to be finished. Finally, my deepest appreciation goes to Reggie and Mel for the horror and the laughs.

Ultimately I have to acknowledge my family. Thanks are due to my Mum for her help and love and the same to Lin, who sadly never got to see the project completed. But the biggest thanks must go to my wife Heather, my sons Ben and Matthew, none of this would matter, important though the issues are, if I didn't have you.

CHAPTER 1

Setting the scene

Introduction

The purpose of this introductory chapter is to set the background for the book. In the first instance the background and structure will be explained. The project began life as an investigation of the possible justification for the use of positive discrimination to improve the position of minority ethnic communities. Due to the modified version of 'grounded theory' employed, modified in the sense that it was not possible to undertake the research free from any preconceived ideas, the emphasis rapidly tilted towards ethnic diversity and its practical implications. The book has three sections, and ten chapters the content of the remainder of which will be set out individually below. The bulk of this chapter is devoted to a discussion about the methods adopted and to explaining some of its more unusual features and limitations.

Background and structure

In view of the substantial evidence available (Ahmad 1993a; Modood *et al* 1997; Alexander 1999; Mason 2000; Parekh 2000), it is reasonable to suggest that minority ethnic communities are relatively disadvantaged compared to their white counterparts on a number of indices. Although it must be recognised that terms such as ethnicity are disputed and that experiences are diverse within and between minority groups (Modood *et al* 1997; Iganski & Payne 1999; Sly *et al* 1999), this does not diminish the importance of the overall patterns identified. Furthermore, 'race relations' has gained a significant profile in public debate recently as the election was fought on the basis of immigration issues to a large extent and little was done to separate asylum from immigration, or to challenge the assumption that immigrant means visible minority (Alibhai-Brown 2005a). This appears to have an electoral trend, as prior to the 2001 election a poll conducted by MORI and commissioned by the United Nations Population Fund indicated that 'race relations' and immigration rated fourth on a list of major concerns for Britain: *'Worries about race relations and immigration have risen from 3% in 1996, to 19% now'* (www.mori.com/polls/2001/unfpa.shtml). This might mean, as the Commission for Racial Equality (CRE) pointed out, that awareness grew rather than hostility, however, in light of the persistence of the Labour government to follow in the footsteps of their predecessors in balancing tough immigration policies with extended legislation (Lester 1998; Branigan 2001a), this seems unlikely.

One potential means of improving the position of minority ethnic people in employment, and therefore in the longer-term in other areas of life has been to positively discriminate in their favour. Although this is unlawful under the provisions of the Race Relations Act 1976 (amended in 2000) there have been examples of its successful use in other countries (i.e. the USA and South Africa[1]). Furthermore it was used by Labour to increase the numbers of women in Parliament prior to the 1997 general election (Brasher 1996) though it was subsequently judged to be unlawful and struck down (Branigan 2001b; Russell 2001). Perhaps it should not be surprising that there are renewed calls for its use, particularly for minority ethnic communities (Hattersley 1997; Dodd 2004).

This project started life as an exploration of the justifications for positive discrimination on behalf of minority ethnic communities, in short, whether it

---

[1] Although both its existence and success in the context of the United States are vigorously debated, see Edwards (1995) and Glazer (1998).

could ever be justified. Consistent with the methodological approach adopted here it grew substantially away from that starting point. The current buzzword in relation to matters of equality of opportunity is 'diversity' and it is in this direction that there has been a seismic shift of late. Despite the inherently inclusive implications of diversity, I have chosen to concentrate on 'ethnic diversity'. Although other aspects of identity are considered whenever appropriate, as Bagilhole has argued: *'There are...stages when one source of disadvantage needs to be separated out so that it can be given due attention'* (1997: 1). This narrower focus has been lent more legitimacy by the recent developments in public policy in relation to the needs and interests of minority ethnic communities. The Labour government since its election in 1997 has stressed the need to increase ethnic diversity in the public sector workforce, for various reasons, some explicit, others less so, which will be dealt with below. Consequently this project is about ethnic diversity and its practical implications.

However, as Dreachslin *et al* (2004) have argued albeit from an American point of view that it is important to be clear about the levels and context when writing about issues of ethnic diversity. From their point of view there are essentially three levels worthy of consideration. The first relates to public policy and the macro-political context. Joppke (2004) for instance has written about ethnic diversity and state policies. The next level is the organisational level, and the one below that the micro level (in their area this relates to clinical competence). The authors maintain that there is a significant deficit written about ethnic diversity and organisational behaviour when compared to public policy and everyday practice. This book seeks to address that gap by placing the everyday practice issues within their organisational context.

In order to ground the research into a policy context it was sited within the National Health Service (NHS), and the issues are explored through the *perceptions* of various actors involved either in the provision of health care, or, given the importance attributed to employment issues, in the operation of personnel policies. A national mail survey of NHS trusts was carried out targeting

Personnel Directors, to gauge the progress of equal opportunities policies, and, to a lesser extent, to evaluate their understanding of ethnic diversity.

To complement this, an in-depth interview survey, taking the form of a case study, was carried out in a major city in the south west (hereafter called Robbinston) with various actors involved in the provision of health care. The region has a minority ethnic population of 2.8%, but areas with 25% or more during the period of data collection (OPCS 1993). It is usual for case studies to provide a significant amount of background information on the area in which the research has been carried out. Unfortunately, this level of information cannot be reproduced here because the region in which the city is located is not ethnically diverse and would be immediately recognisable. Anonymity was promised to the interview respondents, and was also part of the assurances made to satisfy the rigorous ethical clearance procedure conducted by the University of Plymouth. Therefore, despite the fact that this might undermine to some extent the claims towards a case study approach, it is nevertheless unavoidable. The research methods and its limitations and those of the study generally are outlined more fully below.

This book has three sections. The first and second utilise the data gathered via the interview survey, whilst the third is constructed from material also gathered via the questionnaire survey. The first section concentrates on the quality of care provided to minority ethnic communities. Although it is readily acknowledged that *'Any attempts to understand the lives of black people in Britain must incorporate an historical perspective. [T]he history of British imperialism and legislation constraining immigration forms the backcloth against which contemporary race relations are acted out'* (Donovan 1986a: 3), I do not intend to provide such a history of immigration and legislation here, since it has already been covered well by Donovan (1986a), Baxter (1988), Gerrish *et al* (1996), Jordan & Düvell (2003) and others.

Instead, chapter 2 focuses on communication barriers, defined as a combination of language and cultural barriers that influence the willingness of minority ethnic individuals to approach the NHS and the quality of provision they receive if and when they do so (for a definition of culture, as it is used in this book, see the glossary at Appendix 1). Although authors such as Bhopal and White (1993) have criticised the tendency to emphasise communication problems at the expense of other pressing health issues, it was the main area of concern of the respondents, supported by a consultation document provided by the local health authority (HA). The evidence suggests that communication remains highly problematic for certain sections of society, that the consequences can be distressing, even dangerous, and that this may not be adequately recognised by those responsible for providing and administering local services

Chapter 3 is devoted to the question of discrimination. Does 'racial' discrimination influence the treatment of minority ethnic people in relation to health provision? An enormous amount of evidence suggests that this has been an on-going problem for society, and the evidence presented here supports this. Furthermore it seems that the MacPherson (1999) report – argued by many to be a seminal point in British 'race' relations (Johns 1999; McLaughlin & Murji 1999; Parekh 2000) – provides the overarching context in which discrimination and racism are challenged and defended. In line with the wider debates those who work in the NHS generally feel that MacPherson went too far, while those representing the needs of users generally believe that it did not go far enough. The latter mostly view the failures outlined in chapter 2 as the result of what may best be described as direct institutional discrimination.

Section 2 then is devoted to the issue of policy. What can or should be done to overcome any problems in terms of provision? It contains three chapters, primarily focusing on Robbinston although the first is national in scope. Chapter 4 concentrates on the post-1991 reforms (DoH 1990), which were meant to introduce market discipline into the NHS. This was allegedly undertaken in the interests of economy, efficiency and efficacy, but there were specific elements which were predicted to have real potential for improving services to minority ethnic communities (Hopkins & Bahl 1993). This was explored with the interview respondents, and the outcome supports the bulk of the available evidence. It seems that the potential was never realised, and further, that the movement towards Primary Care Groups (PCGs) (DoH 1997), which was happening during the interview survey, would be equally disappointing.

The remaining chapters are locally specific and relate very much to the consultation exercise that was conducted by the HA with local minority ethnic communities. Several things were demanded and corresponding policy promises were made. Chapter 5 concentrates specifically on measures taken to address the problem of language barriers and chapter 6 on attempts to deal with cultural gaps between white health professionals and minority ethnic users, particularly cultural awareness training (CAT). The section underlines the lack of commitment in the region to going beyond a nominal involvement of users and making promises that some considered unlikely to be kept. Furthermore, even if the HA fulfilled or was likely to fulfil its promises it is questionable whether significant improvements would result.

Section 3 forms the backbone of the project devoted as it is to the issues of greater ethnic diversity. There is a widespread assumption shared by the Labour government that achieving greater diversity in general and ethnic diversity in particular within important social institutions would naturally improve the service provided. Chapter 7 sets out the development of this argument and attempts to go further than mere assumptions by trying to ascertain what is meant by ethnic diversity and how it will work in practice. If the respondents of this research are in any way representative it would appear that either it has not been thought through, or, that it is a deliberate attempt to place the burden of responsibility onto minority ethnic communities themselves.

The eighth chapter moves on to consider the best means of achieving ethnic diversity, and specifically the current strategy of the Labour government. This appears to involve mainstreaming 'race' equality issues and regaining centralised control over human resource functions (Carter 2000). Positive action widely viewed as the most radical of lawful equal opportunities activity, has been feted as an essential component in the achievement of ethnic diversity (Baxter 1997; Iganski *et al* 1998; Parekh 2000). Yet doubts have been expressed about the degree of high level commitment to the practice (Iganksi *et al* 2001), although with the raft of measures instituted since the research was conducted this may now be changing. Nevertheless, existing research evidence suggests that this will be resisted (Kandola & Fullerton 1998) and again the research findings presented here support this. In fact, the chapter suggests that a massive paradox exists in which those making everyday employment decisions are both more conservative and more radical than the government. The central problem appears to be (theoretical) individualism and how to overcome it.

Chapter 9 charts the course of a fairly new development in equality theory, managing diversity, which appears to have gained some ground in the personnel function of the NHS. Here we will consider what it means from the perspective of Kandola *et al* (1994, 1995, 1998) and chart its progress and impact in the UK. Although its progress is apparently measured in the labour market *per se* the evidence presented here suggests that its individualistic emphasis might appeal more readily to those making day-to-day employment decisions in the NHS. Furthermore, those who would seem to be natural allies of the government, i.e. Human Resource Directors and personnel professionals (Carter 2000) may prove resistant to any attempt to engage in positive action measures, having already bought into the rhetoric of managing diversity. Ultimately, the central theme of the research is that where services fail minority ethnic communities are apparently to be made implicitly responsible for any improvements or ultimately blamed when improvements prove elusive (as they unquestionably will without immediate and radical action). Before we move on, it is necessary to set out the research methods and discuss the limitations to the findings.

Research Methods

Having outlined the shape of the book and highlighted some themes for further investigation, it is necessary to set out the methods employed to first gather and then analyse the data. This section then is divided into three main parts. The first describes the principal aims and objectives of the research and explains how they informed the construction of the overall project design. Having explained why each method was used, the second section describes the processes involved in conducting the postal survey: the sampling strategy, the development and administration of the questionnaire; the response rate; and the method of data analysis. Similarly, the third section recounts the process of organising interviews for the case study: sampling; response rates; schedule development; interview procedures; and how the data was analysed.

Aims and objectives

As can be readily divined concerns as to the quality of service provided to minority ethnic communities abound in the available literature (Smaje 1995; Law 1996; Mason 2000). This research project was designed to investigate how these concerns have been addressed, focusing specifically upon the deliberate diversification of the workforce. To do this effectively a dual strategy was considered the most appropriate. The first part of the strategy was devised in order to gain some idea of the progress Health Service providers (i.e. NHS trusts) had made in adopting and implementing equal opportunities policies, and to solicit the attitudes and opinions of those responsible for personnel matters about the notion of ethnic diversity and about possible methods of its achievement. It was decided that the only way of presenting a comprehensive enough picture was to organise and distribute a postal questionnaire. The aims of this were to:

- Identify the activity of health care providers in the UK in the context of equality of opportunity.

- Assess the attitudes and opinions of personnel professionals about the notion of diversity, and;

- Tentatively explore their views about the best way of achieving diversity - emphasising the notions of positive action and positive discrimination.

Within these broad aims there were specific questions which the questionnaire was designed to address:

- Did NHS providers have equal opportunities policies?
- What were their specific components?
- Did personnel professionals *feel* that minority ethnic groups were fairly represented in all areas of the service?
- Were positive action measures used?
- Would personnel professionals sanction the use of positive discrimination, if yes, on what grounds?
- Did they believe that positive discrimination was used within the NHS, either currently or at any time in the past?
- Had the notion of 'diversity' entered the vocabulary of personnel professionals?
- How would they personally define it?
- What would they see as the benefits or pitfalls of pursuing diversity?
- Should they approve of diversity as a policy aim, what policy measures would they sanction in its achievement?

An actual longitudinal measure was built into the questionnaire by replicating some of the themes explored in previous national surveys, initially that carried out by the Equal Opportunities Review in 1993 (EOR No.53 1994).

As stated above there were related issues about the quality of service provided to minority ethnic communities which could not be explored using this particular method, nor could the questionnaire provide a comprehensive and sufficiently deep account of the processes and pressures bearing upon providers to meet these needs. Therefore, it was decided that a case study approach would be used in addition to the questionnaire, employing semi-structured interviews with a range of actors in a suitable geographical area (Strauss & Corbin 1998). In order to do this effectively it was decided that those interviewed should include representatives from (two) local NHS trusts, including health professionals, personnel officers, managers and executives; providers of private health services (if possible); representatives of agencies dealing with minority ethnic or consumer-related health issues; user-group representatives; policy-makers at all levels; and academics working in this area (in both a geographical and disciplinary sense).

The broad aims of the case study approach were to investigate through the attitudes, perceptions and experiences of the relevant actors whether:

- There were any problems associated with health provision for minority ethnic communities within their area.
- Local or national policies were, or had been, effective in dealing with any such problems.
- Diversifying the workforce might work - either as an alternative or as a supplementary strategy - to improve the standard of service provided to minority ethnic communities, and;
- Different, and possibly controversial, methods could be sanctioned in the pursuit of diversity.

Again there were specific questions which emerged from these broad themes:

- What form did identified problems take (if any)?
- Were they the result of language barriers, cultural gaps (which are distinct problems as will become clear below) or individual or institutional discrimination?
- Would specific measures such as universally provided interpreting services, cultural or anti-racist training be effective in this context?

- How effective had national policy been in improving the quality of service provided to minority ethnic communities?
- Did the respondents feel that diversifying the workforce might help?
- Did they feel that minority ethnic individuals were fairly represented locally and nationally within the NHS?
- How would diversity be defined?
- What might it achieve in practical terms?
- What methods would respondents sanction in achieving diversity?

Once the principal themes and issues had been identified and a suitable design for their investigation had been arranged, all that was needed was to begin collecting the data using the tools specified for that purpose. The first step was to develop and distribute a postal questionnaire, the process of which is the topic of the next section.

The Postal Survey

Sampling

As the postal survey was meant to form part of the background for the research, by providing details about the policy activities of health providers in implementing equal opportunities policies, and, to solicit the views of personnel professionals about the notion of diversity and its possible achievement, it was decided that only a nation-wide study would be satisfactory. Therefore, a straightforward census approach was taken, and every NHS trust in the UK was included (Shipman 1972).

Initially the *NHS Handbook 1996/7* was used to identify the appropriate trusts and to establish postal addresses. This was not entirely successful because the list only detailed the names of Chairmen (sic) and Chief Executives. As stated briefly above, the aim was to reach those responsible for personnel matters, and so the directory published by the Institute of Health Service Management 1997/8 was consulted. This gave the names, titles and addresses of Personnel Directors (or suitable departments where this information was not available). Officers responsible for personnel/human resource matters were targeted because of their proximity to the subject area, and the competing pressures they might face in achieving a balance in staffing issues between utility, legality and fairness (see Cockburn 1989: 218). Several trusts which were not included in the NHS Handbook were also identified. In all 541 potential respondents were identified - although with several trusts having merged or in the process of merging, the final figure was approximately 461.

Development and administration of the questionnaire

The questionnaire was developed in stages relating to the different themes incorporated. The sections on diversity were designed in accordance with some of the theoretical work carried out during the process of reviewing the relevant literature (which formed the basis for a journal article, Iganski & Johns 1998), and the questions about the development of equal opportunities soon became secondary to this material. That devoted to the subject of positive discrimination was drawn from themes which emerged from the literature itself.

The questionnaire was piloted by taking roughly 5% of the total sample (25 trusts) and sending them a copy of the questionnaire with a covering letter explaining the purposes of the research, informing them of their rights should they participate, and asking for any comments on the questionnaire. Because the survey was to be sent to each of the four components of the UK, a stratified sample was used. Twenty English trusts were to be included along with two each from Scotland and Wales and one from Northern Ireland. Individual trusts were selected using a simple random sampling technique. Only very minor alterations were made to the questionnaire as a result of the pilot study.

A response rate of approximately 44% (i.e. 11 returns) was achieved as a result of the initial mailing, and only one minor problem was evident.

Consequently, the questionnaire was amended and the main survey was launched. The response rate for the pilot ultimately reached approximately 48% (or 12 returns).

The final questionnaire sought factual information on equal opportunities, and personal attitudes and opinions about the notion of diversity and possible methods of its achievement, including the following:

- Were written equal opportunities policies in place?
- Had action plans been undertaken?
- Were recruitment procedures formalised, monitored and the data analysed?
- What measures (if any) existed for combating 'racial' harassment, either committed by colleagues or patients?
- Had an equality audit been carried out?
- Were minority ethnic communities fairly represented throughout the trust?
- Did they think that diversity might improve the service provided to these communities?
- How would they define diversity, and what benefits or pitfalls would they associate with its achievement?
- What methods of achieving ethnic diversity (given six possibilities) would they favour?

For more detail see Appendix 3, this is a copy of the final questionnaire.

A four stage strategy was organised. Stage one involved sending the questionnaire with a covering letter explaining the nature of the research, detailing my home and work addresses, and informing potential respondents of their rights should they wish to participate (Atkin *et al* 1994). It also promised respondents a summary of the findings on completion of the research, and a stamped addressed envelope was included for their response. The initial mailing for the main survey was timed to correspond with the second reminder of the pilot study. Stage two constituted a reminder letter forwarded approximately 3-4 weeks after the first to those who had not responded. This corresponded with the final stage of the process for pilot respondents. Stage three, then, amounted to a final reminder with a duplicate questionnaire enclosed. The final stage involved a letter being sent to non-respondents asking for any details they would be prepared to provide and included some of the more important questions and themes drawn from the questionnaire.

There were of course problems with this method. On the one hand, the policy detail could have been embellished or even falsified, to create a more favourable impression of the level of activity within individual trusts. There is no absolutely reliable way to validate the responses, and the notion of making false enquiries about employment to cross check policies was deemed unethical. To have asked for copies of policy documents might have adversely affected the response rate, and, ultimately, as several studies have shown (see chapter 8) policies often fail to reflect actual practice.

On the other hand, a questionnaire of this type may not be ideal for soliciting attitudes and opinions, even though Likert scales were adopted, because there is no means of probing beneath surface answers (Robson 1993; Fink & Litwin 1995). It is also impossible for the respondent to develop their responses in conjunction with the researcher, which may be important, particularly in relation to a topic to which they might not have given any previous thought. Furthermore, there is considerable scope for respondents to misinterpret questions (one question in particular caused problems, even after post-pilot amendment) and this may not be recognised by either the respondent or the researcher.

A strategy was devised for validating the policy details, albeit imperfectly. As will become clear in chapter 8 a host of similar studies have produced strikingly similar results, and this continuity can be regarded as a limited form of validation. Arguments about the depth of responses and possible misinterpretation of questions can also be countered. Although the respondents might not have thought about some of these issues before, this was part of the strength of the research project as a whole. Because the respondents were guaranteed anonymity in the final report, there is no reason to doubt the veracity of the attitudinal data (Beishon *et al* 1995). Perhaps the most important justification for using a postal survey, however, lies in the size of the undertaking. In no other manner could so much information have been obtained from so many respondents over such a massive geographical area (Bailey 1987; May 1993; Beishon *et al* 1995; Czaja & Blair 1996).

Response rates

The survey began in July 1998, with the initial pilot study, and was completed by the end of November of that year. From approximately 461 legitimate mailings 266 responses were received, a final response rate of 58%; a creditable response rate for a national mail survey, particularly in the context of parallel governmental surveys (possibly contributing to 'research overload').

An interesting point to note is that every effort was made to find the name of Personnel/Human Resource Directors, because it was assumed that this would maximise response rates. If people were named they were likely to feel a greater obligation to complete the questionnaire and return it. At least that was the underlying logic, but trying to reach a named individual in this way can backfire, because recipients sometimes used this as a pretext for returning the survey uncompleted. This happened on at least two occasions. These were promptly sent back making it clear that the post rather than the person was being targeted. Some responses contained job application forms or rejections indicating that the recipient had not read the correspondence attached to the questionnaire, and had probably disposed of them. These were sent back to the named individuals, on the assumption that they had not received the initial correspondence, stamped confidential with their names highlighted on the envelope.

There are several possible reasons for non-response in this instance. Firstly, the NHS was at the time preparing for another swathe of radical reforms in 1999 in the form of PCGs (DoH 1997). Several trusts were in the process of merging with others in their immediate areas. Consequently, policies were either in a state of flux or were being reconstructed. Of course it is impossible to determine the percentage of potential respondents to which this applied, but it does explain to a certain extent their reluctance to commit to a policy agenda which might not reflect the current or the coming reality. Secondly, the survey was sent out at the same time as a similar survey by Hurstfield (1999) on behalf of the NHSE and it is likely that this took priority. Thirdly, the subject matter could be perceived to be sensitive and is therefore more likely to receive a lower response than less challenging issues (May 1993).

There is another possible, supplementary, explanation for non-response. A colleague suggested that in her opinion the NHS is engaged in ring-fencing 'health' as an area for investigation for health professionals involved in graduate and postgraduate social science research. On reflection I believe that this - though clearly not a widespread problem at present (for instance certain trusts were keen to share the results) it is certainly occurring to some extent as this extract from a refusal letter indicates:

> We continue to participate in NHS wide surveys conducted on behalf of the Executive or other professional organisations which give us comparative information. In addition, we support our own employees in their professional/academic studies but clearly, the time available to support others is limited.

Furthermore, in the wake of the second follow-up to the main survey I received a phone call from a personnel professional trying to oversee a merger, asking for my identity and on whose behalf the survey was being carried out. When I told them that this was not government-sponsored research, she said that she would do what she could. No response was subsequently forthcoming.

Whilst it would be easy to overestimate the significance of these occurrences, because the support and co-operation was overwhelmingly positive, allowing such developments to proceed without mention would be unwise if not dangerous. If health research were to be ring-fenced for professionals working in the field this would certainly harm the quality of social research being undertaken, and undermine the credibility of the end-product. How objective would the findings be? What fresh perspectives could be drawn upon? I raise this issue as a possible explanation for non-response in relation to my own work, but also as a barrier which may have to be challenged and overcome in the future.

Data analysis

The resultant data were analysed using a computer package (in this case SPSS, Foster 2001) - though they were collected for descriptive purposes - outlining the progress trusts have made in implementing equal opportunities policies, and assessing official attitudes to the concept of diversity and various means of achieving it - rather than to explore causality or test a hypothesis (May 1993;Ragin 1994).

The Case Study: Organising Interviews

Sampling

For the case study a number of features were important in identifying a suitable area. First, there had to be a reasonably sized minority ethnic community. Second, I wanted an area which had not been 'over-done', such as London or the north west, and one with as local a perspective as possible. Third, it had to be somewhere with a favourable policy climate, which I hoped would become clearer once the completed questionnaires began to come in. Finally, it had to be within striking distance of Plymouth (if at all possible) in order to minimise travelling time and expense.

One area which seemed - at least cursorily speaking - to have most of these features was identified, labelled here as Robbinston. Therefore, returns from

Robbinston were examined very closely and eventually the decision was made to tentatively enquire about its suitability via different sources. As a snowball technique was to be used for each of the various groups of actors, initial respondents were identified and targeted (Donovan 1986a).

First contact was made with an established academic working in this field who also happened to reside in the area. The tripartite aim of this correspondence was to identify similar research projects which had been carried out in the recent past, or were currently being conducted; to ask if he would consider being interviewed personally; and whether he could suggest other suitable academics or research students who might agree to take part. Around a week later he contacted me by phone with information about one past and one present study, suggesting that the author of the former might be worth interviewing.

The next stage was to identify two trusts which were likely to serve areas of high minority ethnic settlement, and which provided mental health services (a major feature of the health-related literature). To establish the first of these criteria census data was used to locate the densest areas of minority settlement, and then the nearest trusts were located using an A-Z map. Three suitable trusts were identified all of which included in their remit the provision of mental health services - as recorded in the *Directory of Mental Health Services* (Mind 1994). One of these selected itself because of its proximity to the densest areas of minority ethnic settlement, the other was selected using a simple random sampling technique - the excluded trust was treated as a reserve should one or both of those contacted prove unwilling or unable to help.

The strategy, once agreement about access had been arranged, was to use the Personnel Director, or as it turned out, the Deputy Director, as a source of information about relevant people to interview (although the intention was also to interview those involved at the policy-making level of personnel matters). Not knowing how the management structure of different trusts had developed since the reforms, this was felt to be the easiest and surest way of reaching them. Essentially, my criteria for selection meant that only those involved in employment policy and practice should be included, and that this should be split as evenly as possible between the directorates - with any bias leaning towards the nursing profession, as they perform most of the one-to-one caring. Interviewing people responsible for the catering and ancillary services was also an aim. Furthermore, it was vital that potential respondents should cover the full range of specialities contained within the trust(s). This comprehensive approach was felt to be necessary because the central focus of the study was the employment culture of the trusts, via the attitudes and opinions of those who make the bulk of the day-to-day decisions.

Out of a meeting about possible access with the Deputy Director of Nursing (my original correspondence went astray) of the trust selected via random sampling, came a further avenue of academic enquiry. As a result of a letter to the suggested individual I was able to obtain a copy of a report on increasing the proportion of minority ethnic students on health awards recently published by a local higher education institution, an interview with the principal author, and the names and addresses of the co-ordinator of a report undertaken by the local HA, and the leader of a relevant project in Bradford - both were subsequently contacted. So the snowball was allowed to roll as freely as possible and led to various areas of investigation which would have been closed had a different sampling technique been employed.

Having determined that the most suitable respondents would be user representatives, and that interviewing was the best means of obtaining data from this group, the next step was to make contact. To do so it was decided that the local telephone directory would be the most accessible means of identifying agencies either involved in ethnic minority issues specifically or consumer issues more generally. Eight such agencies were identified and contacted via mail - each was asked if they could supply a list of user groups in the area, and whether a representative of their organisation would take part in an interview (stating the aims of the research).

Five responded, though only two were able to provide a list of suitable groups in the immediate area. One of the lists was more comprehensive than the other, and so it was used for the purposes stated. Of those who did not provide information, one agency had already liaised with the principal supplier and was therefore able to prevent duplication, while neither of the remaining respondents were able to help with information.

The list provided had been annotated with a double asterisk indicating groups concerned specifically with minority ethnic health issues, and others with a single asterisk, for groups with at least some interest in these matters (in their opinion). Initially the former group were contacted by letter, although as a clearer picture emerged of the policy landscape, one of the latter groups was subsequently approached. Again this provided a further academic avenue of enquiry.

In an attempt to contrast the attitudes and opinions of the public sector - i.e. the Health Service - with a private sector supplier of health care a private company in the area was also identified. Other respondents were identified and contacted for their national political prominence and declared interest in the research topics being investigated. This was not done on any systematic basis, but merely as new possibilities presented themselves.

Although the snowball technique was a very effective way of contacting potential respondents and of identifying different avenues of enquiry which were not immediately obvious there are problems with this type of approach. Perhaps the most relevant is the criticism that initial respondents control future contacts, and can therefore bias the results because they tend to direct researchers to people very much like themselves. There is no doubt that this is a very distinct possibility, but in this case the dangers are very much reduced. As far as the user-groups were concerned, the list was fairly comprehensive and I was in no way bound by the suggestions of the informant, indeed was not bound by them. With regards to the trusts' Personnel Director, this would have been difficult to achieve due to the comprehensive nature of the required sample. On the one hand, it formed a limited validation device, because some stories and accounts could be checked by making comparisons with those provided by others. Secondly, it enabled the exploration of shared values, norms, attitudes and beliefs with different groups of people involved in different aspects of providing health care.

Response rates

The original academic contact agreed to be interviewed as did one of the researchers he had suggested. An interview was also arranged with the author of the report referred to above, an academic working at a different higher education institution that was and is directly responsible for increasing the numbers of minority ethnic students on health based awards. Another potential contact was identified through an interview with a user group/community business organisation. Despite the willingness of the academic contacts to participate, it proved impossible to arrange the desired interviews in the available time frame.

Gaining access to the health providers proved equally difficult. Unfortunately, the trust located in the heart of the minority ethnic community – and therefore the most suitable - refused to take part. Their reluctance was due, ironically, to the state of flux their personnel policies had been thrown into by their adoption of the *Positively Diverse* national development programme (DoH 2004b). Unlike the research conducted by Beishon *et al* (1995) therefore, any bias is likely to be towards the least vigorous in policy-making terms, though the participating trust was confident of its ability to present a diversity-friendly image, a belief reinforced in the initial meeting with the Deputy Director of Human Resources, who informed me that the trust was meeting national human resource requirements by employing 3% minority ethnic individuals, which compared favourably with the demographic profile of the immediate area it served (the criteria used to judge recruitment efforts). He was also keen to stress his belief that more could and should be done to increase both numbers and career opportunities upon recruitment.

The second trust was initially enthusiastic, although I was only in contact with the nursing directorate in the first instance. The Deputy Director of Nursing was very keen to help and at an early meeting she agreed to select a representative sample of respondents across the trust and to make the initial contact on my behalf. However, three weeks later she informed me that the Personnel Director had vetoed my use of the trust. She was not given a reason for this decision, but I suspect that it was made partly because of an imminent health scandal. News bulletins reported that staff would have to undergo immediate retraining which was probably arranged in part via the personnel department. Furthermore, my original contact was fairly new in post and when she informed me that her trust would not be participating, she made it clear that the Director of Personnel was unhappy that my application had proceeded so far without his approval; it would seem internal politics also played a part in the decision.

Once the first refusal had been received overtures were made to the third and reserve trust, they seemed keen to participate, but demanded some material about the research on which to base their decision. I promptly sent them a research summary. Two months later I received confirmation that the trust would be prepared to participate, and suggesting times and dates for a negotiation meeting to take place. At that meeting it was agreed that I would interview forty people involved in employment policy - that is, recruitment, promotion and training - working in six out of the seven directorates (unfortunately the Mental Health Directorate was in the process of being dissolved as these services were being centralised in the form of a new mental health trust). The Deputy Director also suggested that I might like to talk with trade union representatives as a separate body within the trust. To allow me to select respondents effectively a copy of the management structure was mailed to me, and a sampling strategy was devised - including a request that trade union representatives should also be approached. This was then returned to the Deputy Director, along with a summary of what I was seeking to achieve and a copy of my interview schedule, to enable him to identify and contact likely respondents in each area.

It is interesting to note that at the initial meeting he warned that it might not be possible to include clinicians because *'They have to be treated like Gods, because they deal with life and death issues every day'*. Ultimately the list of contacts provided by each directorate failed to include any doctors or consultants, which was regrettable and obviously influenced the results, but was in itself an interesting development. He also assumed that I would not want to interview anyone from the Human Resources Directorate. I took this to mean either that he thought that the personnel were so well versed in equal opportunities and diversity issues that it would be unnecessary to speak to them, or, that discrimination and associated problems could not possibly occur because of the nature of their work. It must be stated that there was no reluctance on his part once he realised that its inclusion was vital for the purposes of my research.

Of the eight minority ethnic and consumer agencies mentioned above, interviews were arranged with three representatives. Three did not respond at all (though one of these no longer existed), one was unable to help and the other would not have been of any value.

From the list provided by one of the agencies, fifteen groups were contacted. These included voluntary sector organisations funded by the City Council and services funded by local NHS trusts. Of these fifteen, six interviews were initially organised, and a seventh from the reserve list as discussed earlier. During the early stages there was no indication that the response rate would be very high, and so when one potential respondent agreed to be interviewed over the telephone this was considered to be an opportunity worth taking - particularly as it furnished the chance to employ a method of data collection which would not otherwise have been contemplated.

Three other groups made contact but were unable to take part. One of these was on the verge of closure, another representative phoned to confirm my interest and then did not phone again, and another left a message while I was out of the University. I tried to contact this latter group several times, but they did not attempt to reach me again. Their reluctance was unfortunate because as far as I could ascertain they were the only group on the list which had complete independence. In fact this might have been part of the problem. One of my respondents had tried on several occasions to form links with the group in question but they were not interested because they saw her organisation as a white organisation and: *'[it's t]he old problem about people wanting to deal with their own problems on their own terms and not wanting to be a minority in a white organisation, or what they see as a white organisation'* (R8). It is altogether possible then that the group had learned - a healthy grape-vine exists in Robbinston - that I was white and this knowledge had undermined their willingness to take part. Of course this is speculation, but not without grounds.

Despite several attempts to reach a major private health provider in the area there was no response, and so the public/private contrast which might have further illuminated the limits or otherwise of ethnic diversity are not explored from this perspective. Likewise the potential respondents in the public eye, who have recently expressed strong opinions on these issues, were not prepared, due to the pressures of work, to participate (this was established through correspondence).

Interview procedures

One-off semi-structured in-depth interviews were conducted with a range of people involved in some capacity, albeit indirectly, with minority ethnic health issues. Essentially the broad themes investigated were:

- The awareness of respondents about possible shortcomings of health care provision for minority ethnic groups.
- How this could best be explained.
- What measures had been taken to improve matters (if necessary).
- Whether national policies mooted as possible ways of dealing with such matters, either directly or indirectly, had influenced health care for these communities.

- How diversity was defined by respondents; whether they supported its achievements.
- What benefits (if any) it would imply.
- What method(s) of its achievement would they be prepared to sanction.

To explore these themes a single interview schedule was used but different weights were given to different topics in accordance with the expertise and interests of respondents, although this was often a matter of trial and error. Some respondents provided material where none was anticipated, whilst others were unable to provide as much material as expected despite their roles/occupations. Still others made clear from the beginning which subjects they were concerned with. Over the course of the interviews, different themes and issues were added or omitted (Donovan 1986a) and the final schedule constitutes Appendix 4. This is a necessary process as data collection and theory development should progress simultaneously (Strauss & Corbin 1998), in an attempt to achieve a narrower focus from a broad-based view of the topic. For analysis to be effective and sufficiently comprehensive a certain amount of distance needs to be achieved between the two phases and so the detailed process of analysis is outlined below.

Before setting out the manner in which the face-to-face interviews were conducted it is necessary to relate the unexpected use of the telephone as a means of collecting data. As stated above this was used only once, and was in no way planned. However, it did provide some interesting contrasts with the other interviews, especially as the same schedule was used for both. It was a quicker and cheaper method of gathering the required data than the face-to-face interviews and reduced the personal discomfort of meeting a stranger in strange surroundings. There is also some evidence to suggest that interviewer effects are minimised (Fink & Litwin 1995; Frey & Oishi 1995) - although in this case the respondent knew something about me because she worked alongside a previous interviewee. There did seem to be more willingness on the part of the telephone interviewee to criticise the quality of health provision, and to attribute this and the lack of ethnic diversity to racism. How much of this was due to the data collection method cannot be established.

There were also many negative features. For example, the lack of personal interaction made it more difficult to direct the interview because there were no visual cues. It was also much harder to clarify what was said and seek detailed responses on certain issues as the respondent seemed unable to follow entirely the more complex questions and to have more control over how and where the interview proceeded (Fink & Litwin 1995). Compared to the in-person interviews the telephone interview was also a little shorter than the average, though not appreciably so; the respondent appeared to lose track of the time (Fink & Litwin 1995). Finally, the inability to record the interview, as appropriate facilities were not available, meant that a huge amount of data was lost because of the interviewers' inability to take notes using shorthand. Therefore, key sentences and words were used to reconstruct what was said. Consequently it was impossible to quote the respondent directly.

Face-to-face interviews were arranged by prior agreement and the dates, times and locations were chosen by the respondents. Each interview began with an informal chat, unless respondents indicated either explicitly or implicitly that this was unnecessary or unwanted, and a brief exposition of their right to anonymity and the right to withdraw from the research at any time.

The interviews were designed to elicit informant views and opinions peripherally on the quality of services provided to minority ethnic communities but centrally on the value of existing and potential measures - principally diversity. Did they approve of the notion? How did they define it? How might it work? What method(s) would they sanction in its pursuit? As stated previously the order of the questions was determined by the informants and the direction that they chose to take after the initial question was posed. After some of the interviews new themes were added to the schedule.

On the whole an 'active' approach to interviewing was taken, whereby the interviews were identified as a source of knowledge production as much as a tool designed to elicit knowledge from respondents. *'In other words, understanding 'how' the meaning-making process unfolds in the interview is as critical as apprehending 'what' is substantively asked and conveyed'* (Holstein & Gubrium 1997: 114). This was deemed to be an appropriate way of interpreting the process and the results because of the original nature of some of the concepts under investigation. Often a respondent would openly state that they had not previously thought about certain issues before, or that they were beginning to see things differently, or from a different perspective.

Consistent with the principles of active interviewing, respondents were encouraged to draw upon and make links between different facets of their experience, in order to produce a richness of meaning that was both relevant to their everyday lives and to the research topic. Their entire stock of knowledge was sought by provoking *'...responses by indicating - even suggesting - narrative positions, resources, orientations and precedents'* (Holstein & Gubrium 1997: 123). Consequently, respondents were given the opportunity to explore various ways of conceptualising the issues and of exerting narrative control by constructing their responses in both substantive and perspectival terms. To put it simply, the object of the exercise was to gain access to substantive data about the experiences, attitudes and beliefs related to the research subject (the 'whats' of the interview process) through the lens of shifting respondent standpoints erected and shifted in collaboration with the interviewer (the 'hows') (Holstein & Gubrium 1997: 121-7).

The question sequence varied because the whole process took on an evolutionary aspect as new questions emerged from the responses given, or as they appeared within the context of individual interactions. A practical expression of 'reciprocal clarification' took place as the original images about the research subject and subjects, which later became categories, influenced the conceptual framework in which it was built and were in turn influenced by that framework (Ragin 1994). To underline the mutuality of the process, and to acknowledge some of the criticisms by feminist researchers (i.e. Oakley 1981), personal experiences were shared with participants, although only where this seemed appropriate (Seidman 1991). This controlled presentation of self, i.e. sharing personal anecdotes, stories etc. (which included attention to personal appearance) was also designed to elicit 'collective' stories as well as 'cultural' stories - where the latter equate to cultural narratives grounded in popular stereotypes (Miller & Glassner 1997: 104).On a more practical note I found that Seidman's (1991) advice to follow-up hunches was extremely valuable as it reinforced the active approach outlined above.

The unique context of each interview, as implied above, far from tainting the findings, was viewed as an additional source of data and significant nuances were faithfully recorded. Indeed the uniqueness of each interview did produce themes and incidents worth recording. One such involved the expressed wish of certain respondents (four in number), during negotiations about their participation, for some written material about the background, aims and procedures of the research. Each was sent a copy of a research summary detailing this information in the briefest and simplest form available. Only one of the respondents appeared to be guided by this material during the interviews, though not to any great extent. It was clear from what most respondents said that they found it inaccessible!

Another interesting point to note was the contention in much of the literature (for example, Czaja & Blair 1996) that interviewing allows the researcher some control over the environmental circumstances. Although there were few problems with this, because the majority of respondents made satisfactory arrangements, in one instance an interview was conducted in an office with the door open maximising background noise from the neighbouring office. It did not provide any great distraction, but I felt that it was a deliberate attempt to illustrate that the interview was unimportant to the interviewee.

Every interview was taped with the agreement of the respondents, but I eventually abandoned *detailed* note-taking due to the difficulty in attending properly. Taping is thought to affect the way that some people react and respond during interviews, and there was certainly evidence of this. For example, one respondent was interviewed as a representative of a voluntary sector organisation, but she was also employed part-time by one of the local trusts. On tape she was very studied in her responses and was careful not to be too critical about the quality of health provision. Once the tape was turned off an entirely different picture emerged, and she was highly critical of both service provision and employment policy. Both accounts have been used here, identified where appropriate (taped material is presented as quotation). Another made clear on tape that certain things should not be reproduced in any written work as it might damage relations with the local authorities.

Despite this, taping was valuable because these actions and attitudes can themselves be considered as valuable data, and demonstrate the level of insecurity people, perhaps minority ethnic people in particular, feel when voicing criticisms of major institutions such as the NHS (Baxter 1997). Guilt might also play a part where important public services are concerned because respondents can feel that criticism aimed at people in such work is unfair. Furthermore, taping enables the researcher to examine every detail of an interview, and with such a wealth of data and emerging categories this is crucial. Interviewers also influence the data by their very presence and in the way that they ask questions (May 1993; Fink & Litwin 1995), but I feel that the comparisons made between different accounts and stories validate, where factual or policy matters are concerned, my findings.

Tapes were transcribed fully and after the first few had been completed patterns in the data could clearly be seen and so the process of category development began early on, enabling further comparison and analysis. Doubts have been expressed about the validity and reliability of data produced via interviews due to the potential for error. For example, respondents may give interviewers the answers they think are socially desirable, or feel too embarrassed to admit that they do not know the correct answer. Apparently this can be accentuated when the research topic is 'racial' where participants are thought to provide researchers from a different ethnic background to themselves with answers they think are socially acceptable (Czaja & Blair 1996). Biases can creep in during face-to-face interviews, but in the context of active interviewing bias is arguably less problematic because the conventional view that a passive vessel of answers lies behind the respondent, waiting to be tapped by an interviewer asking the right questions, in the right order, in the right way, is totally rejected.

In total thirty two semi-structured interviews were carried out with different respondents, each lasting between 35 minutes and 2 hours, and the interview period stretched over four months between September 1999 and January 2000. All were conducted by the author, due to the nature of the research and the financial constraints imposed by that nature. To ease the process of identification for the reader, the designation of the respondents is detailed in Appendix 5.

Data analysis

Before writing up began all the material was thoroughly re-read. All the quotes used are represented faithfully as spoken and recorded, and spellings are phonetically reproduced to match the pronunciation of the informants. Some words and phrases have been excluded - for example, *'um'*, *'right'* and *'you know'* - because they seemed to elucidate very little in terms of meaning. Where words and sentences appear in brackets during quotations, this should not be attributed to the informant but is used to clarify or qualify what was said.

Several software packages can be used to analyse qualitative data, for example N Vivo. Perhaps more than any other method grounded theory demands an intimate understanding of the data in its entirety. As a result data analysis was conducted manually. The conceptual tool bent to the task of data analysis was the constant comparative method initially developed and articulated by Glaser and Strauss (Strauss & Corbin 1998). This was judged to be appropriate because of the nature of the interviews and the resultant data - which did not lend themselves to more traditional methods (Ragin 1994; Strauss & Corbin 1998). It involves four discrete stages: *'(1) Comparing incidents applicable to each category, (2) integrating categories and their properties, (3) delimiting the theory, and (4) writing the theory'* (Glaser 1965: 440). In accordance with these principles, the information was coded by incident into a range of different categories (suggested in part by the interview schedule), and, as part of the process, compared with earlier incidents in the same category (May 1993). Perhaps the principal difference between these categories and those produced in research employing conventional interviews emerged in the consideration of substantive and perspectival factors assembled in collaboration with the interviewer (Holstein & Gubrium 1997).

Memos were taken from the outset to prevent coding by anticipation and to allow cumulative ideas to be grounded (Strauss & Corbin 1997, 1998). Filing was achieved by copying relevant material from the transcribed interviews, which were saved onto floppy disc and transferring them to separate disks designated for that purpose. As these files developed they took on the characteristics of what Berg (1995) calls 'index sheets', though they were highly detailed and inductively rather than deductively constructed. Each was headed by the theme or sub-theme and verbatim items were identified by transcript and page numbers, where passages contained more than one theme, they were entered on all relevant files. *'Cross referencing in this fashion, although extremely time consuming during the coding stage, permits much easier location of particular items during the later stages of analysis'* (Berg 1995: 60).

Once a broader picture of each category had emerged, the comparison switched from *'incident with incident to incident with properties of the category which resulted from the initial comparison of incidents'* (Glaser 1965: 11). This led to a greater integration of the elements within each category as the over-arching theory took shape. One of the advantages of this method is the natural delimiting of the theory as the analysis progresses, leading to both integration and reduction. As higher level concepts emerged to draw together underlying uniformities in categories and/or their properties, and, the delimiting of proposed categories, partly due to their theoretical saturation.

Writing up the findings proved reasonably trouble free, due to the continual note-taking and reflection (Glaser 1965). As Holstein and Gubrium (1997) argue, the data cannot be allowed to 'speak for itself'; rather the discursive procedures interviewees employed to produce meaning - in collaboration with the interviewer - were described where appropriate, using illustrations and examples drawn from the transcripts. Essentially the point was not to summarise, organise or reconstruct what was said, but to deconstruct it and highlight the 'hows' and 'whats' *'of the narrative dramas conveyed'* (Holstein & Gubrium 1997: 127). To indicate where possible that appropriate meanings were created through dialogue, rather than discovered through careful questioning. This is essential if the interview process, as a meaning-making occasion in its own right, is not to be misused or misunderstood.

Explanations and limitations

Before moving on I want to explain certain features of the research, and to outline the more important of its limitations. As the project has been driven by a modified version of grounded theory it changed shape to some extent. In the beginning the principal objective was to investigate the possibility of justifying positive discrimination for minority ethnic communities. A central part of the plan in the early stages was to explore the progress made by NHS trusts with regard to conventional equal opportunities, using existing and forthcoming survey evidence. However, it soon became clear as the interview survey began that procedure was less important than perception. In other words the way in which respondents thought about and defined diversity, and how they viewed it in operation, became more important (for the purposes of this research at least) than charting any procedural progress towards greater equality of opportunity. Consequently the shift in thinking from equal opportunities further towards diversity occurred. The problem with this is that it prevented a comprehensive investigation of managing diversity with the mail survey respondents.

Having said that, it was only in light of the comments added to a number of questionnaires that I was aware of the impact the theory had already made within the Health Service, which enabled me to pursue the matter in greater depth with appropriate respondents during the interview survey. So despite the collection of a great deal of superfluous questionnaire data (at least as far as this project is concerned), a substantial amount has been used to construct the third and most important section of the book. The nature of the research design ensured that the data determined the direction of the study, rather than slavishly following up research questions or hypotheses that ultimately proved irrelevant.

The distinction between equal opportunities and diversity caused many of my mail respondents to express concern at the focus of the research. They insisted that managing diversity should not be lost in the ineffectual morass that typifies equal opportunities policies. Perversely the findings illustrate that it is often such practitioners who threaten its purity and integrity.

A related issue was my concentration on ethnic diversity. Many felt that this undermined the very concept of diversity. Yet, ethnic diversity is in itself a distinct political project, which has recently been given impetus by governmental interest and policy. In fact, retaining an ethnic focal point prevented the research drifting into the meaningless ambiguity that much diversity theory and literature represents (see chapter 9). Taken too far, as this study suggests, diversity can be a dangerous distraction from equalising opportunities for disadvantaged communities.

The structure of the book is also unusual to some extent because the findings and the relevant literature are combined to form discrete but clearly related chapters. This can be justified because

...the literature can be used to confirm findings *and*, just the reverse, findings can be used to illustrate where the literature is incorrect, overly simplistic or only partially explains phenomena. Bringing the literature into the writing not only demonstrates scholarliness but also allows for extending, validating and refining knowledge in the field (Strauss & Corbin 1998: 51-2).

The intention was to provide a more holistic approach to the issues being discussed (Baxter 1988), rather than allowing the literary evidence to act as a simplistic device for validation and negation.

One feature of the research appears to bridge the explanation/limitation divide I have created here, namely objectivity. It is vital to any research project that the author make clear their own perspective before a reader embarks – in some cases credulously – on a journey through the written outcome. I subscribe to Becker's (1967) argument that we are always going to take sides, particularly in the area of ethnic relations. Torkington expresses this same sentiment very ably, *'In the field of race relations there is no room for neutrality'* (1991: 41). Therefore, I wish to state very clearly that on balance my sympathies lay with minority ethnic communities. As a white working class male I have witnessed racism from my earliest years, despite a lack of local diversity, sometimes from people very close to me. This is not to say that I have set out to prove that the Health Service fails, nor that white health workers (who for the most part do an excellent job) are committed racists (or indeed are any more racist than their peers, myself included, see Johnson 2000). Therefore, the findings and the manner of their presentation reflect the continuing anger I feel at the inability and widespread unwillingness to acknowledge much less meet diverse needs.

Having explained some of the features that may cause consternation or confusion, it is now necessary to address some of the limitations of the study. First, no in-depth consideration of mental health issues was possible during the interview survey despite their importance. Statistical representations consistently show that certain ethnic groups are overrepresented in the system, that they arrive via authoritarian means and that they receive relatively harsher treatment than their white counterparts (Bhat *et al* 1988; Littlewood & Lipsedge 1988; Torkington 1991; Law 1996; Skellington 1996; Bhui 2002). Unfortunately, the mental health units were in the process of forming a new independent mental health trust. Furthermore, a local voluntary organisation run by and for black people refused to co-operate with the research possibly due to my ethnicity.

Second, although ethnic monitoring has been heralded by many as an important way of addressing diverse needs (Bahl 1993a; Gunaratnam 1993; McIver 1994; Smaje 1995; Baxter 1997; Parekh 2000), despite some reservations (Ahmad & Sheldon 1992; Sheldon & Parker 1992; Karmi 1993), no consideration of this issue has been included. Although providers have been charged with monitoring in-patients for some time as part of the minimum data set (NHSE 1994) very little useful material was obtained during the interviews. Although the RECs Annual Report for 1998/9 revealed that providers were not systematically monitoring and that the HA had not intervened to force compliance. This confirmed some of the earlier findings of Mwasamdube and Mullen (1998) who conducted a combined mail and interview survey on behalf of the Ethnic Health Unit of trusts (36 from 42) and HAs (12) in the region to identify the sensitivity of services to minority ethnic needs. Although 84% of trusts collected the data, only 67% of HAs monitored compliance and of those only 58% used the information (1998). This is also consistent with the national trend at that time (Jamdagni 1996).

Another regrettable omission from the research was the exclusion of any minority ethnic members of staff. One health professional did take part but primarily as a representative of minority ethnic health users – though the two roles were combined. She was also employed by a neighbouring trust which was unable to participate in the research. The participating trust did provide me with two such contacts but neither eventually took part. One simply could not spare the time the other refused because she *was always being asked to take part in equal opportunities projects*'. Her refusal only serves to reinforce my findings about the meaning and operation of diversity.

I have not focused specifically on gender and class issues and how they interact with ethnicity in structuring individual and group-based experiences of the Health Service because this was not the explicit intention of the research. For one thing it has been done already to some extent (Bagilhole & Stephens 1997, 1998, 1999), and for another as stated above the object was to encourage people to think about *ethnic* diversity. Having said this gender and class issues are identified where appropriate.

A less satisfactory matter was technical in nature. All of the interviews were taped, but unfortunately due to a malfunction, four of the recordings were inaudible. Fortunately, I was able to faithfully reconstruct the data using skeletal notes made during each interview, more detailed retrospective notes, but also from memory (having discovered the problem almost immediately). The views of the respondents have been represented only where they were extremely clear, and they have not been quoted. There is some disparity in the number of times certain interviewees are quoted in the text, this is partly due to the tape malfunction, partly due to the fact that one interview was conducted over the telephone, and, that another was an exploratory interview which proved to be interesting but not altogether relevant (see Appendix 5). However, the disparity is mainly due to the fact that some people were more forceful and articulate than others, and there is some bias towards their accounts. It must be stated very clearly here though that there has been no misrepresentation of the views of the interviewees as they were related to me, and I have made no elaborate claims that cannot be substantiated with reference to the data.

Perhaps time and resources have imposed the biggest restriction of all. With more of both it would have been possible to include the newly formed mental health trust, followed up the new reforms and, respondent willing, have rearranged the lost interviews. What I can say with confidence is that the book is the product of my best and faithful efforts to pursue the truth.

SECTION ONE:

Meeting the needs of minority ethnic communities

CHAPTER 2:

Communication barriers: the produce of ignorance and ideology

'One is not superior merely because one sees the world in an odious light'
— Vicomte Francois-Rene de Chateaubriand

Introduction

The purpose of this chapter is to explore the quality of service provided to minority ethnic communities by the NHS via the perceptions of the interview respondents. In the first instance the neglect of minority ethnic health issues will be briefly reviewed, and the evidence that the Health Service has failed to provide a sensitive service to minority communities will be presented. As will become clear the user representatives had an entirely different view about the quality of provision than those responsible for providing services or for training future health workers. Although one of the trust's employees was prepared to accept that the service was not entirely adequate the majority were quite satisfied, though there were evident contradictions, i.e. that the service has always been adequate but has recently improved. Ultimately, the trust employees considered any difficulties experienced by minority ethnic users to be 'their' own responsibility and this will be framed within a discussion of the prevailing dominant ideologies. Minority ethnic communities must shape themselves to the needs of the service rather than the other way around.

Background

Although an enormous amount has been written about the relative health status of minority ethnic communities (Donovan 1984; Calman 1992; DoH 1992; Smaje 1995; Nazroo 1997) we will not venture too far in this direction though the two things are of course indivisibly linked (Skellington 1996; Nazroo 1997). Ultimately the rationale for this research project was framed within the belief that *'Researchers... should be concentrating upon the sensitivity of general service provision...'* (Johnson 1987:133).

That the Health Service fails the general public to some extent is all too apparent, and there is evidence to suggest some dissatisfaction throughout society (Judge & Solomon 1993; Airy *et al* 1999). This is particularly evident at present due to on-going hygiene issues, continuing labour shortages and a series of embarrassing scandals (i.e. the illicit harvesting of body parts) (Meikle 2001). However, the dissatisfaction of minority ethnic communities has been arguably greater than their white counterparts (Judge & Solomon 1993; Airy *et al* 1999) and this ought not to be surprising. Until the early 1980s, in keeping with the general laissez-faire approach to social policy (Sivanandan 1976, 1982; Williams 1989; Penketh & Ali 1997), there was virtually no recognition of diverse health needs.

> ...the history of policy responses to the changing nature of British society following the migration of New Commonwealth settlers to Britain after the Second World War has been characterized by a lack of positive action and of laissez-faire, coupled with issue-specific response when unavoidable (Johnson 1987: 128).

During the 1950s and 1960s the primary health concern was the perceived degenerative effects on health and morality of large-scale immigration – what has been labelled *'Port Health'*, and this association between immigration and population controls has continued (Kushnick 1988; Bhopal & White 1993; Johnson 1993; Law 1996; Batty 2005). In fact the primary responsibility for needs identification and provision until this time lay with the voluntary sector (Johnson 1987; Ahmad 1993b). The ground breaking Black Report contained only three pages on the subject of ethnicity (Townsend & Davidson 1982: 58-60).

At around the same time another ground breaking report produced by Brent Community Health Council (CHC) (1981) identified very clearly that the Health Service – albeit locally and anecdotally – failed to acknowledge much less meet diverse needs. Interpreting services were inadequate and different cultural needs were overlooked, sometimes contemptuously. The report also accused the NHS of acting as an arm of the immigration service by acting to control minority ethnic numbers. Allegedly *'more leaflets [had] been produced in Asian languages on birth control than any other topic, and some women from minority ethnic groups reportedly felt that they had been offered abortions and sterilisations more readily than white women'* (Brent CHC 1981: 13-14).

Shortly after, the Department of Health (DoH) launched an initiative to challenge the perceived growth in rickets amongst the 'Asian' community. The *Stop Rickets Campaign* was designed to raise awareness about rickets and prompt health professionals into providing appropriate advice on vitamin D deficiency. The central theme of the campaign however was that services were not appropriate and that language and cultural barriers were hampering effective service delivery (Bahl 1993a). In 1984 the *Asian Mother and Baby Campaign* (AMBC) was launched in part to deal with the communication barriers identified (link working, one of the resultant innovations, will be discussed in chapter 5) (DHSS 1987; McNaught 1987).

Despite dedicated policy measures (albeit victim-blaming in nature, Kushnick 1988; Johnson 1993; Stubbs 1993; Gerrish *et al* 1996; Mason 2000) and the implicit hope that language barriers in particular might dissipate with length of residence (Fletcher 1997) it would appear that communication remains problematic for many members of Britain's minority ethnic communities (Rawaf 1993; Lambert & Sevak 1996); particularly for women from certain communities and older people (Torkington 1991; Jay 1992; Nazroo 1997). The research for this book followed a survey funded by the NHS Ethnic Health Unit (Mwasamdube & Mullen 1998) and an extensive consultation exercise, in the form of a series of specially arranged public meetings, workshops, focus groups, work groups and individual interviews, carried out by the local Health Authority (HA) during 1996/7. The principal causes for concern as expressed by the local communities very much mirrored what many have come to expect (McIver 1994), i.e.

- Continuing language difficulties.
- A general lack of cultural awareness amongst health professionals.
- Inappropriateness of services and treatment.
- A lack of minority ethnic health workers in the area.

Communication problems are the central theme of this chapter because they were also strongly identified by the respondents, particularly the user representatives. As Sheldon and Parker (1992) argue, communication is a widespread problem for all users, underlined by research carried out for the DoH (Airy *et al* 1999), so it is important not to focus simply on language. Communication is here defined as a composite of lingual and cultural factors, again, as recognised by most of the user representatives.

Although a lack of information on the availability of services, and to support appropriate health promotion has been identified within this framework (Bahl 1993a; Bhopal & White 1993; McIver 1994: Ch.4) this did not emerge as a major issue. Therefore, we will concentrate exclusively on barriers that hamper direct patient/professional interactions. The importance of this is obvious, as Smaje observed *'Few would deny the need to enhance communication between ethnic minority patients and health professionals'* (1995: 28). In reporting the findings of the fourth Policy Studies Institute (PSI) survey Nazroo said, *'The data show that communication, which is the central feature of a consultation with a doctor, is a significant problem for a large number of ethnic minority patients'* (1997: 142).

Whilst acknowledging the importance of communication barriers it should be noted that certain commentators (see Bhopal & White 1993, for example) have suggested that too much attention may have been levelled at them to the detriment of more important priorities. It is perhaps as much to do with the way such problems are constructed as to how they are prioritised. Indeed Johnson (1987) and Ahmad (1993a, 1994) have warned that such tendencies have been part of a conscious strategy to emphasise the deviance of minority ethnic cultures and to shift responsibility onto those communities (see also Sheldon & Parker 1992; Bradby 1995). As this chapter - and indeed this book – unfolds, the resonance of these assessments will become apparent, as the dominant theoretical perspective of 'ethnic sensitivity' (Stubbs 1993), the idea that difficulties are caused by cultural differences and a corresponding lack of awareness on the part of white health workers, informed by biomedicine, the tendency for health workers to treat illness and disease as a feature of a dysfunctional machine (the human body) (Torkington 1991; Ahmad 1993c), appear to enable health workers and administrators to construct different needs as deviant and thereby undeserving.

The shape and consequence of failure: user representatives

There was a distinct contrast between the views of those representing the needs of users and the employees of the trust. The vast majority of the user representatives felt that the Health Service did not fully meet the needs of minority ethnic communities. However, there was a clear contrast between those employed in and around the Health Service with a formal responsibility to represent the interests of users, here labelled official representatives, and unofficial representatives, those whose loyalties were primarily assigned to the communities (at least as far as this study was concerned).

Official representatives

One respondent headed the local Community Health Council (CHC), and, while his work did not involve direct contact with minority ethnic communities, he was aware of some dissatisfaction. The actual complaints that had been made were fairly specific:

> We occasionally pick up stuff via complaints work, but not sufficient to have any statistical significance. We do occasionally get somebody who is, who is from a black or other minority ethnic group making a complaint, but that complaint may just be because they're a user who's had a bad service. Where we do get issues, what we do hear about is...I've had specific concerns raised with me through public meetings around access of Asian women to services because of the gender issue of doctors. I'm told, I have to say I'm told by Asian men that their wives sometimes don't use services because the GP, particularly the GP, is male and that they have not got access to the choice to be able to say they want a female GP. So that's a concern. We are aware of course that there are issues in terms of language, interpretation, translation and so on (R12, p.1, para.1).

It was clear that his official role in the Health Service influenced his views about the nature of such problems. He went on to express some sympathy for health commissioners faced with diverse needs and scarce resources, but putting himself in the place of minority ethnic users, illustrating the value of active interviewing (Holstein & Gubrium 1997), he would not be as sympathetic.

The other respondent was actually responsible for representing and meeting the needs of minority ethnic communities from within the HA, and, as a result of the consultation exercise, had direct knowledge of service shortcomings.

> The issues were much more the broad issues about understanding, people in the NHS understanding cultural diversity... So as I say the specific service issues were relatively limited and everybody I think unanimously identified the main barrier to good health care is a mixture of language and cultural misunderstandings...cultural and linguistic misunderstandings if you like (R11, p.1-2, para.2).

So the issue of gender in relation to GPs etc., identified as an issue by the head of the local CHC did not materialise (though this is unquestionably a problem for certain sections of the minority ethnic community, Nazroo 1997), but communication barriers did. In fact the report published in the wake of the local consultation exercise stressed this very strongly.

One of the recommendations contained in the report was that local health professionals ought to receive instruction in different cultural needs in relation to health (see chapter 6):

> Yes, and for all health workers to have an appreciation...that that's how they have to work. Now, that does mean that they do perhaps need to know more about some cultures...and they bring all that with them; and good health workers do try and do it, but it's very patchy. And what black communities say to you is that we ought to be able to depend on that fact that every health worker...will understand enough about what they don't know about our communities to ask the right questions... (R11, pp.5-6, paras.15-18).

The implication here is clear, that any failings in relation to communication are largely due to individual ignorance, and in order to rectify this health professionals should be given a general awareness of different cultural beliefs and practices, even if that simply allows them to ask pertinent and sensitive questions. The dominance of this approach variously labelled 'ethnic sensitivity', 'cultural pluralism' and 'multiculturalism' will be outlined and evaluated below.[1]

Unofficial representatives

In contrast the unofficial user representatives were much more critical of services, and the possible reasons for this are obvious. They did not have the same investment in the system, and were closer to the communities in question. Seven out of eight respondents were certain that communication presents a substantial barrier to access and the quality of service provided to minority ethnic communities.

---

[1] For detailed discussions of the development of theories relating to 'race' relations see Brent CHC (1981); Sivanandan (1982); Penketh & Ali 1997; Parekh (1998, 2000).

Whereas the official representatives had taken the view that communication barriers were due to a lack of awareness, their interpretation was less charitable. The problem was one of competence. One respondent argued that health professionals are frequently culturally incompetent in their dealings with minority ethnic groups (R5, p.2, para.6). This was a structural issue, not simply the outcome of individual ignorance or prejudice.

Another respondent, with responsibility for organising a mental health charity in the area, provided a good illustration of this process in action. On the subject of disproportionate rates of mental illness amongst *'Black people'*, she referred to conclusions drawn from the discipline of Transcultural Psychiatry (Stubbs 1993):

> There have been various theories suggested, like cultural concerns. When people display certain behaviours it might be just part of their culture, and they're misinterpreted by people in the white population (R8, p.1, para.2).

She underlined this by sharing her past experience as a member of a Mental Health Act Tribunal:

> ...watching people come through that system, you know, I could see that people from different races have a lot more trouble putting their case over, and really needed black advocates to be with them and to advise them. So I mean they were coming up against a white culture really (R8, p.7, para.26).

According to these respondents then, cultural incompetence has more to do with the prevailing culture of the Health Service and the society of which it is part, than a lack of awareness on the part of individuals. Although she draws implicitly upon Transcultural Psychiatry – which itself derives from 'ethnic sensitivity' – to make her case, she emphasises the exclusive structural edifice presented by 'white culture' rather than individual ignorance.

Interestingly a third respondent picked up on these themes in echoing the need for advocates:

...my Step-Dad's from Jamaica and he's been here for years and year's but he's still very Jamaican in the way that he speaks and his culture, and he had to go to the Eye Hospital for some tests and I asked my Nephew to go with him as an interpreter. Now he speaks English but he speaks Patois and I know that he says things to me that I understand, but I know that the medical profession won't. And the doctor put some drops in his eyes and said: Can you see? And my Step-Dad said, Well it's a bit foggy, and the doctor looked outside and said, Oh well, no it's clear outside. But he meant his eyesight was foggy. And I've heard like my friends have said things like that to me before, so if the doctor asked them a question about indigestion, they don't use terms like 'indigestion' they use terms like 'gas', you know? (R6, p.1, para.2).

This incident was cited as evidence of the 'cultural incompetence' of white health workers when faced with minority ethnic clients. Yet it might have been less to do with culture, than class or geography. The terms suggest a misunderstanding based in the class disparities between doctor and patient (the latter actor being clearly working class according to the respondent) (Torkington 1991; Ahmad 1995; Saunders 1996), or, possibly, a misunderstanding deriving from regional dialect. This illustrates the caution that needs to be exercised when cultural issues are being considered. However, specific failings were identified and their consequences set out.

Failings and consequences

Communication barriers, as stated earlier, are viewed here as a composite of lingual and cultural barriers, but both were identified in isolation with their attendant consequences. Although we may expect language barriers to decline over time and many individuals also register with GPs from similar backgrounds (Donovan 1986b; Farooqi 1993; Fletcher 1997) such barriers persist (Jay 1992; Karmi 1993; Rudat 1994; Nazroo 1997). Nine out of ten 'South Asians' and eight out of ten Chinese respondents who took part in the fourth PSI survey used a different language than English in at least some circumstances. The research interpreters also found difficulties amongst other participants (Nazroo 1997; see also Alexander 1999: 24). It was reported in the local consultation report and action plan that one in ten Pakistani women spoke English slightly or not at all.

This clearly impacts upon the access to and experience of health provision. Nguyen Van-Tam *et al* (1995) in a survey carried out in Nottingham with the Vietnamese community found that between 43% and 69% of respondents experienced lingual barriers at some stage in the health process, from making appointments with GPs to reading medicinal information (1995: 107). Leiston & Richardson (1996) revealed a similar pattern in Milton Keynes and Aylesbury in a questionnaire survey involving 40 minority ethnic individuals attending GP surgeries; 73% (29) reported difficulties at some stage in the process.

Language barriers are often more than inconvenient they are potentially disastrous. For instance, white midwives who participated in Bowler's (1993) study reported poor relationships with women who spoke little or no English. To illustrate this she related an incident during a home visit in which a midwife left a bottle of paracetamol with an 'Asian' woman in the full knowledge that she had no idea how to use them.

According to a representative heading a Chinese voluntary organisation such barriers and their adverse consequences are mirrored in Robbinston. Along with a colleague she had taken on much of the interpreting burden, but the consequences were, according to her account, sometimes disastrous.

> My people die in hospitals unnecessarily and they haven't been told why they died, and misdiagnosis because of language, lack of language provision and cultural insensitivities...and just this year [1998] three Chinese died unnecessarily (R4, p.24, paras.90 & 91).

Furthermore, added to the grief caused by such incidents, she argued that friends and relatives had also been dealt with very insensitively:

> ...I think it's got to take a few unnecessary deaths in the community to shake them up, and it happens, it happens because of lack of communication and lack of language sensitivity in hospitals. There are Chinese die unnecessarily and I have had a 75 year old mother who came to me and holding a death certificate in

English, and she was in tears, she came to my office and she said: "...Please tell me what did my son die of? All he had was tummy upset, I took him to hospital they took him in for observation and he was there 5 days and the next thing is he die on me" (R4, p.13, para.48).

Whether in this case lingual or cultural factors had any bearing on the patient's death is impossible to say, but the alleged treatment of his grieving mother was neither acceptable nor appropriate.

In relation to culture, the specific concern appeared to be about inadequate dietary provision in local hospitals, and this had been raised during the local consultation exercise. The importance of food cannot be overstated,

> It is not just a question of serving 'curries', vegetables or salads. The diets of different black groups vary a great deal and familiar food is important if a person is feeling ill. Not only do they need to eat in order to get proper nourishment so that they can recover, but food that is enjoyable also helps to make people feel better. Many white people are vegetarian or appreciate foreign food, so more variety would be of benefit to all patients (McIver 1994: 76).

This has not always been recognised by the Health Service (Brent CHC 1981; Gerrish *et al* 1996; Parekh 2000; Gunaratnam 2001), and although it does affect the majority population to some extent (Airy *et al* 1999), it has been a very long standing problem for minority ethnic communities in particular. The Brent CHC Report (1981) identified a significant lack of provision for different religious and dietary requirements, and this has subsequently been supported by empirical research (Joyram 1994; Gerrish *et al* 1996). Yet despite this body of evidence dietary provision apparently continues to be culturally inappropriate for minority ethnic communities:

> Culturally there are differences in, like meat in hospitals isn't halal, food isn't prepared properly or anything like that (R1, p.1, para.7).
> Yes, I think one of my greatest frustrations apart from the language problem is the dietary in hospitals (R4, p.2, para.4).

The latter respondent went on to illustrate the source of her frustrations thus,

> I had an elderly lady who had a stroke and who can hardly speak....And she doesn't eat cheese, most Chinese will not eat cheese and beef, beef is for the religious reason. Most of them are Buddhists, so they don't eat beef. But you see the hospitals not aware of that at all... [A]nd this lady she doesn't eat any cheese, and yet she always had cheese omelette put under her nose, and she was so hungry, and yet when we actually write a list down to say please do not give her cheese...in Chinese and English so that she point out to the nurse, we actually provide that for the hospital and put it on her dining table, and yet...They still give her cheese. And she was so hungry she just had to eat it, and when we raised these questions with the senior nurse, a staff nurse, and the hospital authorities, and the nurses who were serving her, because...they change shifts...they don't even understand it. So the instruction didn't pass on from one to the other, I was told, what's the fuss, she eats it! (R4, p.3, paras.8 & 9).

Although the respondent links beef with religious prescription, it is also recognised that many Chinese people will not consume milk or milk-based products, such as cheese (Abdussalam & Kaferstein 1996). According to the respondent, the provision in local hospitals is often so inadequate that family and friends are encouraged to bring appropriate supplies during visiting hours (R4, p.3, para.6). This reflects activity in other parts of the country, but has been discouraged by health professionals (Gerrish *et al* 1996).

Again there were felt to be highly negative consequences. One potential result of ignoring the dietary requirements of certain minority ethnic groups might be the creation or perception of additional health problems. In relation to mental illness, for example, failure to eat can be seen as a symptom of depression and result in extended sections and harsher treatment. Torkington (1991) recounts the experience of a young woman refusing to eat due to inappropriate dietary provision and the misinterpretation of the attendant health professionals. The Chinese respondent outlined another way in which health can be affected:

> [It was] either cheese omelette or nothing. And you know she has to eat it, but she told me...I can't stand cheese I feel sick afterwards. Because Chinese do not eat cheese a lot, a lot of them do not eat cheese (R4, p.4, para.10).

51

Quite aside from the indignity of having to eat something that is generally avoided - in this case cheese - it is possible that an illness might be prolonged or even exacerbated.

Worse still is the prospect that people will not seek help when they need it because of lingual and cultural problems (Jay 1992; Ahmad 1995; Smaje 1995; Nazroo 1997). Of course there are various factors involved in the usage of available services, including their geographical distribution, the attitudes of individuals towards the Health Service and differences in health beliefs and knowledge (Smaje 1995). For example, Nguyen Van Tam *et al* found that over a third (36%) of their respondents preferred to use Chinese remedies (1995: 107) and the preference for traditional and private medical services is also a feature of other communities (Donovan 1986a; Thorogood 1989; Ahmad 1992). Indeed evidence suggests that white people consult with 'alternative' practitioners more than any other group (Nazroo 1997).

Generally speaking consultation rates have been consistently higher for 'Asians' and 'Afro-Caribbeans' than for their white counterparts, allowing for a gender bias towards males in the former community (Farooqi 1993; Culley 1996; Nazroo 1997). Though secondary analysis using various statistical techniques has shown very little difference overall (Smaje & Le Grand 1997). Nevertheless, this should not be taken to mean - as the evidence here and elsewhere suggests - that access to and quality of services is satisfactory. Furthermore, the Chinese community has a much lower rate of consultation than any other community (Smaje & Le Grand 1997), and it would seem that inappropriate service provision is a key issue (Kushnick 1988; Torkington 1991; Nazroo 1997). Nguyen Van Tam *et al* reported that Vietnamese users often chose to defer visiting GPs due to lingual and cultural problems. Of the 130 who provided information, 61 (47%) had done so.

To illustrate this same process, the same respondent recalled a conversation with a hospital worker in an area with a fairly large Chinese community, when asked how the hospital dealt with the needs of Chinese patients he said,

> "No problem, we don't get Chinese clients. I don't think we...I've been here twelve years I've only had one". It makes you wonder why [they] don't get Chinese clients (R4, p.2, para.5).

Her own view was that people either cope alone or look elsewhere for help:

> Now as a result of that the Chinese rarely use the facilities and the amenities of the hospital in this country, most Chinese, because the majority of them still have, and very often they still go back to Hong Kong, and they got their own place sometimes. Most of them still have, and very often they still go back to Hong Kong now and again to visit their relatives and friends and at the same time they will go and try to use the hospital in Hong Kong to get their treatment.... And sometimes if they can't afford it they borrow money, they'd rather do that, or their children pay for it if they're working. This is mainly due to reason language problem, they feel like fish out of water, and the dietary, the food, and it's very, very insensitive to our needs (R4, p.2, paras.4 & 5).

In essence she argued that some Chinese people from Hong Kong would rather travel despite ill health and/or risk financial difficulties than trust local Health Services. This reflects the findings of Leiston & Richardson (1996: 29): *'For some the language barrier is so large that when serious health issues arise they would prefer to consult privately a GP who spoke their own language or even go to a doctor in their country of origin'.*

Disputed causes: Employees of the Health Service

Although the strength of criticism levelled at the Health Service and the location of culpability varied according to the relative position of user representatives to the system, there was nevertheless a consensus about the existence of communication barriers. However, this was not a view shared by the trust employees and others associated with the NHS on a professional basis.

The initial response was generally to question the notion that the Health Service, and in particular the participating trust, had ever experienced any problems providing services to minority ethnic communities. Yet as the interviews progressed paradoxical beliefs emerged, i.e. that although the service had always been adequate there had been recent, and significant, improvements. Ultimately though where problems were grudgingly acknowledged they were firmly laid at the feet of the victims.

What problem?

Only one employee of the trust accepted the possibility that services did not fully meet the needs of minority ethnic communities.

> I mean I'm sure that there is always masses that needs to be done about improving communication, and also looking at health care staff's knowledge about cultural practices in health care...Yes...and also practices around particularly health care issues...sort of blood transfusions, care assistants, diets, practices around death, and I mean I'm sure there are lots of issues there that need to be improved and looked at and developed, and staff better trained, better aware (R24, p.2, paras.5 & 6).

This acknowledgement might have been based on a number of factors. Firstly, she was the Disability Co-ordinator for the trust, and was therefore heavily involved in pursuing equality of opportunity and better access albeit on behalf of a different community (which is not to dismiss the experiences of disabled people from minority ethnic communities). Secondly, because she was not responsible for front-line services, her role was subject to a certain amount of ambiguity – representing both users and the trust.

The overwhelming majority felt that the service provided was for the most part satisfactory. One respondent accepted the possibility that there might be weaknesses in provision, but that all that could be done was being done:

I'm not aware of any particular problems, but I would probably think that we don't do enough. We offer an interpreting service, but not all our literature is in minority ethnic languages, and we have discussed it in various forums and departments. But we can come up with this problem. If you put it in this minority language and then somebody phones up you don't have somebody at the end of the phone who can take the call...? And so you're always going to have to need an intermediary, but yes I'm aware that, you know, we cater to a certain extent, but I think I'm not quite sure how we could do more, but we probably could do more (R23, p.1, para.1).

Others were more confident about service quality,

No, as I say, I've been very lucky in my life, but I've never...had any problems or seen any problems in my time...as I say in the operating theatres, I've worked there for a long time (R16, p.1, para.4).

Not as far as I know. I know there are policies for the monitoring of... So locally, here in the department I haven't got a problem, no (R25, p.1, para.2).

Several reasons were produced to support this position.

Demography was reported to be a major factor - the trust was located outside the inner city away from the residential areas of most minority ethnic groups.

No I don't because I think we're sort of, almost a rural general hospital, we don't have many problems in that respect... I don't think we have any great focus because it's a fairly mixed cultural area, and I think our catchment area is much less so, but there are no great issues there (R15, p.1, para.1).

There are some diets, but it really in [the city] it hasn't been raised as any major problem. Like my colleague has worked in hospitals in London, and like the menus, their first language is Bangladeshi or whatever and that actually English is their second language, and the food is very much for the ethnic groups. Now obviously in here because we don't have so many it's the other way around, so it is English... (R19, p.9, para.29).

This is a common response to issues of ethnic diversity (Gerrish *et al* 1996; Iganksi *et al* 2001) that is becoming less sustainable in political terms (Straw 1999). Even taken at face value it was only relevant to the main hospital site and one of the community clinics. Even then, one of the respondents was employed in a unit designated a *regional* centre of excellence (R29), and a District Nurse thought it possible that the hospital was failing to refer minority ethnic patients to the clinic (referral being a particular problem for 'Asian' communities, Farooqi 1993). In light of the findings produced above, it is essential to consider the impact of inappropriate services on the numbers of minority ethnic people accessing available services (Jay 1992; Smaje 1995; Nazroo 1997). This did not occur to the majority of trust employees.

Another factor in the perception that problems were absent was that ample provision was made for lingual and cultural needs. This was strongly argued in relation to language barriers:

> No we've got, I would say it's very good because we do have an interpreting system, which we follow quite closely. And all wards have a very comprehensive and up-to-date list of interpreters, so if there is a problem with patients or with staff, but normally the staff, we actually look at them before they come to us, so it's not a problem. But certainly staff are aware and they have support (R13, p.2, para.3).

> I mean from providing a service the biggest obvious one is language, but again, we have things like interpreters on site, so they can be called on if we have problems (R15, p.1, para.3).

This was by far the most common response to the idea that language barriers might exist. One respondent felt that, due to a lack of communication between the trust and community more widely, that people might not be aware that interpreters are on hand, but they are (R30).

Yet, there was substantial testimony to the contrary. It became clear that the claims of the Chinese respondent, supported by other research (Torkington 1991; Nazroo 1997), were based in fact. The trust often relies upon friends, voluntary workers and relatives to provide interpreting facilities:

> The only problems we would have is if someone came down that didn't speak English. But usually they bring a relative with them that does speak, and we do

> have interpreters that can come along if need be... But usually if there's someone
> with a different culture someone always comes down with them, a member of
> their family and that comes down to the anaesthetic room (R16, p.1, para.2).

> Because we do often have a language barrier, we do try and let the relative or
> language person come into the room so that the doctor can actually communicate
> with them so that then it can be passed on (R.25, p.1, para.2).

That health workers have traditionally relied upon informal language provision is well-documented (Baxter 1988; Parekh 2000). For example, Nguyen-Van-Tam *et al* (1995: 108) reported that of the 70 Vietnamese people who provided information on interpreting, 14 (20%) called upon adult relatives, 25 (36%) used child relatives and 27 (40%) required assistance from community workers and/or others. Similarly 75% of those reporting language difficulties as part of the PSI survey used family members or friends as interpreters (Nazroo 1997).

The reality and inadequacy of these *ad hoc* arrangements has been well covered in the literature (Ahmad 1995). For one thing, voluntary workers are often unable to offer the level of services that are required. Sometimes, it was suggested by one of the respondents (R4), people die as a result. It is equally unacceptable for friends and relatives to provide interpreting services (Torkington 1991; Gerrish *et al* 1996). Aside from issues of confidentiality, male relatives may censor information during translation for cultural reasons, or, may choose not to pass things on due to personal embarrassment. Six (15%) of Leiston & Richardson's (1996) respondents reported feelings of embarrassment about being accompanied. Furthermore, it is extremely likely that informal interpreters will have an insufficient vocabulary to convey everything professionals say - a particular problem where children are expected to translate (Joyram 1994; Bothamley 1996). Ultimately, 40% (16) of the respondents in Leiston & Richardson's (1996) survey preferred formal interpreting arrangements, and the 'Asian' respondents in the study by Gerrish *et al* (1996) confirmed the importance of formal interpreters.

There were times when neither professional interpreters or friends, relatives or voluntary workers were available, and it was then that the spirit of improvisation really came into its own. Torkington (1991: 93) reports the comments of a GP's receptionist about the use of informal sign language. She said *'This is quite satisfactory. We understand each other well'*. Predictably the Somali women who recounted stories about language difficulties did not agree. Unfortunately the trust employees in similar circumstances also rely on gestures to communicate:

> But I think she said 'yes' and 'no' but I think that was about it, but I mean we could communicate by gesture and everything but they [the woman's family] were worried that if there was anything serious she couldn't communicate (R13, p.13, para.36).

These examples were produced in order to illustrate the ability of the service and its staff to adapt to challenging situations, to underline the spirit of improvisation. Instead they expose a dangerous complacency at the heart of the trust, or perhaps something much worse. The representative of the REC recalled a conversation with a doctor who described a situation, in which he had been forced to improvise,

> I was talking to a health care professional who told me that he used to work in an area where they had a high proportion, I think it was Bangladeshi women, for example. And his frustration that these women would come with wasn't even their first child, their second or third child, and that they still couldn't speak English. So I said, Well how did you manage if you didn't have interpreters? And he said, Well it was like a vet relationship. And I had this horrible chilling feeling in my gut that he was saying that literally these women were like bitches (R5, p.21, para.64).

While it would be wrong to attribute this kind of attitude to the employees of the trust, it is reflected in the relevant literature (Henley 1986) and there is an implicit sense of illegitimacy about the needs of minority ethnic communities apparent in the attitudes of the majority of the trust's employees, which will become clearer as the chapter progresses.

The language of improvement

Despite the common response that the service provided was already adequate, and the evidence to the contrary, many of the respondents adopted the contradictory position that things were improving. For example, a nurse trainer at a local university with institutional links to the trust said:

> The service is getting better I think. There is perhaps a growing awareness that the service has improved and I think there are...And I'll give you a good example here: the Race Alliance Group that I'm on certainly made me more aware that it's high on the trusts' agenda to try and improve (R20, p.1, paras.1 & 2).

From within the trust a respondent, a health visitor located in an inner city clinic, acknowledged that the service was not perfect, but gave an example of the evolutionary nature of improvement. She mentioned a newly settled refugee community to make her point.

> For example, we do have a Somali community locally in the area. And until we all understood that actually in terms of making appointments or turning up on time for it wasn't actually necessarily something that would be part of their culture. Then we need to have that information so we can actually try and: a) make our service more accessible to them, and b) understand that if people aren't actually going along with what's offered it's not necessarily because they don't want it but because their culture is different. And we need to have some understanding of that...It was to do with the fact that we would say for example, but the practitioners would say: I can give you an appointment at 10 '0' clock on Tuesday morning is that convenient for you? Yep. And you'll come here to see me? Yep that'll be fine. And they didn't. Language didn't seem to be an issue, but then 10 '0' clock on Tuesday people wouldn't arrive and when that was followed up: it was: Oh such and such happened and I did that. So it was actually around the fact that they, some of the groups were more used to being able to, if there was an issue, they would tend to present with that particular concern that they had as and when it arose, rather than having to make an appointment for a day or two's time perhaps (R18, p.1, paras.1 & 2).

In sympathy with the views expressed by the HA representative, she clearly felt that awareness was a key issue. However, although she later argued that structured training would be useful, ultimately it was simply a matter of exposure and time.

One of the central areas of identifiable improvement had been in relation to dietary provision. The general manager responsible for support services on the main hospital site said,

> Let's say it could be important in areas like catering...Particularly with some religious requirements that some cultural groups have. But as I say that was very apparent years ago when we were unaware of requirements. But things, as I've said, have very much moved on now. And I think everyone, and I mean the whole workforce, let's say in the catering department...have become very aware of each ethnic group. White, black, yellow, whatever...And I think we've got to the point now where we recognise it, and we realise the seriousness of not being able to provide the appropriate dietary requirements. And I think we've gone a long way to satisfying the need...(R21, p.5, para.17).

This was supported by the catering manager, who argued that 'cultural meals' had been provided on request for some time, but a group promoting minority ethnic issues had approached the trust and advised them to publicise the fact:

> They were sort of what did we do and everything and it showed that we were doing it but we weren't publicising the fact, so they said write it on your menus, show that you do do it; which by the next week they were on the menus and have been ever since. That's about 5 years ago...And so we've always done whatever was needed. We can't have it here ready because we get so few. It really is. Yes, I could have food here all the time, but it would be a total waste because it really is few and far between, but it is on the menus and everybody is aware of it (R19, pp.10 & 11, paras.32 & 33).

'Cultural meals' had been available for some time, but the improvement came when information was provided to users. Dietary provision on another hospital site had also improved, but only very recently:

> And I'm on a nutritional group and we've discussed that actually at practically every meeting whether we can actually provide that. And I know that our catering manager is very strong on that, and that has increased, you know, a lot... Our catering manager, he said, he can actually provide that now he's got that built into his budget, so it's not being used fantastically but it is there, so that's a good thing (R13, pp.7 & 8, paras.21 & 25).

On the whole then the tone was generally optimistic. The only potential problem that the catering manager could foresee was a breakdown in communication with the nurses responsible for relaying the needs of the patients. In the event of such an occurrence unusual, though perhaps in the circumstances sensible, steps could be taken:

> It's not a big part of our diets, vegetarian is accounted for on every meal anyway, so a lot will go with that, but if it's going one stage further then we'll go and visit the patient and sort out what they can and can't eat. And no one has ever not had a meal, ever, in any form of diet, and so we've always done whatever was needed... (R19, pp.10, para.33).

The ideas of adequacy and improvement do not sit well together. The notion that things are adequate certainly is not shared with users (as discovered by the HA through the consultation process) or user representatives, and with respect to dietary provision, even the nurse trainer identified a lack of sophistication. As for the concept of improvement it appears to rely rather too heavily on improvisation, muddling through rather than being adequately prepared. Although demography was repeatedly used to explain either the absence of problems or the impossibility of providing adequate services, it seemed that something more fundamental was at work.

It's 'them' not 'us'

There was a discrepancy between the views of those who represent minority ethnic communities and those who deliver services. Essentially, the majority of trust employees blamed minority ethnic groups for failing to access or to obtain the most from the Health Service, and this would seem to substantiate the claim that the dominant approach to the needs of minority ethnic communities has been and remains 'ethnic sensitivity' or 'cultural pluralism' (Brent CHC 1981; Ahmad 1993a; Johnson 1993; Stubbs 1993; McIver 1994; Gerrish *et al* 1996). A theoretical development of the 1970s, which was central, according to Culley

(1996), to such professional guidelines as the Code of Professional Conduct for nursing established by the United Kingdom Central Council (UKCC). Although Baxter (1997) argues that the Code and guidelines published by the English National Board for Nursing, Midwifery and Health Visiting (ENB) embody the professional duty to challenge 'racial' inequalities, she nevertheless agrees that 'ethnic sensitivity' is a dominant ideological feature in the NHS. Furthermore, unlike education and social work the pre-eminent concept has allegedly gone unchallenged (Culley 1996; Mason 2000).

Cultural differences are emphasised as the source of any difficulties in providing sensitive and appropriate services. Unfortunately, difference too readily, though generally implicitly, translates to deviance or inferiority (we will discuss cultural pluralism more fully in chapter 6). In the words of Mason: *'This emphasis on **difference** is not, it should be noted, one which **celebrates** diversity. Rather it emphasizes divergences from some presumed norm that can all too easily resonate with ethnocentric beliefs and racist prejudices'* (2000: 99). On the contrary it is widely argued that the culture of health professionals and the Health Service is problematic. For example, Torkington (1991) argues that the medical ideology which informs health provision derives from the eugenicism of the late nineteenth and early twentieth centuries. Therefore, culture along with class and other characteristics are used to distinguish between the deserving and undeserving, a common feature of bureaucracies (Lipsky 1980) including Health Services (Strauss & Corbin 1998).

It is apparent from the material presented here that perceived ethnicity and culture are being used to some extent to establish whose needs are 'normal' and therefore legitimate and others whose needs are 'abnormal' and by definition illegitimate (Kushnick 1988; Ahmad 1989, 1993a; Stubbs 1993; Kelleher & Hillier 1996; Mason 2000). Reflecting the attitudes and actions of the midwives in Bowler's study the majority of the trust employees appeared to use *'stereotypes to help them to make judgements about the kind of care [visible minorities] want,*

62

need and deserve' (1993: 157). There were a number of distinct aspects to such cultural victim blaming.

Cultural proficiency or deficiency

Although it is well documented that certain communities retain strong familial ties and obligations (Henley 1991; Parekh 2000), perhaps one of the most well worn myths about minority ethnic groups is that they do not use services because they rely on the family (Donovan 1986b; McFarland *et al* 1989; Chevannes 1991; Torkington 1991; Bahl 1993b; Patel 1993; Penketh & Ali 1997). There is substantial evidence to counter this, for example Counsel and Care produced a report – *More than Black and White* (1996) - based on 100 interviews with minority ethnic elders in four major cities. Whilst the respondents did not want to enter residential homes (partly due to communication barriers), they also reported an unwillingness to burden their families (Brindle 1996a). Similarly, in research into the responses of health and social care workers to self-harm and those attempting suicide, there was a belief that it could not happen to certain groups because of the cultural stigma attached (Batsleer *et al* 2003). The danger of perpetuating such stereotypes is that people will not get the help or care that they require (Joyram 1994: 8).

Nevertheless, it appears that such stereotypes remain in circulation (Nazroo 1997; Alexander 1999). A survey carried out on behalf of the DoH with 84,000 patients with coronary heart disease across 194 trusts, revealed that on being discharged from hospital 53% of white respondents reported that their family circumstances were taken into account, but only 41% of 'Black Caribbeans' and 39% of 'South Asians' (Airy *et al* 1999: pp.28-29). It is not possible to state with any conviction that assumptions were made about familial support networks from this evidence, but it is possible to make an informed guess.

Several of the trust employees articulated this same assumption:

...although there hasn't been a lot of take-up [of 'cultural meals'], because we don't get an awful lot of coloured people who are actually patients here, surprisingly, we've got quite a few nurses for some reason. And whether that is because of the way their family structure is formed and they actually look after each other...? Yes, although that of course is breaking down so we might well see some coming through... (R13, p.7, para.23).

Yes...they are selected by the in-patients at the hospital, so therefore, that's why I'm...it might sound like I'm actually ignoring the ethnic minorities. But the fact is that they're not being brought to our attention. So whether it is that when they're in hospital, they're tending to look after their own to look after themselves and they don't want the interference, or whether it is that they're not being offered services I don't know (R31, p.2-3, para.18).

There is some recognition that things might be changing, and that the staff based on the main hospital site are not referring people on, possibly due to the same stereotypical notions:

The assumption is made by hospital staff that an Asian patient will not require any information about community nursing services or any other community-based services that may be available because 'they look after their own' (Bothamley 1996: 22).

However, the respondent quickly moved beyond this explanation and posed the following question:

...is it just that they prefer to treat their health their own way? So I think we've got to look at this traditional, staying at home looking after themselves, using the family network and the relations and everybody else. So it's very difficult to say that would they use the service more because what are the reasons for them not using it in the first place, or, why are we not seeing them? As is pretty evident at the moment (R31, p.3, para.19).

On the strength of her certainty about the preferences of minority ethnic communities, she felt that the further shift in resources to community-based care occasioned by the introduction of PCGs (discussed briefly in chapter 4) was a welcome necessity. The point was reiterated by one of the ward Sisters:

> But I do think if one of the ethnic groups were going to a GP or something like that they might want to see a female, a lot of them do, especially Bangladeshi ladies and things like that do want to see maybe somebody of their culture because they have a very strict culture. I don't know much about it, but they do, and I feel that it's going to be out in the community and places like that that you need someone who can be there for them, and stay and be with them (R16, p.10, para.36).

This suggestion was based on the assumption that minority ethnic communities could be better supported in their preferences (Jayaratnam 1993). Despite the fact that the bulk of the available evidence supports this claim (Rudat 1994; Gerrish *et al* 1996; Nazroo 1997) such assumptions have been questioned (Donovan 1986b; Farooqi 1993) and these respondents confessed to having very little knowledge about, or contact with, minority ethnic communities. Therefore, minority ethnic communities can be the victims of assumed cultural *proficiency* in the provision of health care.

Minority ethnic groups can also be blamed for causing problems due to cultural *deficiencies*. A key issue here revolved around the issue of hospital visiting (Jayaratnam 1993; Baxter 1997). For instance, a manager responsible for the out-patients clinic had this to say:

> I mean I've never heard any particular comments or, any particular issues. I mean we do have concerns because in certain cultures when you come to outpatients you come, as a family unit. You know, come with the whole family...which is a problem for us because we don't have space, but I mean it's not, I mean it happens not necessarily on a cultural, in ethnic minorities. It happens across the board, but there is perhaps a greater tendency, because you need interpreters, or you may need support, or you may need a chaperone. Or, you know, for all those issues. But it's not a major problem, and we would certainly not stop people coming for that reason, but obviously we say to all our patients, don't come with everybody because we just don't have enough seats. But that applies to everybody, not just to minorities (R23, pp. 4 &5, paras.15 & 16).

Although she stretched the point to include other communities, minority ethnic communities were the biggest transgressors. This was supported by other respondents a Ward Sister recalled an incident in which a *'lad of mixed parentage'* became angry when challenged about his extended family *'taking over'* the day room (R29, p.4, para.25).

The trust's Head of Nursing recounted a similar experience because 'Asians' did tend to get between twelve to fourteen family members visiting them at any one time. In one particular case the family in question felt victimised until it was made clear that they could all visit only at different times (R27, p.1, para.2). Although Baxter (1997: 46) claims that *'...this can seem unduly harsh where there is a cultural tradition of the extended family visiting members who are sick'.* So the perceived cultural proclivities of certain minority ethnic communities were identified as problematic, making the entire task of health provision more difficult.

The deficiency of certain cultures was carried by some into the realms of cultural weakness. Many of the health problems identified in minority ethnic communities have been linked to these same cultural deficiencies:

> Although the overt scientific racism that explained the mortality and morbidity in some peoples as resulting from their inherently weak constitution is now eschewed, similar notions exist in an updated form (Bradby 1995: 406).

According to several of the respondents the weaknesses are not only physical they also manifest themselves in ways that impede health provision. For example,

> There are cultural differences obviously and we find that there are some male or female patients who accept things more than others. For instance, if we have an investigation and there are certain cultures that do actually find it difficult and so in that case we, if you like treat them differently. Inasmuch as we encourage them to bring relatives with them into the investigating room, partly as chaperone, partly as a hand to hold when they need moral support. Whereas other cultures sometimes think well we've got to grin and bear it, and if we need it done it's got to be done this way (R15, p.3, para.9).

So while some 'grin and bear it' others have to be treated with kid gloves. Another respondent echoed these sentiments:

> ...some females prefer to see females, some people don't mind they're a doctor and that's it. But I know a lot of the ethnic ladies do not like seeing male doctors, they are very, very frightened of them (R16, p.11, para.39).

By her own admission she did not have a great deal of knowledge about minority ethnic issues, but here their generalised cultural preferences are asserted and in the same breath presented as weakness. It is not just that their culture precludes them from consulting with male doctors (speculation becomes truth) they are *terrified* of them.

In the final analysis, whether minority ethnic groups access services or not, whether they get the best out of them or not, is entirely down to them. On the one hand different cultures are seen as proficient, in other words willing to be self-sufficient and look out for their own. On the other they are deficient. As Batsleer et al (2003: 106-7) write:

> Whether this 'difference' is seen in positive terms ('They/We have strong families') or in negative terms ('They/We have extremely patriarchal families in which women are excessively passive), the formulation of difference distracts attention from the interconnection and potential fluidity and openness of culture. More specifically it distracts attention from the challenges of diversity and from the problems, difficulties and responsibilities that lie within the culture of large, predominantly white, often multi-cultural health and welfare organisations.

We will now explore these issues through the construction of certain minority ethnic requirements as 'special needs'.

Special needs

So the failure to access services, or to maximise them once accessed, was often due either to cultural proficiency or cultural deficiency. However, there was a much deeper issue lurking far below the surface. One respondent, who had initially argued that the trust was failing to communicate properly with minority ethnic communities, ultimately said:

> I think perhaps cultural expectations as well make it difficult, the perception of a
> need might be different; and an expectation about what an organisation like a
> health care trust can really provide. So expectations may be different between
> cultures, as to what a need is and what can be provided (R30, p.1a, para.3a).

Others took up her theme:

> So I think our expectations, what we often expect of our cultures are perhaps not
> always acceptable to the ethnic minorities. But not having a great deal of contact
> with them I couldn't say (R31, p.1, para.2).

The implication is clear, the main problem is that minority ethnic communities expect too much of the Health Service. More than that, the central question is legitimacy, whose needs *should* be met?

The conclusion must be that minority ethnic needs are not of central concern to the Health Service, to use the language of the managers it is not viewed as the 'core business' (Carter 2000), even though repeated references are made officially to counteract this perception (Johnson 2004). In 1995 Ahmad stated that:

> While the rhetoric of *special needs* and special provision remains strong its
> impact has been to marginalise health needs of minority ethnic groups to 'special
> projects', without making mainstream services more accessible (1995: 418, my
> emphasis).

Unfortunately, this notion also appears in the unlikeliest of places (see Rawaf 1993: 40 and Karmi 1993: 51.) Every operational member of the trust employed this concept of 'special needs', for example,

> But certainly like providing special meals, and when people die that you have to
> lay them out in a certain way. That's been highlighted quite a lot...The past sort
> of couple of years, we've had highlighted the *special needs* of patients.
> Especially when they die, you know what to do, this is the special thing that they
> need to be buried on certain days and this sort of thing, and a lot of issues have
> been highlighted quite heavily (R13, pp.7 & 8, paras.23 & 24).

> I mean...right down to a patient on a ward might need a *special* diet, which is of course a cultural thing (R17, p.3, para.7).

> Just by virtue of the things that an organisation does, it doesn't take on – I mean like diets. I mean we do have *special* diets. I can't say what they're like (R24, p.7, para.27).

This is disturbing because this use of language, in concert with phrases like *'cultural meals'*, only serves to illustrate the 'otherness' of minority ethnic requirements, enabling their needs to be neglected, portrayed as peripheral and marginal. If they are *special* then they are not *normal*, and if they are not normal they do not need to be considered as a central part of the business of the Health Service (Fletcher 1997).

At times it felt very much as if the trust employees were trying to underline the nature of their core business. During several interviews, cultural issues were deflected in the following way:

> And a couple of our staff have done sign language, so if there's someone there who's deaf then we can bring them, and you know, they're not experts, but they could do their little bit and it assures the patient that there will be some form of communication (R16, p.1, para.2).

> It's obviously mainly the Asians that we have a problem with language, we did have one person who was actually trained to do the deaf and dumb signs. We do have booklets for blind people in the unit so that they read Braille of what the [unit] offers (R25, p.1, para.2).

It could be argued that this was an attempt to turn the discussion onto more familiar territory. Yet the manner in which these diversions were employed, it seemed as if the interviewees were trying to underline the core concerns of the Health Service, demonstrating the irrelevance or illegitimacy of different cultural requirements. One respondent actively informed me that ethnicity was not an issue for the Health Service, and that I ought to have been researching issues of gender discrimination (R28).

One recurrent theme, which has emerged in relation to the illegitimacy of minority ethnic needs, involves the inability or refusal of minority ethnic individuals to learn English. *'There is a remarkable amount of prejudice directed at people who cannot speak English. Studies have shown that many health professionals feel black patients should know how to speak English and that if they don't they must be stupid'* (McIver 1994: 69). One of the midwives in Bowler's study said *'It's disgusting not to speak English after so long in Britain'* (1993: 160). A Ward Manager provided a very clear example of this in relating the following story involving an Indian family:

> ...but they were specifically saying that because of the language, because when they went away, went home, she couldn't communicate because she'd never, I mean she'd been here for *thirty years*, but she'd never spoken English, and I don't know how they get on but obviously they do. But I think she said 'yes' and 'no' but I think that was about it, but I mean we could communicate by gesture and everything but they were worried that if there was anything serious she couldn't communicate (R13, p.13, para.36).

Although the emphasis placed here on the phrase 'thirty years' appears in the text as neutral, denoting either sympathy or condemnation, during the interview itself it was very clear that the sentiment was *not* sympathetic. The consequent willingness to risk someone's health and well-being by relying upon gesticulation, simply because they were 'negligent' enough not to learn English is in itself very disturbing. It conveniently ignores the difficulties of learning a language, particularly for many who have received no formal education (McIver 1994). Such matters are clearly used to deflect attention away from the service and onto the communities themselves.

Conclusion

In this chapter we have talked about the possibility that communication barriers adversely affect the access and quality of service once accessed, offered to minority ethnic communities. Amongst those representing the needs of users there was a consensus that such barriers exist; although official representatives were more inclined to sympathise with health providers than their unofficial counterparts.

Those directly responsible for services, however, largely rejected this. They framed their views in several ways. Some dismissed the possibility of problems due to demography – there could not be a problem because the trust was located beyond the inner city. The numbers issue has been a recurring excuse for inactivity and inadequate service provision for some time (Smaje 1995), particularly in the south west (Jay 1992). Many argued that existing provision was adequate, although the evidence to the contrary was compelling. Similarly, the notion that things were improving was not entirely reassuring, it smacked a little too much of muddling through.

A common feature of the accounts produced by the health workers was the tendency to lay the blame for any problems at the door of minority ethnic communities. It was not entirely negative. For example, any underrepresentation of minority ethnic people accessing services might be due to cultural proficiency, the willingness to take responsibility for the health of one's friends and family. Though this has consistently been questioned, and has just as consistently been used to justify inaction (Patel 1993).

When people do access services they apparently create problems rather than experience them, an implication that Jay (1992: 27) detected across various statutory agencies in the south west region. 'They' colonise waiting areas and as a result of the weaknesses produced by deficient cultures 'they' make the lives of (exclusively white?) health workers more difficult. Kandola and Fullerton detail the way in which the private sector has approached such issues (1998: 101). However, the essential feature of such a response works on the basis of changing the organisation rather than cultural mores.

It became clear that the central problem was illegitimacy, minority ethnic communities expect too much of a service that was not set up to meet their 'special' needs (Brent CHC 1981). Although they are citizens, living, working (frequently in and for the NHS) and paying taxes (Donovan 1986a; Patel 1993) their needs are not considered by those who really count to be part of the core business of the NHS. There is an implicit belief that the service should not have to bend to the needs of minority ethnic groups. 'They' (visible minorities) ought to adapt to the shape of 'our' (white) service (Brent CHC 1981; Jay 1992; Bhopal & White 1993; Fletcher 1997).

This has been recognised more recently in the context of health provision (Hiscock 2004) and the need to challenge these views and refocus ideas about the core business receives considerable attention in material and policies emanating from the Department of Health (DoH 2003a, 2004c). Nevertheless, it may be a difficult challenge to bring home as the beliefs that inform it are deep-set and appear to be based in the cultural practices that underpin much health care work.

The implicit racism identified here would appear to derive from an ideological cocktail composed of biomedicine and cultural pluralism (Ahmad 1993a; Stubbs 1993). Health provision has been dominated by the medical professional who, through the channel of biomedicine, draw upon eugenicism to distinguish between the deserving and undeserving (Torkington 1991). Cultural pluralism, although explicitly an attempt to make white individuals aware of cultural differences to eradicate ignorance, all too often leads to those differences being constructed as abnormal or deviant. It became clear that the majority of the trust employees felt that different cultural requirements were therefore illegitimate and that the onus lay with minority ethnic communities to either assimilate or take on the responsibility of improving or providing services (Ahmad 1993b). In the next chapter we will explore more openly the concept of discrimination and racism in relation to health provision.

CHAPTER 3:

Institutional racism in the NHS

'The price one pays for pursuing any profession or calling is an intimate knowledge of its ugly side' – James Baldwin

Introduction

This chapter explores head-on the notions of 'racial' discrimination and racism and their impact, through the perceptions of the interview respondents. Baxter (1997) suggested that racism is rarely investigated, at least explicitly, in the context of the Health Service. Echoing the material contained in the previous chapter, there was a distinct contrast between the views of the unofficial user representatives and the rest of the respondents. Although the trust employees and those involved in a professional capacity with the Health Service acknowledged the existence of prejudice, few were willing to accept that this was ever translated into action (with the exception of interactions between 'elderly' white patients and minority ethnic health workers). However, this was not borne out by the evidence, particularly with regard to procedural matters.

The majority of this constituency argued that the MacPherson Report (1999) had provided minority ethnic communities with the opportunity to attack important societal institutions, such as the NHS, and encouraged individuals to deflect justified criticism or to seek unfair advantages. The unofficial user representatives argued on the contrary that the Report had not gone far enough and were able to provide clear examples of discriminatory actions and outcomes.

The majority considered racism to be a central, and conscious, component of British society, and therefore, by logical extrapolation, of its major institutions.

Background

The reluctance of the NHS to address much less deal with issues of discrimination and racism has been much commented upon in the relevant literature (Brent CHC 1981; NAHA 1988; Ward 1993; Snell 1996). For example, Law (1996: 150) maintains that the *'...recognition of the importance of ethnicity in health policy has increased, although questions of challenging racism and racial inequality have yet to arrive on the national policy agenda'*. Evidently such claims are based on more than simple conjecture.

A framework for dealing with 'racial' discrimination has been in place since 1978 with the publication of *Health Circular (36)*, which outlined the requirements of the Race Relations Act 1976 for the Service, and several subsequent circulars have dealt with specific aspects of health provision in relation to minority ethnic health and also employment issues (Law 1996). Yet there has reputedly been very little response from NHS employers (Baxter 1988; Ward 1993). The CREs 1984 *Code of Practice* has not been influential (Ward 1993), and its 1992 *Race Relations Code of Practice in Primary Health Services* has not been widely taken up. A follow-up survey by the CRE showed that a mere 29 from 600 HAs had any plans to implement it (Law 1996). The fact that the CRE has issued 108 notices to NHS employers since the passage of the Race Relations (Amendment) Act 2000 illustrates that this is a continuing problem (Harding 2005).

In keeping with the low profile of discrimination and racism in the NHS generally (Bhopal & White 1993; Ward 1993; Baxter 1997), the report produced locally by the HA did not include any reference to the existence of either. Despite concerns raised about this issue by one of the working groups, the report merely acknowledged that certain groups – i.e. women of 'South Asian' origin – are subject to significant levels of racial abuse and violence in the community. Insensitivity on the part of a small minority of NHS staff in isolated incidents was acknowledged, but communication barriers were seen as the principal cause of inaccessible and inappropriate treatment. Statutory agencies in the south west, including NHS employers, have tended to dismiss the existence of discrimination due to numbers. Apparently this is a common and long standing belief, i.e. that there is not enough ethnic diversity in the region to create a problem (Jay 1992). The silence that surrounds racism is a constant source of frustration to many minority ethnic professionals (Batsleer *et al* 2003).

There is also some reluctance amongst those involved in caring professions to recognise anything that might call that role or their commitment into question (Brent CHC 1981; Baxter 1997). A point raised by the representative of the local HA below. It may also derive from the desire to see major social institutions such as the NHS as ideologically neutral (Ahmad 1993d). Judging by the material presented in the previous chapter it must also have something to do with the ideological cocktail composed of 'ethnic sensitivity' and biomedicine, which appears to justify the discriminatory attitudes and actions of white health workers and others involved in the planning and delivery of care, without their having to acknowledge them. As Bowler suggested with reference to the white professionals who participated in her study, the *'Midwives could employ a stereotype to allow them to practice discrimination based on ethnicity without having to admit to themselves, or appearing to others to be racist' (1993: 174).*

In many ways this is reminiscent of the 'New Racism' identified by Barker (1981); see also Gordon & Klug 1986), whereby scientific racism and notions of biological superiority/inferiority are displaced by an emphasis on cultural difference to the point of incompatibility. However, the underlying motivation for the 'New Racism' was ethnic segregation and ultimately the repatriation of people from visible minorities (even where repatriation was physically impossible, see Barton & Johns 2005).

To some extent, as Younge (2000) has argued, things have moved on since the late 1960s/early 1970s and the place of visible minorities in Britain is no longer explicitly contested, except by right-wing extremists. Consequently it would not be appropriate, or I think accurate, to attribute such aims and objectives to the trust employees and others involved in this research project. As mentioned previously they were more concerned about the inability or unwillingness of certain groups and communities to adapt to fit the shape of the existing service. This would support the contention of Culley (1996) and Mason (2000) that assimilationism, the desire to see minority ethnic communities accept indigenous culture and to be eventually absorbed, has been more resilient in the Health Service than in virtually any other public sector organisation.

Despite the reticence of health workers there can be no doubt that prejudice and discrimination have shaped the service provided to minority ethnic communities at both an individual (McNaught 1988; Ahmad *et al* 1991; Bowler 1993) and structural level (Brent CHC 1981; Bryan *et al* 1985; Kushnick 1988; NAHA 1988; Anionwu 1996; Baxter 1997; Alexander 1999; Parekh 2000).

It was partly as a response to the claim by Baxter (1997) that racism and discrimination have rarely been explored explicitly with regards the Health Service, and partly due to the implicit racism identified earlier that the issue was raised so openly with the interview respondents. The discussions were initially structured around the broad notion of 'discrimination' allowing the respondents the opportunity to present their own definitions, drawn, where possible, from their experiences. This was framed in a much more far reaching way for the trust employees and others associated professionally with the Health Service, in order to take account of their breadth of experience:

> Two areas of racism in the NHS that act as barriers to health care for ethnic groups are health workers own racist attitudes and prejudices, often unconscious, which have shown to have an adverse effect on professional/client relationships; and black and *ethnic* staff suffering discrimination and racial harassment at work (Bothamley 1996: 22).

Perhaps unsurprisingly, considering the seminal importance attributed to it (Parekh 2000), the interviews generally flowed around the aftermath of the MacPherson Report (Macpherson 1999). The notion of institutional racism, which has gained renewed academic currency and has attained a higher profile in public discourse than ever before, was extremely resonant with the interview respondents.

Just as in the previous chapter there was a sharp contrast between the views of unofficial user representatives and those employed in and around the NHS. A very small minority of trust employees accepted the provisional definition of institutional racism established by MacPherson and felt that it was applicable to the NHS, i.e.:

> The collective failure of an organization to provide an appropriate and professional service to people because of their colour, culture, or ethnic origin. It can be seen or detected in processes, attitudes and behaviours which amount to discrimination through unwitting prejudice, ignorance, thoughtlessness and racist stereotyping which disadvantage minority ethnic people (MacPherson 1999: para.6.43).

The overwhelming majority, however, echoing the immediate response of the Metropolitan Police Service and sympathetic sections of the right-wing media (Kundnani 1999; McLaughlin & Murji 1999) felt, as representatives of a major public institution, both undermined and under attack. In their view the Report went too far and has subsequently provided minority ethnic individuals with the means to ward off justified criticism and to gain unfair advantages. As this suggests, and as was intended by the open-ended nature of the questioning on this issue, they tended to branch out from discrimination between patients and staff to consider relations between staff members. Substantial evidence suggests that minority ethnic health workers face as much abuse and discrimination from white colleagues and managers as they do from white patients (Baxter 1988; Beishon *et al* 1995), but we will consider this in slightly more detail in chapter 7.

For the majority of the unofficial user representatives on the other hand, MacPherson clearly did not go far enough. Reflecting the criticisms of McLaughlin & Murji (1999) they inferred that the definition outlined above allowed individuals to avoid identification and censure. Far from labelling every white employee as inherently racist, which was a central concern in the immediate aftermath of the publication of MacPherson, the definition allows racist individuals to hide behind terms like 'unwitting' and consequently behind a nameless, faceless edifice.

The unofficial user representatives paint a much more complex and far-reaching picture of racism in the NHS. As Bowler (1993) maintains the use of stereotypical assumptions is discriminatory regardless of the intentions of the perpetrator, however, the majority of the unofficial user representatives believed that the outcomes were consciously produced. The model they employed relates closely to that produced by Patel (1993) and more recently (in relation to the public sector in its entirety) by Parekh (2000).

Without categorising minority ethnic communities as passive victims or overlooking the challenge that they and their organisations have posted (Stubbs 1993; Gerrish *et al* 1996) there remains an urgent need to explore, openly and honestly, the role of discrimination and racism in the planning and delivery of services. To quote Ahmad (1993b: 214), *'The focus…needs to shift away from 'ethnic differences' to racist constructions of black needs, and racism in service provision at individual and institutional levels'*. How this is to be initiated when many of those responsible deny not only the existence of discrimination and racism, but also their consequences (i.e. inadequate, inappropriate and insensitive services) remains to be seen.

Pride and prejudice

Baxter, in making the distinction between prejudice and discrimination acknowledged that *'Prejudice is the property of all people...'* (1988: 3). 'Racial' prejudice remains a significant problem nationally as demonstrated by the *British Social Attitudes Survey* (Cartice & Heath 2001). In fact there was pretty much a consensus amongst the respondents about the existence of prejudice. In the previous chapter we provided evidence that trust employees do make assumptions about minority ethnic communities, i.e. that underutilisation of services is the result of families and communities taking the strain. While this is not in and of itself always based on explicitly negative assumptions the consequences have the potential to be very damaging (Gerrish *et al* 1996).

There was also evidence of overt prejudgements based on negative generalisations and stereotypes, amongst the trust employees (echoing the findings of Donovan 1986a; Ahmad *et al* 1991 and Bowler 1993). For example, one respondent expressed his frustration at the apparent unwillingness of minority ethnic people to seek employment in the NHS in the following way:

> Why aren't you? Well we all work in my Dad's shop. Well okay fine that's the reason is it? (R21, p.17, para.57).

Another argued that:

> ...it's a known fact that it is a sign of femininity in Asian cultures that your pain threshold is low, and so naturally, certain individuals can accept less than others as far as treatment is concerned (R15, p.7, para.19).

Although it has long been recognised that certain minority ethnic groups seek familial or self-employment to a relatively large extent (Modood 1997) the 'Asian' shopkeeper stereotype is so well worn that pop groups have even reclaimed it. Little thought is given by the respondent as to why people *might*, if indeed they do, prefer this employment option.

As for claims about lower pain thresholds amongst certain minority ethnic groups, these were made in the training literature provided by authors such as Henley (1982; 1986), and although much evidence exists to suggest that health professionals adhere to them (Brent CHC 1981; Atkin *et al* 1989; Rawaf 1993), there is substantial evidence to suggest that they do not bear close scrutiny (Donovan 1986b; Bowler 1993; Calvillo & Flaskerud 1993; Anionwu 1996).

The purpose of such arguments would appear to be, on the one hand to blame the trust's perceived failure to attract minority ethnic recruits on the communities themselves (Younge 2001), and on the other, as also mentioned in the previous chapter, minority cultures are being defined as inherently weak or weakening (Pearson 1986; Torkington 1991; Ahmad 1994). In order to illustrate the dangers inherent in such attitudes, Kushnick (1988) recalls a conversation with a white woman who witnessed the neglect of an 'Asian' woman crying out in pain during labour, she asked the Sister whether something ought to be done and was told that this was normal for 'them'. Her baby was stillborn, but *'The point is not that there is evidence that earlier medical intervention would necessarily have saved the child, but that such "truths" about black people's cultural characteristics have profound professional behavioural implications'* (1988: 463).

Having said this, the trust employees and the official user representatives were prepared to accept that prejudice is a central part of human existence:

> ...that's assuming that every organisation is kind of prejudice-free, no organisation is prejudice-free, and no person is, but you're not overtly racist, or sexist, or discriminatory in any way (R23, p.20, para.61).

> Inevitably we're all racist (R11, p.13, para.45).

Despite this acceptance they were not prepared to admit that prejudice is translated into action. On the subject of discrimination then there was another chasm separating those employed in and around the NHS and those representing (albeit unofficially) user interests.

Attitudes without action

Negative attitudes are not the principal source of the problems faced by minority ethnic communities in the UK. As Sivanandan argued:

> People's attitudes don't mean a damn to me but it matters to me if I can't send my child to the school I want to send my child to, if I can't get the job for which I am qualified and so on. It is the acting out of prejudice itself that matters. The acting out of prejudice is discrimination... (1983: 2).

The majority of the trust employees refused to accept that prejudice necessarily influences action. Yet it is extremely unlikely that strongly held negative views, based on gross stereotypes, are never translated into action. In other words prejudiced people in a position to discriminate are likely to do so (Clements & Spinks 2000). For example, Ahmad *et al* (1991) found that white GPs systematically discriminated against minority ethnic patients, and Bowler (1993) revealed a similar pattern amongst white midwives. The Coronary Heart Disease survey carried out on behalf of the Department of Health found that minority ethnic patients were significantly less likely to report having been treated with dignity and respect by hospital staff (Airy *et al* 1999: 24).

Despite the common sense nature of these arguments and the supporting evidence, those employed in and around the Health Service largely denied that prejudice can translate into discrimination. The most common response to the question of discrimination amongst trust employees was as follows:

> I think the majority, certainly the people I've come across, I don't think I've ever come across any outward signs of being discriminatory (R19, p.12, para.37).

The representative of the HA shared this view:

> By and large people don't, most people I've seen, certainly at middle management level don't discriminate (R11, p.23, paras.84 & 85).

As discussed briefly above the report published by the HA omitted any reference to discrimination. This would certainly run counter to the expectations of Baxter (1988) and Fernando (1993: 19): *'I have no doubt that many people of African, Caribbean and Asian communities would ask for strict controls on racism within our current institutional practices'*. I asked if any of the minority ethnic communities consulted complained of discrimination:

> No they didn't. What I found is that quite a few activists will emphasise discrimination and will...In fact discrimination seems to be one of the...The terminology changes in this area so fast, you know? And I think you have to be up front with people and say well what do you want to call this issue at the moment? And the thing that seems to come up more than discrimination as such is institutionalised racism. That's a phrase that's thrown around quite a lot, but not by ordinary people... It was important to get beyond the groups who represent people. You've got to talk to people themselves. The NHS has tended, because it's easier, and there aren't many of us here at the health authority, it's easier to talk to somebody who says I represent the black community and I'm a black mental health expert. I'm the Asian, the expert on Asian problems, or I'm from the Racial Equality Council I can tell you all you need to know about black health in [the city]. It's not true because when you talk to real people what they tell you, and this is the same for white people as well. I do a lot of work in areas of high health needs, which are entirely white. You've got to hear from real people what their issues are, and they're not the same issues that professionals identify (R11, pp.2 & 4, paras.3 & 11).

In short, discrimination is a problem identified by activists but not minority ethnic communities themselves. I suspect that she would dismiss much of the evidence presented here on this basis, yet it would be difficult to attribute the label of 'activist' to the majority of my respondents, assuming that she was using the term in a revolutionary sense, because they were generally Fabian in their beliefs (Williams 1989). The system must change, but it can and should be changed using evolutionary rather than revolutionary tools.

Furthermore, she fails to acknowledge the power dynamics involved in such a consultation process. It would, as several of the user representatives maintained, be very difficult to challenge and criticise face-to-face the service on which your life and the lives of your loved ones might depend, particularly from the basis of discrimination and disadvantage experienced by many minority ethnic people (Baxter 1988; Ahmad 1993d).

Where discrimination was identified users were rarely identified as victims, at least where staff were the perpetrators; the most common example offered was discrimination against minority ethnic health workers by white users, a significant feature of much of the relevant literature (Baxter 1988; Beishon *et al* 1995). For example:

> Oh yes, I mean there are...I've heard certainly instances of staff from ethnic minorities receiving abuse, verbal abuse, maybe worse I don't know from white Engl...You know white people because of their race. So certainly staff experience discrimination, and I can't remember the other part of your question – oh yes, whether it occurs the other way around. Oh I'm sure it must happen yes (R24, p.7, para.26).

The main perpetrators were reported to be older white patients,

> Yes, I'd say that because the catchment area that we work in is predominantly elderly and also because the structure of the patients that we have is obviously elderly and that is 65 now rising to 70 and above, up to 110, that's our age group. And if you think that in that age group they've gone through two World Wars, a lot of the people have probably not left the area and are not culturally absorbed. And as aware as some of our younger patients, and we have had some quite sort of confrontations between staff that are black and their white patients. And also we haven't had anything with staff, I must say, the staff are extremely good in that way. It's probably because they're a younger generation and so on. But certainly between black nurses and white patients are very vitriolic in some cases (R13, p.4, para.11).

However, this doesn't seem entirely convincing particularly in light of the findings of Bagilhole and Stephens (1999). During a similar interview survey they found that

> ...the perception of most [white] managers was that sexual and racial harassment were not common at the hospital and that when they occurred – especially in relation to racial harassment – they came mainly from elderly patients, both of which perceptions contrast with the views of many ethnic minority women and their union representatives (1999: 240).

Their study showed that white colleagues perpetrated the bulk of the harassment (see also Carter 2000). Even if the trust employees were painting a fair reflection of reality, why would involvement in two World Wars predispose older people to 'racial' discrimination? This carries even less explanatory weight when we consider that so many people from the Caribbean and the Indian subcontinent, and many others, fought in those conflicts – though of course that history has been submerged (Tully 2005). It would seem to be one device amongst many to distance the Health Service from racism in general, and indeed to confine it to one small section of white society (Gilroy 1987; Torkington 1991; McLaughlin & Murji 1999). Conversely, as we shall see, parts of the Health Service procedurally encourage and condone racism.

In spite of the claim that relations between white and minority ethnic staff were very good in some areas in others there was some recognition of discrimination against minority ethnic staff members by white colleagues

> No I can't...Yes, no...I'm not aware of any amongst my staff but in the past I have encountered it in a consultant. An extremely strong discrimination against black people, which I found very offensive at the time. Because we were talking about recruitment policies and this person was saying well, you know, I wouldn't even want to repeat it, but I was quite horrified. That someone in that position could be so open about their views, or the fact that they held those views, let alone be open about them. So yes it does exist. I'm talking there about being racist... And in fact the issue was this member of staff, we were talking about recruitment and we were talking about black doctors, and he said we have to hold a consultants post open for the white boys... Anyway, so yeah I have come across it amongst medical staff. But I'm not aware of any specific, for example nursing staff that I manage... (R23, pp.3-4, para.s10, 11, & 15).

So where discrimination did occur it apparently never affected minority ethnic users, either older patients harassed minority ethnic staff members, which was understandable due to their life experiences, or, it was confined to isolated employment decisions (objectionable though the consequences may be to this respondent).

Various reasons were given for this perceived harmony. Again a central issue was the notion of improvement. There was generally less discrimination in society, due to evolutionary processes, communities learning to live together, and that as a major part of society the NHS reflected that improvement:

> I think the population in general have hopefully, have gone away from that attitude [of racism] anyway. But it certainly existed, as anyone will say... It has been tough at times I do believe and I think that we've all learnt an awful lot...So I think we've got to the stage now where I think everything is becoming fairly equal (R21, p.5, para.18).

Yet there was reason to suspect that any improvement might not last. The same respondent continued:

> ...the days when you thought: oh an Asian person, an Afro-Caribbean person, gosh that's unusual! Those days are gone. It's a candidate now. They've come for an interview and thanks very much for coming. You're grateful. So I think that's the situation we're in... And I'm not saying that there haven't been interview panels that wouldn't discriminate. Can't say. Possibly. But the opportunity to discriminate was there (R21, pp.4 & 21, paras.15 & 72).

In recruitment at least any improvement has been based on pragmatic grounds rather than moral ones. While this would be consistent with recent developments in equal opportunities theory, i.e. the business case (see chapter 7) it does not take into account the problems associated with a change in circumstances.

One need only think about the position of women in the economy during and after two World Wars (Hancock 1992; Butler & Landells 1994). A laundry firm in Sheffield fell foul of the 1976 Race Relations Act because it made six black employees redundant in difficult economic circumstances using stereotypical notions about 'West Indians'. They were targeted on the assumption that their sick records would be relatively worse than their white colleagues and that their 'happy-go-lucky' nature would lead them to reapply when things improved. The assumption proved to be wrong on both counts. (Wainwright 1999: 21). The lesson to be learnt here, and one which must be kept in mind when setting forth a business case for equal opportunities (see Section 3) is that any gains, however significant, might be lost when economic circumstances change.

Another barrier to discrimination was the notion of professionalism. The HA representative argued that:

> By and large people don't, most people I've seen, certainly at middle management level don't discriminate. I mean it's just, well, I've not come across specific cases of it. But there's no doubt that discrimination exists at the base, at a much more basic level (R11, p.23, paras.84 & 85).

It was just accepted that middle managers in particular, presumably those making employment decisions would not, indeed could not, discriminate; a position not dissimilar to that of the Scarman Report in relation to policing (Scarman 1982).

> I also think and this is something quite close to my heart, I think everybody is an individual and has their own thoughts. They have all their own baggage from when they're young, and they have their own prejudices and you are never, never going to get rid of them, and I'm completely convinced of that. That's my own personal feeling okay? So I just want to be clear on that. But I think if you're in a responsible position you will actually be able to work professionally, and you should be able to sort of get over what you've got, and you can actually still have it inside yourself, but you know how to control it and you know what the boundaries are. Sometimes it never appears, but I think you've got to have that willingness and awareness. But as you said by raising it I think it does start to get people thinking or whatever (R13, p.14, para.37).

As intimated above though, it is extremely unlikely that a sense of professionalism would be sufficient to prevent someone from discriminating (Clements & Spinks 2000). Indeed the very notion is in itself highly culturally biased, hailing from white Western rationalism. Central to this is the highly contentious notion of objectivity (Becker 1967; Strauss & Corbin 1998).

Therefore in explaining their scepticism about the existence and impact of 'racial' discrimination the respondents were not entirely convincing. There was another identifiable trend in this denial in which the victims, as in so many other instances, were blamed for a general decline in 'race' relations.

The aftermath of MacPherson

According to the majority of the trust employees the issue of discrimination was only really an issue because of the aftermath of the MacPherson Report, and there has been widespread recognition of its seminal importance (Johns 1999; McLaughlin & Murji 1999; Carter 2000; Parekh 2000; Younge 2001). One consequence has been a heightened sensitivity amongst minority ethnic communities particularly when major institutions such as the NHS are involved:

> Because obviously we're aware that we have to treat everyone equally and if they accuse somebody else of not treating them equally, then we have to be very impartial and we have to look at both sides. But it was strange that both times, it was the coloured person and there was no justification we did investigation into both times and it wasn't. So I just feel that the sensitivity is very much on the coloured person's side sometimes. But as a manager I have to be sensitive to their sensitivities if you see what I mean, because they've probably had antagonisms before (R13, p.11, para.33).

Several trust employees argued that minority ethnic people, whether patient or employee, are too ready to see racism around every corner. This echoed the findings of Baxter (1988), Carter (2000) and Jay (1992: 22). During the latter's pilot study of racism in the south west, for instance a 'black' professional told him, *'You are constantly made to feel responsible if you raise the question; it is you who are making it an issue'*. For the majority of the trust employees this was in no small part due to the aftermath of Macpherson. Apparently there was an even greater problem.

Not only are minority ethnic communities hyper sensitive they are also using the prevailing political climate to their advantage in various ways.

> ...you see we've got this employee who is black and there have been issues in the past about performance, and I know of instances where those have not been taken up because of the potential of being accused of being racist (R23, p.11, para.37).

> I must say, I've been thinking about it, that I have had two very, how can I put this, very hard issues to deal with, with two members of staff. They were both Jamaican and they both are on, were concerned about issues on different wards. Trained nurses, one of them was a ward manager, and felt that she was being victimised because of her colour. Now this wasn't brought up as an official complaint, but it was something that was brought in with other things that were going on in the ward. There was no justification for actually bringing up the colour, and it struck me as very odd that nobody had mentioned it except the person themselves. So it sort of, you wonder whether sometimes and as a manager you have to be fair, to say are they using that as an excuse for non-performance, and that's a very hard thing for a manager to look at. (R13, p.11, para.33).

Instances of such abuse were reputedly widespread. The head of nursing reported that a 'black' nurse had complained about facing disciplinary charges on just such grounds (R27, p.1, para.1), and a general manager argued that medical secretaries are often accused of racism – by minority ethnic patients - for effectively failing to push them to the head of the appointments list (R22, p.1, para.1). Carter (2000) in research carried out in a trust in the west of England revealed a similar pattern of perceptions amongst white ward managers.

This analysis would seem to have been borrowed, to some extent at least, from the alleged effects on the Metropolitan Police Service in particular and the police service in general. Street crime was reported to have increased because officers were unwilling to stop and search minority ethnic groups for fear of being labelled as racists (Kundnani 1999: 6-7). McLaughlin & Murji (1999) are concerned that we now have a climate in which any and every claim regardless of its legitimacy might be dismissed as the machination of a small minority to gain unfair advantages. They use this extract from *The Daily Telegraph* to underline their claim: *'It is already being reported by front-line officers on patrol last night that black youths were taunting them, saying that they would not be able to arrest them now. There will be much more of that, and worse'* (1999: 378).

Of course it would be unrealistic to suggest that some individuals will not take advantage if they can, or that minority ethnic people are never oversensitive in their dealings with white people (Gerrish *et al* 1996). Indeed Proctor and Davis

(1994) assert that past experience has imbued some sense of *'healthy paranoia'*. It is the degree to which the trust employees identified people taking advantage and being guilty of heightened sensitivity which was disturbing. As McLaughlin and Murji (1999) maintained any and every instance and incident might be dismissed in these terms, yet there is strong evidence to question these attitudes.

In a similar context Bagilhole and Stephens (1999) wrote, *'It is interesting to note that they [minority ethnic women] ignored racist remarks from other staff and argued that they were careful not to make an issue of them'* (1999: 240). Similarly the Joint Chair of the Health Visitors Association Race and Equality Sub-committee said, *'There is a widespread feeling that black nurses have a chip on their shoulder, and they don't want to be labelled and so tend not to complain'* (Cohen 1995a: 484; see also Jay 1992: 19; Kandola & Fullerton 1998). It could be that rather than minority ethnic people using discrimination as an easy source of unfair advantage, it is being used by white employees to silence legitimate claims and perhaps restrict the subsequent career opportunities of minority ethnic communities (Carter 2000: 78-80).

Furthermore, the argument that minority ethnic communities are exploiting the post-MacPherson political climate provides an implicit explanation for the non-existence of discrimination on the part of health workers. In other words, white health professionals do not discriminate against minority ethnic groups because in the current political climate in which emotions and sensitivities are running high they fear the potent label of 'racist'. Therefore, white health workers will not discriminate due to the dangers of being caught in the context of a hostile climate. I would refer to this explanation as the 'Bishop Brennan defence'. In one episode of *Father Ted*, an alternative comedy programme about the exploits of three Irish Catholic Priests, Father Ted has to kick Bishop Brennan 'up the arse' to honour a forfeit. He does so and when challenged manages to convince the Bishop that he is so terrified of him and that the consequences would be so severe that he simply would not have done it in the first place.

The logic is powerful without being persuasive. The evidence suggests not only that racism and discrimination are alive and well and hampering service provision and career opportunities, but that the most hostility is reserved for those who dare to complain. There is a distressing lack of awareness about the strength and locus of power relations within society and institutions such as the NHS.

The reclamation of MacPherson?

While many of the trust employees clearly blamed the MacPherson Inquiry and subsequent Report for providing minority ethnic people with a stick with which to beat the white community, two respondents actually supported its findings,

> There is institutional discrimination. I think some of the definitions that have come out recently with the Stephen Lawrence Report about the definitions of institutional discrimination are really quite good, and apply to the Health Service. It's there in the warp and weft of the organisation, and I think that probably what we don't do enough is to actually look at it and challenge it and see how it's affected us... Oh yeah, but it's to do with stereotypes again isn't it? I mean it's all part of discrimination... Yes it's unwitting a lot of the time, I'm not saying a lot of it is overt, it's unwitting but that's the bit about institutional discrimination is that often it's there but I mean we don't even realise it's there... It's about culture isn't it? It's everywhere, it's insidious isn't it? It's in our schools it's in our institutions. And it's about trying to break down those barriers between people (R24, pp.7, 8 & 14, paras.26, 31 & 57).

> Yes I think it is institutional discrimination, most definitely. And I think that can also spread across the other groups that you're talking about as well, and it's quite difficult to change...It's about values isn't it? Your decisions about what's appropriate come from your basic values, and if it's a completely different culture that's making those value judgements how do they know if it's right or not? (R30, pp.10 & 14, paras.36 & 52).

This notion of institutional discrimination also appealed to the representative of the HA. She said:

> But there's no doubt that discrimination exists at the base, at a much more basic level, and it's built into the way that certain services are delivered...It's indirect.

The structures don't really match community structures. (R11, p.23, paras.84 & 85).

Although the nurse trainer was firmer about locating the blame for inadequate service provision at the door of the NHS itself he also adhered to the definition contained in the MacPherson Report. According to a minority of those employed in and around the Health Service institutional discrimination does exist and has been ably identified by MacPherson.

As discussed by numerous commentators institutional discrimination is difficult to identify (i.e. Richards 1994; Mason 2000), and we need to be careful about attributing every service shortcoming to racism, as recognised by Kurtz:

> Where services are poorly developed as in certain instances for sickle-cell disorders, there is also an unhelpful tendency to consider that this is due to racism, whereas the present level of provision may well be explained as a stage in service development, as was the case for haemophilia services not so long ago (1993: 82).

Nevertheless, there was evidence of what could only be labelled institutionalised discrimination. For example, one of the unofficial user representatives was responsible for running a sickle cell and thalassaemia clinic and she argued that it was undervalued and at times denigrated – a consistent theme in the relevant literature (Kushnick 1988; Torkington 1991; Johnson 1992, 1993; Anionwu 1993, 1996; Law 1996; Baxter 1997). On numerous occasions she had been told by local GPs that the money could be better spent elsewhere, echoing the findings of Donovan (1986a). Her main concern was the lack of support from within her employing trust, it was poorly funded and low profile work:

> I'm the only one doing this and there is money put into the service but it's like £10,000 short, and they're pushing me to move into, to expand the area, and I've produced report, after report, after report. And I just said to my manager, I'm not doing any more reports. I've given you all the evidence this is what I require to make this service effective. And nothing is done. Yet I have colleagues who started if you like at the same time as me, and they're fully funded, you know, they can go off on training days without any problem at all, they can order

equipment; little things like paper, stationary. Whereas I'm beg, stealing and borrowing. You know, I hear that a company's closing down, they've got folders going and I went down there to... You know it's ridiculous (R6, p.6, para.16).

She further underlined the perceived unimportance of the service she provides with an illustration:

...every year the chairman of the trust has...this lunch thing and I was invited. I thought God I don't even know him I don't know why he's invited me...So I went along and there was myself and another African-Caribbean worker, who was an officer within the trust, and we were talking and he said to me, Oh what do you do? And I said what I did, and it was obvious that he didn't know what I was talking about, and I said to him, You did a really good report on the services that I provide in your annual report... (R6, p.33, para.112).

That services remain patchy and inadequate for those who suffer from these haemoglobinopathies can scarcely be doubted (Bowers 1993; Anionwu 1996), but the question is why?

When asked whether things would be different if the illness was more prevalent, though similarly rare, in the white community she said:

Oh God definitely. Oh without a doubt, without a doubt (R6, p.7, para.23).

This opinion is supported by much of the available literature (Kushnick 1988; Ahmad 1993b, 1995; Davies *et al* 1993; Bassett 1994; Bothamley 1996). Of course this could be due to the tendency encouraged by the advance of 'New Managerialism' in the NHS for managers to limit the response to 'special' needs in the context of scarce resources (Bhopal & White 1993; discussed more fully in chapter 4, see also Carter 2000 for a discussion of its impact on equal opportunities). However, as discussed in the previous chapter, we need to consider the processes by which some needs rather than others are constructed as 'special'. The comparative response to hamaeglobinopathies that predominantly effect white people (i.e. cystic fibrosis and phenylketonuria) coupled with the relative neglect of the local service suggests deeper issues are involved.

The clearest example of institutionalised discrimination involved catering for the stated preferences of white patients for white health professionals. It would appear, from the available evidence, that this is not a rare occurrence, or at least it is not a wish rarely expressed. For example, 26% of the white respondents who took part in the fourth PSI survey said that they would prefer a white doctor, 60% of those cited language problems, but the majority of expressed reasons were implicitly and often explicitly racist (Nazroo 1997: 123). Furthermore, such preferences are facilitated, although as Alibhai-Brown recently stated: '...we never hear about the large numbers of black and Asian health care workers rejected by patients who are exercising their choice not to be touched or treated by them' (1999: 4). She reported that several minority ethnic workers had contacted her not only to illustrate the level of abuse they receive from white patients, but also the limited support offered by their colleagues and managers (see Beishon et al 1995).

The reality of this was evidenced by one of the ward managers in the trust who outlined what she called the 'non-attendance policy':

> The patient one is always quite difficult and how I deal with it as a manager, I always sit down with the nurse, talk it through with them, but the nurses are quite on board... They know...And what we do is, we have a policy of non-attendance for the staff to the patient, so they will actually withdraw and another nurse will actually go and see to that patient. I mean we treat it in the same way as if a female patient didn't want a male nurse to see to her, which we have to abide by if that is their choice; because we have to give patients choice and we do so. There is a male nurse seeing to you but we could get somebody, a female, but they'd probably be a little longer to come. So we do give them that choice and I think we do have to be fair and we have to give them the choice. But the nurse needs to be counselled very carefully, and needs to be followed up. That's how we deal with it (R13, p.5, para.14).

Although this was not a trust-wide policy, as the situation had been dealt with entirely differently by a community clinic based in the inner city, to the extent it does occur the trust is actually complicit in the racism of white patients. This policy of non-attendance sends a very clear message to the nurse, one that counselling will do very little to salve – that racism is perfectly legitimate. This would again chime with the findings of Jay (1992), Beishon *et al* (1995) and Bagilhole and Stephens (1999: 240), who argued that: *'The respondents [female minority ethnic employees] cited...being moved to other parts of the hospital and being isolated without proper support as examples of racial discrimination'*. A general lack of awareness about the nature and extent of discrimination amongst managers, and an informal approach to it could only serve as a signal to staff and patients that such behaviour was acceptable.

This is certainly the link drawn by Alibhai-Brown (1999) in discussing an incident in which a kidney was allegedly donated with a racist qualifying condition. She argues that people are entitled to express their views – no matter how distasteful – but that there is no excuse for allowing racism to thrive in a public setting. Thus she argues that the life of the white patient was more important than the principle involved, however, that the incident occurred is simply one facet of the racist culture at work in the NHS. Since the Patient's Charter (PC) was produced in 1992 (discussed in chapter 4) she asserts that (white) patient choice has been enabled to such an extent that morality has been obscured, and minority ethnic staff are just expected to put up with the most appalling racism. Although there are areas in which this problem has been taken seriously (Greenwood 1996), it would seem that the 'non-attendance' policy described above is part of a much wider development within the Health Service.

Despite the belief amongst a minority of those involved with or employed by the NHS that it is institutionally discriminatory, and clear evidence of institutional discrimination at work, the problem with the MacPherson definition of institutional discrimination is that it arguably allows individuals off the hook, and, locates racism in the hearts and minds of an extreme minority. *'The five prime suspects have been transfixed into the racist 'other' where their witting racism is presented as a totalizing condition of their being'* (McLaughlin & Murji 1999: 375). This would fit with the coat of paint theory of racism articulated by Gilroy, in which racism is viewed as a thin layer covering an essentially healthy culture (Gilroy 1987). This interpretation did not satisfy the unofficial user representatives, but before we consider why this might be the case in more detail, first we should consider what was said about discrimination.

Sites of discrimination

The stories that emerged about discrimination were quite distinct. For instance one respondent recounted her early experiences of nursing

> And it's like when I was nursing on the wards if a patient from a different ethnic minority group came in, I would, it's awful to say, but I would give them special treatment. Because I would know, because what I found was that other staff would just be, Ugggggh, like this. I'd think, God, this person deserves to be treated with respect. And I do, I'd go out of my way to make sure they had whatever they wanted, that they knew exactly what was going on (R6, p.26, paras.84 & 85).

In order for minority ethnic patients to receive a reasonable standard of service she felt obliged to positively discriminate in their favour. There is evidence to suggest that the relative neglect she was trying to address continues; asked whether any staff went out of their way to help only 17% of respondents from the Coronary Heart Disease Survey agreed. However, 27% of 'Black Caribbean's', 40% of 'Indians', 45% of 'Bangladeshis' and 46% of Pakistani respondents stated that no staff went of their way to help (Airy *et al* 1999). It may be that the tendency of allowing or expecting minority ethnic employees to deal with patients from minority communities goes beyond the *ad hoc* provision of interpreting services outlined in the previous chapter, and, that they are made to feel guilty for doing so (George 1994). This is a subject we will explore in much greater depth in chapter 7.

More specifically some of the user representatives clearly felt that the discrimination, as discussed since at least the early 1980s (Brent CHC 1981, Bryan *et al* 1985), is partly designed to achieve ulterior outcomes. In other words the NHS is used as means of controlling minority ethnic populations. In her official capacity as a user representative one respondent outlined the development of a health programme to improve the plight of local refugees. She said:

> ...we've got an interagency refugee forum, which was started up four years ago. We approached health whose immediate interest was about tracking and screening refugees and asylum seekers, which to some degree is understandable from the public health perception, but unfortunately it adds to the stereotype about what black people/refugees are (R5, p.17, para.52).

The health needs of the refugees were secondary to the threat that they seemingly posed for the rest of the population, and this approach was in turn based upon stereotypical attitudes. In many ways the 'Port Health' mentality continues to find expression (Donovan 1986a; Smaje 1995; Law 1996), and the Health Service can serve to inflame public perceptions and is allegedly being used as a supplementary means of immigration control (Batty 2005).

The authors mentioned above also accused the NHS of practising internal methods of population control, reflecting the claims made about the pre-eminence of eugenicism in the ideological tradition of health care. Minority ethnic women have allegedly been offered birth control advice more readily than their white counterparts, and, more ready access to abortions and sterilisations (Bryan *et al* 1985; Kushnick 1988; Torkington 1991; Bowler 1993; Stubbs 1993; Skellington 1996; Baxter 1997). A similar process among certain white health professionals was detected during this survey. For example, one of the unofficial user representatives who was also a health professional described this incident from her recent experience:

> ...the letters that I get from GPs, and the phone calls, they're terrible, I mean they really are very, very racist...I mean one consultant, she's retired now, she'd never met me I'd just started the job and a woman contacted our voluntary group...to say that she's pregnant, she went to see the doctor they told her she had to terminate the pregnancy because her partner already had a child with someone else who had sickle cell disease. So she rang up to say what can I do? What should I do? So I said, Look you need to get yourself tested first of all to find out whether you do have the trait, and if you do we can actually test your baby early in pregnancy, and you can then decide whether you want to continue with it or

not. No, this hadn't been put to her by her doctor; they told her that it was imperative that she terminate. So I rang the consultant concerned and said, you know, that I'd had a conversation with this woman, and her response was: Oh well you know what these black women are like don't you? This is what she said, seriously, I was gobsmacked. I'm on the phone and she said, They put it about a bit, and they sleep with so many different men, I'm sure she doesn't even know who the father of the child is. And she carried on talking, and she said: Well of course you and I know what we're talking about don't we? And I said, Actually I'm a bit disturbed by what you're saying here, and she said Oh no, no, no, she said It's common, she said, Of course she's got to terminate, there are too many of them anyway. And I said, Look I'm very busy at the moment, look I'd love to continue this conversation with you, can we meet up? This time, sometime this week? And of course she'd never seen me before you see, and I wanted her to see who she was talking to. And we arranged a meeting but unfortunately she went off sick and then retired (R6, pp.8-9, para.26).

Here the negative attitude towards minority ethnic people, based upon unfounded generalisations and stereotypes, is translated very clearly into action. So in contrast to the views of trust employees the unofficial user representatives were able to provide explicit evidence of discrimination, and, examples of discrimination with the eugenic undertones described by writers such as Bryan *et al* (1985) and Kushnick (1988). These stories were extended to form a coherent explanation for the failure of services to meet the needs of a diverse society.

The personal is political

As stressed above most of the trust employees were unable to identify any evidence of discrimination, except that aimed at minority ethnic health professionals by 'elderly' white patients. A small minority accepted the definition of institutional discrimination established by the MacPherson Report, with the emphasis on unwitting racism. Similarly, some of the unofficial user representatives initially accepted these notions of indirect discrimination or unwitting racism. The Chinese respondent was a classic example of this, though towards the end of the interview she said

> I'm forever voicing my frustration and anger about the lack of provision for the Chinese, especially the elder, especially the isolated, and the frail and terminal illness people, and especially culturally they're very, very insensitive. Yeah, and ignorant (R4, p.30, para.121).

When I asked her in what sense she was using the word 'ignorant' – as it can either mean rude and insensitive or simply being unaware – she replied:

> A lot of them don't want to know (R4, p.31, para.123).

Ultimately only one of the eight respondents consistently argued that racism and discrimination is faceless and institutional. It is possible that the initial reluctance of the rest to identify racism as an individual rather than an institutional problem was based on the fear that such an accusation might affect the standing or even the funding of their organisations. This would further question the belief, underlined by the reluctance to complain about racism identified by Bagilhole and Stephens (1999), that minority ethnic communities are exploiting the post-MacPherson climate to gain unfair advantages.

In fact the outcome of the report may prove to be detrimental to improving relations in general and services in particular. As McLaughlin and Murji (1999) and others have pointed out the provisional definition of institutional racism is highly problematic because it invites the tendency to treat it as the last word on the subject, contrary to the intentions of the authors, and lets individuals off the hook. The unofficial user representatives dismissed the idea that no one was to blame. Authors like Richards (1994) and Donovan (1986a) suggest that institutional discrimination emerges naturally out of direct discrimination because majority groups organise institutions to suit themselves. Thus the resultant exclusion is not deliberate or conscious but evolutionary. Baxter (1988: 4-5) identified various ways in which racism can influence the operations of important societal institutions:

1. It ignores the reality of diversity and continuing to do things in traditional ways.
2. White people in powerful positions are unconsciously influenced by racist stereotypes.
3. Rules and regulations though intended to be, and indeed applied, neutrally have the effect of disadvantaging minority ethnic communities (see also Baxter 1997).

None of these interpretations would sit well with the views of the majority of unofficial user respondents, rather they argued that racist institutions are *consciously* created and maintained by the active or inactive racism of individuals; what might be termed direct institutional discrimination or racism.

Health workers are as much a part of societal racism as anyone and the Health Service reflects that. One respondent argued that this is inevitable:

> ...if we have a culture where being racially and sexually and impairment discriminatory, you know, the people, then it becomes their [specifically health professionals] way of life, their culture (R5, p.14, para.43).

Certainly the actions of the ward manager in instituting a policy of 'non-attendance' illustrate this most clearly. Although she clearly felt that her responsibility was to support the preference of patients, and that working with older people racism was only to be expected, she only accepted responsibility where the patients were white. She was far from sympathetic when an Indian family requested an Indian nurse for their mother, even though there was a genuine reason for this. It is this kind of inexplicable inconsistency of attitude and action that can only really be attributed to racism (Mavunga 1992).

These respondents linked the communication barriers identified in the previous chapter with racism. One respondent in particular stated very clearly that language barriers and cultural gaps are used as an excuse to conceal the fact that the Health Service refuses to see different needs as anything other than 'special' needs (R2, p.1, paras.1 & 2). This enables the needs of minority ethnic groups, along with other disadvantaged groups, to be seen as illegitimate and unworthy of attention. She further argued that institutional racism is just one aspect of an exclusionary culture which is white, male middle-class, heterosexual and able-bodied, and that the Health Service, as with every major institution, is geared to meet the needs of those who satisfy these criteria. That is why it serves the most demanding and articulate, and, therefore, the least in need, most effectively (R2, p.2, para.2; Titmuss 1962; Le Grand 1982). There is then a conscious element to institutional discrimination, as individuals operate within and help to sustain the status quo.

The majority of unofficial user representatives argued that the NHS fails minority ethnic communities because it was designed by and for the white majority, and, that there is a conscious element to this (Bryan *et al* 1985; for a full discussion of the location of the NHS in the context of the racist origins of the welfare state and of its place in supporting state racism see Baxter & Baxter 1988, Kushnick 1988; Williams 1989). The model developed by Patel (1993), whereby 'racisms' (both personal and institutional) interact via the medium of an internalised colonialism would perhaps best describe the perceptions of this group of respondents, for it would also account for the central part played by occupational cultures (the eugenic roots of biomedicine etc., see also Parekh 2000: Ch.5). Consequently the arguments raised by authors such as Flew (1986) to undermine the notion of institutional racism, i.e. that racism must by definition be conscious would find some sympathy amongst these respondents, because they view the institutionalised nature of racism in Britain to be consciously constructed.

In fact it was even argued, in sympathy with the early literature on this subject (Brent CHC 1981, Bryan *et al* 1985 etc.) that the NHS has and is being used to control minority ethnic populations. Individuals are both the product and producer of the society in which they live, and institutions such as the NHS are a fundamental part of any society. Change is slow because it goes against the underlying principles of major institutions and because it is resisted.

Conclusion

It should be noted here that the unofficial user representatives were not dismissive of the services provided to minority ethnic communities, and recognised that some insensitivity and apparent indifference on the part of health workers is related to scarce resources and overwork (see also Gerrish *et al* 1996). However, it became apparent not only from their accounts but also through the material obtained generally that racism and discrimination is a central factor in the continued failure of the NHS to meet diverse needs adequately.

Despite this the report and action plan produced as a result of the consultation exercise carried out by the HA did not mention racism or discrimination at all, a consistent theme in official reports according to Baxter (1988). However, '*...racism is so central that any report which does not discuss it as a fundamental starting point is invariably going to end up offering a superficial analysis of the experience of black people in organizational settings or society in general*' (Baxter 1988: 21). This would be a fair reflection of the value of the work carried out by the HA. One of the authors, indeed the person responsible for representing the interests of minority ethnic communities within the HA, was eager to dismiss any such claims as the work of activists out of touch with the needs and interests of the community. When Spokespersons for the Department of Health maintain in public forums that racism is a problem but is only the product of a few bad apples (Johnson 2004), then it is not difficult to see why acknowledging the extent of the problem and then challenging it at the grass roots level can be so problematic. The principal issues in Robbinston were identified as communication and the subtle refinement of existing services, devoid of any wider political context.

In a similar though more extreme mode the trust employees argued that although prejudice is normal discrimination is not or at least it is not inevitable. This was held to be the preserve of 'elderly' patients who did not know any better because they had 'been through' two World Wars; though it was also more plausibly argued that they were simply unable to adjust to their diverse new reality. A number of restraints operate to prevent white health workers from discriminating against minority ethnic people – whether colleagues or patients – although none of the propositions were very convincing.

The central theme was that minority ethnic groups have exploited the aftermath of the MacPherson Report to protect themselves from justifiable censure and to secure unwarranted opportunities, even though there is substantial evidence to the contrary (Bagilhole & Stephens 1997, 1998, 1999; Carter 2000). It may well be that this is being used by white people to protect themselves – what better way to silence minority ethnic individuals than to accuse them of trying to gain unfair advantages? The rhetoric and the fear that surrounds positive discrimination suggests that this is eminently possible.

In 1993 Sharda wrote: *'Health professionals and administrators tend to underestimate seriously the extent to which racial discrimination creates additional barriers to equality, both of opportunity in the labour market and of access to services. It also creates poor quality services, suffering, discomfort and alienation for individuals, families and communities'* (1993: 21). The respondents did not underestimate the extent of 'racial' discrimination they mostly dismissed it. Clearly it is not possible to underestimate what does not exist.

This illustrates the gulf of perception between those who oversee and provide services and the majority of those who unofficially represent minority ethnic users. Far from accepting the claims about the MacPherson Report they argued that it had not gone far enough because it allowed individuals off the hook (McLaughlin & Murji 1999). In their eyes institutional racism or discrimination stands as an aggregation of the prejudice and discrimination of individuals. The NHS fails minority ethnic people because it was never designed to meet their needs, and the reform required to address that will be actively resisted. This resistance derives from the perception of a shift in the power relations of society, it threatens both individuals and institutions and this is recognised if never acknowledged (Torkington 1991). In the next section we will move beyond service quality and possible explanations for specific failings to consider what has been done, or was being planned, predominantly at the local level to improve matters.

SECTION TWO:

Improving service provision to minority ethnic communities

CHAPTER 4:

The internal market

'[The socialist] pleads for the changing system. He (sic) advocates Co-operation instead of Competition: but how can he co-operate with people who insist on competing with him?'
– Robert Tressell

Introduction

From the preceding chapters we can see that the Health Service continues to experience difficulties in providing an appropriate and sensitive service to minority ethnic communities. The purpose of this chapter and the others in this section is to address the question, what can, has been, or should be done to improve services? From a national perspective Smaje (1995) produced a comprehensive account of the development of health policy directed to this end. That is not the purpose of the chapter, though Smaje has given some direction to what follows (1995: 123-130). Here we will first explore the impact of the internal market established in 1991 (DoH 1990), one aspect of the 'New Public Management' paradigm introduced during the 1980s (Carter 2000), and associated measures on the general health needs of minority ethnic communities. In the remaining chapters in this section we will consider localised responses to communication barriers.

On the question of the impact of the reforms there was very nearly a consensus amongst the interviewees that they had made either little or no impact or had failed to deliver despite, in the eyes of a minority, having a certain amount of potential. During the interview survey preparations were being made for the PCG to take over the commissioning role from the local HA (DoH 1997). This was finally achieved in April 2000, despite fears about the rate of reform and active opposition by GPs in particular. Although it was not my intention to explore this issue in any depth, due to the speculative nature of the exercise, several respondents were anxious to share their experiences and concerns. The general feeling was that, just as with the internal market, there was potential but that it was not likely to be fulfilled. To a large extent the findings support the contention of Rao & Ramaiah (2000) that statutory agencies in general, and HAs in particular, are paying lip service to the needs of minority ethnic communities.

Background

In the 1988 report, *Action Not Words*, the National Association of Health Authorities (NAHA) accused HAs of failing to integrate minority ethnic health needs into training, planning and service delivery (NAHA 1988), and there were allegedly few opportunities for participation for minority ethnic communities in the provision of health care. Law (1996) argues very strongly that market mechanisms have done more to promote the employment prospects of minority ethnic groups than liberal equal opportunities policies. Therefore, for Law the introduction of market mechanisms in provision may well have done more to improve health care than the *'socialist expansion of public sector bureaucracy epitomised by the NHS, often characterised by consumer insensitivity and supposed 'universalist' provision* (1996: 154).

It was hoped by many that the 1991 reforms would improve health care for minority ethnic communities in a number of ways (Bahl 1993a, 1995; Baxter 1997; Fletcher 1997; NAHAT 1996/7). In a survey of NHS purchasers, Jamdagni (1996) found that a third of respondents (15) had recognised minority ethnic needs more fully since 1991. The reforms separated out the function of purchasers from providers. The independent health trusts would continue to provide services as before, alongside GPs in the primary sector and, where economically viable, through providers in the private sector. Those with responsibility for purchasing, primarily District Health Authorities (hereafter HAs) and new GP fund-holders, would purchase the appropriate services for those in their immediate areas or practices. HAs were charged with assessing the needs of their service population to inform this process (a number of publications offered guidance on this, i.e. NHSME 1991a, 1991b; CRE 1991; Hopkins & Bahl 1993; McIver 1994; Rawaf & Bahl 1998 (indeed Gunaratnam 1993 offered guidance to Health Service managers in every capacity). To oversee the system, Regional Health Authorities (RHAs) were eventually replaced by eight regional offices of the National Health Service Management Executive (NHSME, later the NHSE).

The development of clinical audit and the use of business plans, performance monitoring and contracting, it was assumed, would improve the service provision to minority ethnic communities because purchasers, having identified local needs, would then be able to pressurise providers into meeting those needs. Central to this process was consumer participation because *'Those who commission and provide services must be more responsive, help empower the individual and community in making decisions, and provide the right to redress, advocacy, and protection from unfair discrimination'* (Sharda 1993: 25).

As a minimum, commissioners were called upon to focus on waiting times, monitor complaints and insist on the provision of appropriate information, diets and, where necessary, link workers. Where providers failed to meet their obligations purchasers were given the power to remove contracts and place them with alternative providers. Their role was to be overseen by the Ethnic Health Unit (Jamdagni 1996).

Consumer choice and increased participation would increase the ability of minority ethnic communities to actively intervene in the provision of health care (Gunaratnam 1993; Law 1996). Indeed the local HA had stressed in the report which emerged from its consultation programme that it wanted to achieve a better and on-going dialogue with and between all sections of the community. One of its aims set out in the final report was to *'Work with representatives from black and other minority ethnic groups to look again at the quality specifications for the services we buy from NHS Trusts'*. From the user perspective, associated initiatives like the Patient's Charter (DoH 1991) would set down a standard of provision by which users could evaluate their treatment, and, which could be used to secure their rights. Although it has been argued that Charters cannot guarantee such rights (Butcher 1998)

However, there were also fears that the internal market might lead to the marginalisation of minority ethnic health needs due to competing pressures (Smaje 1995; Bagilhole 1997) and continuing hostility to any positive policy development (Law 1996). As for consumer participation Ahmad (1993b) suggested that the success of market-based mechanisms requires *'active well-informed consumer[s]'*, but minority ethnic communities, along with other disadvantaged groups facing discrimination do not necessarily fit that bill (McNaught 1987, 1988). Furthermore, as consumer involvement is rare across the general population, additional fears were expressed that this phenomenon might be used to portray minority ethnic communities in particular as disinterested, incompetent and passive (Law 1996). Therefore, a range of opportunities and risks were identified in relation to the internal market.

The provider's perspective

There was really no consensus amongst the employees of the trust about the impact of the reforms. Only one respondent felt that they had been actively detrimental. Initially she said:

> Well it depends on how you define success. It's certainly not been equitable, and I don't think there's any doubt about that. It's not been equitable and I don't think it's provided equal opportunities (R30, p.4, para.14).

Her main concern lay with the role of purchasers rather than providers, and fund-holding GPs in particular:

> Well there's been in the purchaser area of that split, there's been as you know, they've been looking at primary care. For example, there's been fund holding practices and non-fund holding practices and the latter have been provided for by the Health Authorities and their priorities are set with all the sorts of national and locally inherited targets etc. But services have been a little bit more at the whim of fund holders. So it might be that you have a particularly creative, powerful, interested partner within that group whose view is that the need is for one particular service to be developed. And that may well be right, and that's been developed for that fund holding practice, for that group, for that user population. So it may be that if you live on this side of the main road you easily get access to, for example, physiotherapy services. Whereas if you live on the other side of the road you don't either because you are in another fund holding practice, or you're in a non-fund holding practice and the priorities are different. So I don't think it's been equitable, and I don't think there's been any real attention paid to any kind of rational needs assessment, but it goes back to what I was saying before: who defines the need? (R30, p.4, para.15).

In her view, GP fund-holding might have enhanced the sensitivity of the contracting process (Sharda 1993: 27), but it had only served to increase postcode inequity (ONS 1999).

There was some support for her views outside the trust, though the respondent in question was employed in the NHS. One of the user representatives argued that fund-holding had actually retarded service sensitivity due to overt racism. She referred to the attitude of GPs to the local sickle cell clinic, who considered it a waste of resources. She also argued that GP fund-holders had actively prevented the enhancement of services. When she had tried to organise training on sickle cell and thalassaemia for community nurses etc. their attendance had been blocked (for similar experiences see Torkington 1991).

From the specific perspective of service provision, a few respondents argued that the reforms had produced positive outcomes. For example, it was argued that they had stimulated a keener awareness of minority ethnic needs, and that this was due to greater accountability:

> It did yes, because probably a long time ago, those things weren't looked at, and I think with the new legislation that's been brought in, those things have to be looked at now. And I think all the policies that have come in, and now people are more aware. And I think now the NHS are trusts and not the whole thing that we used to be. Nobody saw anything that happened in the hospital. Nobody knew about anything, but now everybody is accountable. I mean we were accountable before but the trust was not...the needs of different communities were not governed by anybody if you know what I mean, but now they are (R16, p.2, para.5).

In fact it was even argued that it may have had made a positive impact on service provision within and beyond the trust:

> I'm not aware of any specific services that have been changed or introduced specifically...Actually that's not true, no I am aware, for example, we do now have a travellers project which is [regional], which all the trusts contribute to. Two workers who specifically work with the travelling community, so that they can learn and have a good understanding of this group of people's culture and particular health needs, of which there are many. And actually inform and educate other professionals as to how best to approach these people in offering a service, and providing a service. To have an awareness of some of the issues that there are. So actually that isn't true we do actually have some services. Now whether that's been a direct result of that or not I could not say, but we do have something (R18, p.6, paras.18 & 19).

There was a minority view then that the reforms had made at least some impact on service provision.

The majority were not aware that there had been any change in the quality of provision offered to minority ethnic communities.

> I wouldn't say that we've come on leaps and bounds since we introduced the internal market, or that will change things over night (R28, p.15, para.58).

The implication, drawing on the material presented in the first section, was that little change was needed anyway because services were perfectly adequate. One respondent argued that the reforms had never been intended to improve services, but were really designed to ease the way for privatisation:

> It sort of backfired it allowed us to prove that it was a good service. So I think politically as well as practically, there will still be certainly principles let in. I don't think competition is a bad thing, don't get me wrong, I think it does make sure that people stay aware of what they could do, or the penalties of not doing, and I think that was a good thing. But I think there was too much invested in non-health providing factors (R15, p.23, para.64).

According to this respondent the reforms were politically motivated, and their only real benefit (at great cost) had been to underline the quality of existing provision.

In summary, there was no consensus about the impact of the reforms, although the majority argued that in terms of provision, particularly in relation to the trust, there had been very little impact one way or another. Primarily, again reflecting back on the material presented in the first section, this was apparently due to the fact that provision for every section of the community was already adequate.

The Patient's Charter (PC)

Where there was a near consensus amongst trust employees it concerned the innovation of the PC (DoH 1991, amended in 1998). It was printed in nine languages and was designed to act as a bill of rights for patients, underlining the importance *'...that all Health Services should make provision so that...your privacy, dignity and religious and cultural beliefs are respected'* (DoH 1991: 12). If the care provided did not conform to the published standards then patients were entitled to seek redress. It was as a result of this that the NHSME published guidance to the NHS on meeting diverse needs and the importance of consultation (NHSME 1992a). Johnson (1992) and Bhopal and White (1993) argued that Charters would provide communities with some ammunition in a climate where the will to improve service provision is largely absent. Although the ability of ensuring citizenship rights through consumerist means (such as the PC) has been questioned (Butcher 1998).

In the region in which Robbinston is located Mwasamdube and Mullen (1998) found that 56% of trusts had set PC standards on cultural needs and 70% on religious practices. However, she said very clearly that the lack of activity to meet these needs brought the figures into question. The findings of this research further support her conclusions and the attitudes the trust employees displayed in relation to the PC would perhaps undermine any established standards. For it would appear that support for the PC amongst health workers is also largely absent.

There was some limited support from predictable quarters. The disability co-ordinator said that it had provided campaigners with a weapon with which to beat reluctant managers, and had enhanced the willingness of patients to complain:

> ...and again I'm sorry to go on about the disability field, we've actually used, people were doing this access work and then the Patient's Charter came out which said that services must be accessible to everyone. So everyone said right, great, we're going to hammer the managers... So it empowers people at the bottom. It's giving us extra ammunition (R24, p.23, paras93 & 95).

Another argued that it had made a slight difference:

> Yes I suppose it is slightly, I suppose it is more patient-focused now, but that sounds as if it was never patient-focused. But yes, there is more emphasis on it. And certainly about waiting lists and people not having to wait more than 18 months before they're admitted to hospital. And if they cancel or are cancelled then it has to be done within a month or something like that, all of these things have focused, and I think...Yeah it has helped (R15, pp.5-6, paras.14 & 15).

However, it was seen to have only marginally increased the user-centred ethos that had always characterised the Health Service.

Otherwise the trust employees were highly critical of the PC, reinforcing the belief that the level of professional resistance would be high (Johnson 1992). They agreed that it had encouraged patients to be more demanding, but in doing so had aroused unrealistic expectations. The resources to make it viable had never been made available,

> I think there is a problem with expectation, and I think with the [Patient's Charter] as was, and is at the moment, that people have an enormous expectation. They expect to come to clinic and that they will be seen always within 30 minutes, that they will have their first appointment within 13 weeks and the reality is not that. We're not funded to that level to provide that service, and we do our utmost to ensure that those things don't happen where we can actually have an impact. But at the end of the day if there is no control on referrals, you can't actually achieve it, unless you've got unlimited funding (R23, p.7-8, para.23).

> That highlighted very, sometimes a little to our detriment, because it did I think, it gave the public some false hopes as far as what we could offer actually. Because it was just a guideline, but people thought it was the law and forgot it was a guideline. So I think the public's sort of anticipation I think escalated, and we didn't quite marry up with the services and resources that we had (R13, p.7, para.21).

Furthermore, it had raised expectations without encouraging users to think about the resource implications or the problems faced by providers in the context of scarce resources:

> That everyone understandably as an individual thinks that their need is the greatest. But it may well be that if you're on the other side of the fence looking, for example, at the nature and number of the calls that you've received this week with a certain level of resources to provide for that. That you have to take into account other considerations like what the clinical needs are and how urgent they are (R30, p.6, para.24).

Secondly, and more worryingly, it was perceived as having increased the tendency of patients to complain with ulterior motives

> I think the PC is a good idea, but I also think that somewhere along the line it went too far because it's getting a little bit like America now. With patients suing for things that in my opinion may have happened anyway...But a lot of people are jumping on the bandwagon I think, suing trusts and hospitals...And demands are much more extreme now. And I feel that a lot of people don't understand anything that goes on, that they go away and read about it and they think they never said that to me and everything is blown up (R16, p.3, paras.8 & 9).

This was something of an extension of the argument that minority ethnic communities had used the post-MacPherson climate to gain unfair advantages. Thirdly, it was perceived as having increased the number of verbal and physical attacks on health workers. The Head of Nursing argued that a staff charter was now required, echoing suggestions by Rowe (1995). The PC promised something that could not be delivered and was seen to have brought out the worst in patients. The result was a more cynical and litigious society.

Several respondents felt frustrated by this new consumerist culture. One effect had been to increase the working hours of staff in the context of a labour shortage

> I think from the staffing situation it has put an increased pressure on everybody not just the nursing staff. When we first opened we didn't have as many lists; there certainly weren't as many consultants as there are now. I mean we've taken on quite a few in each speciality, and we have increased probably 50% of our workload, that they're actually talking about working Saturdays now. So we are working harder and it is obviously putting more constraints on the nursing staff from my point of view (R25, p.3, para.21).

It was thought that the work it occasioned was often unnecessary. One respondent was tired of telling people the reason for lengthy waiting times, when it was obvious that they were busy. It also encouraged more non-health related work for front-line staff, because they were now encouraged to read every policy statement thoroughly to minimise the risk of legal action. The trust had even instituted written tests. So in the context of a labour shortage, with user expectations spiralling out of control, already over-stretched health workers have to work through a considerable amount of written material to prevent malicious claims. As per previous chapters, those outside the trust had a different view of the PC and its efficacy.

A backlash running ahead of schedule?

For the most part the user representatives and others had much less to say about the PC. What they did say however was in direct conflict with the views expressed above. Far from the politicised and self-centred population portrayed by the trust employees, the remaining respondents argued that if anything the general public is reluctant to complain. One of the user representatives argued that:

> Yes I would say yes and no [that the PC is a positive development], because some people don't know anything, some people can't be bothered. And the other side thinks it's important and want to know, a bit more about it. But again I would say you have to make people want to do this and that's hard (R3, p.9, para.40).

In other words the public are sometimes too ill-informed or too apathetic to complain and often need a push from interested organisations.

The principal issue though was thought to be the power differential between users and health professionals. For example the disability co-ordinator outlined the partnership model she had adopted for work with disabled people:

> ...the down side of that is that [it] is quite a culture shock for some people. And the public need to be educated too. Because sometimes in rehabilitation if we try and give this sort of partnership approach that's actually quite a shock to the patient. They think hang on a minute I'm the patient here. I thought that you were going to sort me out. I want a prescription, I don't want to be told to go away and change my lifestyle, I want the doctor to sort it out for me. So there are issues about actually working together (R24, p.10-11, para.40).

For similar reasons she felt that minority ethnic communities might also be reluctant to take on a more active role in health provision:

It can disable people who are used to being oppressed by other people coming and knowing best, speaking for them and doing things to them, and that's...some of that's probably true. That minority groups have not had access to good information to be able to make choices, and information is power, so other people take the power from you (R24, p.10, para.40).

For various reasons, but primarily due to social exclusion, this being *'...a shorthand term for what can happen when people or areas suffer from a combination of linked problems such as unemployment, poor skills, low incomes, poor housing, high crime environments, bad health and family breakdown'* (http://www.cabinet-office.gov.uk/seu/), it was unlikely that minority ethnic individuals would be able to provide the level of challenge articulated by the majority of the trust employees (Ahmad 1993b). Furthermore, according to one of the respondents certain sectors of the minority ethnic community would be even less likely to complain:

In the past I had a reason, if you don't shout it suits them, one less to worry about. That's the impression I got. Many, many mainstream providers, Chinese do not say, oh Chinese are okay they never complain, they're all right, they're not troubling anybody (R4, p.16, para.58).

The user representative from the Chinese community argued that services like the NHS actually exploit such cultural factors (see McIver 1994: 28 who presents literary support for this claim), and though things were now improving the reluctance to complain was proving hard to overcome

In addition to cultural issues, it was also argued that the power differential between patients and professionals is as pronounced as ever:

And a lot of ordinary people say they don't want to voice their concerns to doctors and nurses because they know what a hard job they're doing. And they don't often want to be critical of their doctor or nurse, to make a complaint, because that's not the culture of most patients to complain; in case it affects the health care they receive... It's often the suffering in silence. We held a recent open forum, and we had an internal working group running, a consultation structure, and we held an open forum, and I mean there was not that many there, but I mean there was a lot of discussion going on, and a very marked point made was that people felt they were suffering in silence. And they continued to suffer in silence because they would need their elderly patient cared for, their child cared for, or be pregnant yet again, they were looking after their ends (R5, p.5, paras.16 & 17).

Users from minority ethnic groups allegedly fear the repercussions of enforcing their rights. It was implied that the complaints outlined above were part of a backlash by the trust employees that was running ahead of schedule:

I think in some sense doctors and nurses feel that they are the educated ones and that the patients should be told what to do. They shouldn't ask questions, they shouldn't be given the information, because they shouldn't question their treatment. They should put up and shut up (R6, p.21, para.69).

It was felt by a majority of the unofficial user representatives that any challenge to the power differential between users and professionals would be strongly resisted and it was felt that the sort of complaints above were part of a concerted effort to preserve and reinforce it. To illustrate this it is appropriate to reiterate here the Deputy Director's warning that doctors would not participate in this research because they expect to be treated like Gods (Torkington 1991).

The PC then, in common with many of the issues already discussed, was the source of significant disagreement. While the trust employees mainly felt that it had gone too far in empowering consumers, the bulk of the remaining respondents argued that it had not gone far enough. Health professionals retain enormous power in their interactions with users. One user representative actually maintained that the PC was a brilliant device to shift the responsibility of improving services onto the general public. If no one complained then the assumption was that services were okay, but if not and people did not complain, then that is their responsibility (Law 1996). This would certainly suggest a confirmation of one of the central themes of the research – that the system and its

120

representatives seem keen to push responsibility onto minority ethnic communities.

Alibhai-Brown (1999) argues that the NHS has actually allowed the consumerism stimulated by the PC to facilitate the racism of white patients, a reality we can identify in the context of the 'non-attendance policy'. She argues that the PC has created professional automatons unable to make ethical decisions for fear of public disapproval, and there is some agreement from within the service. The Assistant Director of Equal Opportunities for Bradford Hospitals Trust said:

> We have a loyalty to our employee who should not be subjected to racism and also the patient who is entitled to a choice of practitioner under the PC. Our other difficulty is that unlike a shop or a pub, which could bar a customer for racism, we have no such powers (Greenwood 1996: 13).

The difficulty here is obvious and yet the views of the majority of unofficial user representatives would suggest that white managers within a white health system are facilitating the racism of patients. In the case of 'non-attendance' policy it would be hard to disagree.

One issue that both parties could agree upon however was that the PC was unlikely to significantly improve the quality of service provided for anyone. Unlike the trust employees, the user representatives were at least as much concerned about the role of purchasing as provision in the context of the internal reforms.

The role of the HA

The most resonant feature of the reforms for the user representatives was the role of the HA, which was identified as one of their crucial components (Ahmad 1993b; Johnson 1993; Smaje 1995). This may well have been underlined by the findings of Mwasamdube and Mullen (1998) which were then being disseminated locally. Of the 12 HAs in the region that took part in the study,

- 2 (17%) had developed a health strategy for minority ethnic communities.
- 3 (25%) had included minority ethnic needs in service level agreements.
- 4 (33%) had included minority ethnic needs in primary care strategies.

She concluded that '...*a significant number of health authorities are failing to exercise leadership nor are they steering the strategic direction for the purchasing of health care for people from black and minority ethnic communities*' (1998: 6). The limited numbers included in the study do not effect the conclusions substantially as it was a census-based initiative, including every HA and trust in the region.

Although the expectations of providers are clearly outlined in the HAs report and action plan including sensitive dietary provision and appropriate interpreting services, there was little faith that they were monitored or enforced. The respondent from the CHC argued that the main problem had been in organising the relationship between purchasers and providers:

> So in theory the health authority could have done that but in practice I haven't seen it. Partly because they've been so desperately trying to figure in the early stages their role, and their modus operandi. But they'd didn't have the opportunity, and they actually don't have the staff levels sufficiently high enough to do a lot of this stuff. Now having said that they have worked with this CHC. For example, they fund [us] to the tune of 30,000 a year to run what we call the local voices project. And we employ basically a community development worker. He works out in the community on issues of concern to local people, and he's done some work with Asian women in the inner city. So the potential's there and some bits of work have been carried out which have been quite effective but not in terms of an overall blanket approach (R12, pp.5-6, para.18).

He continued in this vein:

> So most Health Services are provided on an historical model. We're doing that because that's what we did... And changing from what we do now, which is based on what we did then is hard because you've got to be able to justify what you're changing it to. Now to do that you've got to know what's going on, and it's a resource issue as well. It's partly resources and it's partly new roles and coming to terms with them (R12, pp.6-7, paras.19 & 20).

According to this respondent a combination of factors had served to minimise the potential of purchasing, namely the historical model of provision, role confusion and a lack of resources (Ahmad 1993b; Karmi 1993; Rawaf 1993).

Even if the HA had developed a strong sense of mission, it would have been difficult to apply pressure to providers. Crucially the internal market had decentralised responsibility and this weakened its control:

> No they don't appear to have done. I'm not aware of any. I mean I could not see why they would either. In some respects they may have made things more difficult. The purchaser/provider split instead of having one health authority in terms of secondary care with an overview and a control of recruitment and access to services, you've got a number of different organisations. And those organisations...in this area we've got 4...combined trusts: acute, mental health and community services...And they've all got different employment policies, different access policies, different access procedures and so on (R12, p.3, para.7).

Even if the HA had retained the level of control it previously had over providers, it would not have been able to discipline errant trusts anyway:

> You can't take the contract away because that could destabilise the trust, and undermine a number of other services. It's got to be done more cautiously and carefully than that (R12, p.7, para.21).

He accepted that the HA wanted to do better but was constrained by the structural implications of the contracting process.

Another respondent agreed that pressure had not been actively applied by purchasers, but argued that:

I would say from the purchaser's point of view I feel that a lot of them are very frightened of rocking the boat. And when certain problems are brought to their attention it's very much like, oh God what do we do with this? Things are very sensitive politically, we don't want the community to hear about this, so therefore the funding will carry on to providers although they may not be providing the services that they're supposed to be providing (R6, p.13, para.44).

The commitment to improve services to minority ethnic communities and to withdraw contracts has never been there. It is not so much a fear of destabilising services, but rather about keeping the alleged failings of the providers quiet and hoping that users and their representatives would not find out. She said:

And there was a problem within the community that was brought to the attention of the health authority, and it would have huge implications to money they were providing for a particular service and the money was not being used effectively, it was not used for what it had been intended. And from my point of view I could see that patients were suffering as a result of this, and I'm very much well, if they're not providing the service let's take the money back, give it to someone who will do it. And that didn't happen. And that's just carrying on and on, it's very much like, Well if the public get to hear about it, how are we going to look? (R6, p.14, para.46).

The other side of the coin was the relative strength of providers:

And I think a lot of people from the provider's point of view they have a lot of clout. They're very, very strong... Oh yeah they have a lot of clout and if they say they will not do, it's not very much, Well if you won't do it we will take it away (R6, p.14, paras.46 & 47).

The fear of negative publicity and the relative strength of providers effectively hamstrung the HA; although mostly, as argued by the majority of the unofficial user representatives throughout, there has been a genuine lack of commitment.

Consultation versus participation?

That there has been a lack of commitment can be detected to some extent in relation to the level of participation achieved in the region. As stated earlier this was central to the ethos of the reforms (Balarajan & Raleigh 1995) and has been an on-going priority since the Management Inquiry headed by Sir Roy Griffiths1988 (McIver 1994). There is evidence of participation and collaboration working on a localised basis, for example in Leeds (Cortis & Rinomhota 1996) and Manchester (McIver 1994). However, it would seem that in the south west region even consultation has been difficult to achieve.

For example, Mwasamdube and Mullen (1998) found that only 50% of HAs had processes in place to obtain feedback from minority ethnic communities, and still less, 42%, had consulted minority ethnic communities on their annual purchasing plans. Similarly, only 26% of the 36 participant trusts had surveyed their local minority ethnic communities, and only 39% reported any consultation on service use and quality. Consultation had begun in Robbinston, but had there been any real improvements?

Most of the respondents accepted that the consultation exercise organised by the HA had been a positive development. Even the most vehement critics of the Health Service appreciated the consultation undertaken by the HA:

> They seem to be more sensitive, opened up to the black and ethnic minorities, and having said that we've had a lot of consultation meeting for the last 3-4 years, we've had various consultation meetings. It's until about 18 months ago, or 2 years ago, things are beginning to take off. And things are beginning to improve, and they're becoming more sensitive to our needs, but in the past it's just lip service (R4, p.5, para.14).

The HAs representative echoed this. She explained that the consultation had been community-led and had spanned a 6-9 month period. The positive aspects of this were evident, it had enabled an on-going dialogue, as the previous respondents had suggested between the HA and the local community:

> Specific things that I feel we've made progress on, are in terms of better working relationships with some of the community groups, and also that we have joint meetings with some of the city council services, who work in the inner city. Like social services community development. And we've brought them together with

some of the GPs and health workers, so that there's much more of a sharing in some areas – particularly with regard to the Somali community because they're quite a large unassimilated community. So we've put a lot of time into them. Everyone agreed that they were a priority really. And we've got this steering group together, and that seems to be one of the first times that you've had people like me who've got a kind of strategic overview in the same room with people from the communities, and people who actually deliver services to the communities personally. That seemed to be a gap that certainly the workers felt had not been bridged before, that all the people who had an interest were in the same room, rather than me writing a document and sending it out and saying this is how you should deal with black and minority ethnic people. So the things I feel most pleased about are those kinds of practical things (R.11, p.6, para.19).

In essence the consultation exercise had enabled the HA to develop a better awareness of the needs of minority ethnic communities, and, to establish an on-going dialogue with those communities and health providers in the interests of involvement and accountability. Doubts were also expressed by some respondents about its aftermath.

A major criticism was that the drive for change had come from the voluntary sector and was not genuinely supported by the HA. For instance,

I haven't seen any evidence of it put it that way. No, I haven't seen any evidence of it at all. I think a lot of it really, if any changes have been made it really has come from the patients, well, from people within the community, form voluntary organisations. I mean a lot of it really is from the voluntary organisations (R6, p.11, para.36).

She argued that without community pressure there would have been little commitment to on-going dialogue, and that any small improvements in services have come about through the same source. In short, the real drive and commitment for change has come from the voluntary sector and without this even the limited achievements of recent times would not have materialised. Not only is this consistent with the birth of provision for minority ethnic communities, i.e. led by the voluntary sector (Johnson 1987, 1993; Patel 1993), it further questions the willingness of the NHS to improve services for minority ethnic communities. The HA was clearly happy to provide short-term funds and allow the voluntary sector to bear the brunt of the service responsibilities (Ahmad 1993b; Bagilhole 1993; Smaje 1995).

The limitations of allowing the voluntary sector to bear too much of this burden has been clearly identified in the relevant literature. The funding provided is often limited and short-term which means that needs cannot be met adequately and the status quo remains untouched, needs deemed illegitimate are kept on the periphery (Johnson 1993; Alexander 1999). According to Patel *'Such projects are often financially supported and positively viewed by mainstream health and social services because they provide a 'buffer' against direct criticism of failure to provide mainstream services'* (1993: 131). Placing the responsibility for providing important services on to the voluntary sector also reflects the institutional desire (underlined throughout this study) to see minority ethnic communities addressing problems that they create (Ahmad 1993b). Funding by HAs etc. can also be used to create divisions within and between minority ethnic communities, because they *'...are in competition with each other for state handouts, and are therefore easier to control'* (Ahmad 1993b: 213). As will be discussed in the following chapter, such divisions were only too apparent in Robbinston.

Consistent with the tenor of these arguments there was a firm belief among certain respondents that the HA had deliberately forced minority ethnic interests off the agenda during the first phase of the reforms:

> They, the health authority, actually had a group called Race and Health, when I first started. They were funded by the Health Authority basically to act as a link for people from black and ethnic minority groups. And when I started I met with the woman who was co-ordinating it and at the time things were changing, and I think GP fund-holding was coming into play, and there was a whole sort of change within the Health Service. And she rang me up one day and said they're not going to fund us any longer, and they would be doing the work that when the doctors ring me to say can you help with this situation, that was what the organisation was doing. So the funding was stopped, they applied they appealed and all the rest of it. And it was No we don't need you any longer, we need to channel the money elsewhere (R6, p.11, para.37).

Furthermore, the consultation process though valuable had not proved entirely fruitful in terms of outcomes, which is likely to undermine credibility for the process in the longer term (McIver 1994). The Chinese respondent maintained that the expressed needs of the community had been brushed under the carpet, when the Chinese community demanded a Chinese health clinic a long period of obfuscation had ensued before they were eventually informed that it was not viable. Consultation all too often obscures the reality that local communities do not have the power to ensure that their demands are met. Thus although dialogue is important, so too is outcome, and it is in this direction that progress seems to have been limited.

Even the HA representative accepted that actual progress had been fairly limited. She referred explicitly to the Chinese community:

> And we're increasingly saying to them: Well yes there are specifically Chinese health issues, yes there are specifically African health issues, but by and large the things that you all talk about are quite similar and we haven't got the resources and we never will have to tackle, to provide a Chinese Health Service, and Asian Health Service. I mean we've got to provide a Health Service that's accessible to everybody who lives here. And so what we need is the groups to talk to each other (R11, p.7, para.21).

The ability to provide separate services to individual communities is beyond the current level of resources available to the local NHS. That the issue of resource constraints was a common theme throughout (see also McNaught 1988), is extremely common in terms of managerial logic. Indeed Lipsky (1980: 33) argued that '...*street level bureaucracies, with certain other government agencies, chronically experience resource constraints. These agencies are virtually never adequately provided for, and perhaps cannot be adequately provided for'.* Demand always outstrips supply, and in many ways the notion of separate services does seem unrealistic.

At times it appeared that even reasonable demands were dismissed in this way, and, referring back to chapters 2 and 3, this is more to do with the way that different needs are constructed as deviant and outside the core business of the Health Service. Smaje (1995) warned that *'the geographic distribution of minority ethnic groups will lead to a residualisation of their needs in newly emerging structures of health provision'* (1995: 123), and this appears to have been prophetic.

It quickly became clear what the consultation exercise had really been about. The HA representative had already said that it was important to get the people *involved* in various aspects of health and she continued to press the idea of involvement over consultation:

> This government in particular is moving heavily towards public involvement in direct delivery of services...Involving communities is very time-consuming, and I think the government haven't realised quite how long the time-scales are. Now I've only come to this over the last 2 or 3 years, but the community development work, public involvement work, is very long-term. And, I think with this project and other projects we're 2 years down the line and I'm only just beginning to get to know people, who are only just beginning to trust you. People from black communities now will ring me up – they actually know my name – and they'll ring me and say such and such happened, or did you know? Or what would you do about this? And lots of other things are the same, particularly disadvantaged communities feel very reluctant to start, and building up all that trust takes a long time (R11, p.21, para.77).

So the drive came from the government, but despite this she does see that consumer/user involvement is vital to the provision of health care. However, the purpose appeared to be as much about winning sympathy for the Health Service as improving services

> It takes a lot of explaining to local communities, and the only thing that I've found that works is to get local people actually working with trust managers on specific detailed issues. Because they need to understand the difficulties that trusts face (R11, p.24, paras.87 & 88).

The object may have been less to give minority ethnic communities a say in how services are run, or to stimulate health workers to identify and meet different needs more effectively, but to buy off discontent. She argued that this had already occurred in relation to a new telephone interpreting service (discussed in the following chapter); at first user groups and activists had denounced it, but as they were now nominally involved and could see the difficulties involved in language provision, they had learnt to accept it.

To some extent this reflects the experience documented by McNaught (1988) in West Lambeth, where the local HA tried to formulate a 'race' policy through just such a process of consultation. Although the process had been lengthy and inconclusive, this was not the view of the District Management Team, which was reputedly satisfied with the outcomes. The interests of minority ethnic communities were also seemingly exploited, though more in the interests of securing greater funds in the face of the restrictions recommended by the Resource Allocation Working Party, than to co-opt communities *per se* (McNaught 1988: Ch. 4).

Although the rationale for co-option was different the outcomes might prove equally ineffectual in the longer term. The HA representative explained quite clearly why the outcome of the consultation exercise in particular and the internal reforms in general had been so limited. It was basically a problem of numbers:

> [Has it been effective?] No. Not at all. And we're equally in [this region] there's no way you can justify targeting huge resources at that very small proportion of the community except in one area... In the inner city area. So having contracts with trusts about culturally diverse services, I mean I was a trust general manager here...for years, well you would only see such a rare number of people from each ethnic group that it would hardly present as a problem. Now you can call that institutionalised racism, okay, fair enough, but it doesn't help you in dealing with it really (R11, p.10, para.30 & 31).

In her view, as became clearer the longer the interview progressed, minority ethnic communities are too small to justify any more expenditure than they already receive (for literary evidence of similar sentiments in the NHS see Smaje

1995). This reflects the findings of Jamdagni (1996) who found that the size of service communities is central to the extent of local activity, and of the six trusts that refused to take part in Mwasamdube and Mullen's (1998) study the most common explanation was demographic. Ultimately though, scarce resources were identified as the biggest single barrier to progress (see also Carter 2000).

As discussed in the previous chapter, this sits very well with the concept of good management defined in the context of New Public Management (Carter 2000). However, the processes by which some needs are seen as peripheral in the context of scarce resources were also identified. Mwasamdube and Mullen (1998) detected a genuine lack of commitment amongst Health Service managers to providing accessible and equitable services. As Torkington (1991: 184) argues, *'If you really want to do something you will find the resources with which to do it'*.

The urgency of a policy response should not be entirely determined by numbers. As the representative of the REC argued, there would be no tolerance of the idea that child abuse is relatively rare therefore it should be ignored. If 5% of the population of a city are having difficulties in accessing services and experiencing inadequate treatment when they do, then this should be seen as a major problem (Jay 1992). It undermines the consistent argument put forward by the HA representative that people are individuals first and foremost. In fact, it seems that minority ethnic individuals are first and foremost seen as group members.

The 1997 White Paper, *The New NHS: Modern and Dependable,* stated very clearly that minority ethnic communities ought not to be disadvantaged on the basis of demography (DoH 1997). In the words of Mwasamdube and Mullen (1998), *'There needs to be equity of access to Health Service provision and health care delivery for all people from black and minority ethnic groups regardless of the region in which they live and the diversity of their population'* (1998: 25; Gerrish et al 1996). Although the HA had carried out a valuable consultation exercise and increased its contact with the local community, its role as a purchaser had not been fulfilled. In the words of Sharda (1993: 21) '...*when consultation has taken place it has been marginal, and often addressed only in relation to language, culture and disease'*. Although various reasons were proposed for this, the allegation that it lacks sufficient political will seems to be justified. Would the next round of reforms prove more effective?

Primary Care Groups

As the interviews were progressing local PCGs were preparing to take over many of the functions of health purchasers, as fund-holders have been dispensed with and HAs are to take on a new role overseeing the work of PCGs and take a lead on the establishment of Health Improvement Programmes (DoH 1997). PCGs are comprised of different health workers based in the community, including GPs, practice nurses, health visitors etc., representatives of social services and user representatives. Many of the respondents were keen to extol the potential of PCGs on the grounds that they would be inclusive. User representation should be much more effective in getting across the views of local communities than was possible in the previous system.

One respondent, a district nurse, had argued throughout that the NHS was poorly focused, because it adopted a curative approach rather than a preventative approach. PCGs appeared to be a step in the right direction: prevention before cure -

> I think it is coming that way, in that they are talking about primary care and care in the community, and everything coming back to the community and they are closing hospital beds. So I think it's coming around that way...I think the government is looking more and more at primary health care in their projects, so I mean hopefully the change is already underway (R26, p.5, para.32).

Several other respondents agreed that PCGs have the potential to make a real difference for patients and minority ethnic communities in particular:

> I think that one of the benefits potentially of PCGs, here is an opportunity for them to actually be looking at their local primary care group, and addressing their needs, because one of the key government agendas is equality of health. So there is an opportunity to address that, or to attempt to address it. I don't think we can accept that there's a panacea for everything... My understanding is that one of the things that PCGs will be doing will actually be profiling their populations and the health needs of the populations. And I think that could be part of what you were describing. Actually getting the various elements within the PCG to say what it is that you particularly would like to see and then taking it back, looking at the way that all other agendas are, and seeing what we can do. Sometimes it's actually fine tuning a service that you already offer that makes it more acceptable to people so it doesn't always necessarily cost a lot of money, sometimes it's a change of attitude which isn't always easy to achieve is it? (R18, p.15, paras.53 & 54).

PCGs were meant to enhance consultation and greater involvement, profiling the health needs of the user population and commissioning care in accordance with the findings; in a similar though more effective vein than the internal market. Yet many felt that this potential would never be realised.

The disruption caused by a new set of reforms might see equality issues pushed off the agenda yet again, as had previously occurred with the internal market:

> I do believe it's still marginal and that with all the changes that we're currently facing with primary care groups, and the massive sea of change, again one gets the feeling that with equality issues, particularly racial equality, has fallen off the agenda yet again (R5, p.4, para.14).

One respondent argued that the constant upheaval was partly designed to ensure that minority ethnic issues remained a low budgetary priority for the Health Service (R2).

So the very process of reform, consciously or unconsciously, may serve to relegate important matters such as equal opportunities and access and retard further progress, rather than providing the basis for great improvements in these areas. It was not simply administrative reform that might prevent the potential of

PCGs from being realised there were also substantive reasons to fear that this would be the case.

One area of concern was the power imbalance built into their construction. Even the respondent who was unreservedly enthusiastic about the development posed the rhetorical question –

> Whether the ethnic minorities are being suitably represented within that? I don't know (R26, p.5, para.32).

Two respondents argued that the membership of the local PCG was (unhealthily) dominated by clinicians:

> But I would hope that with regards to one of the things I was a bit confused about with the primary care groups. For example, they were saying that within this area you could only have 2 nurses on the group, and I think 7 GPs. Talk about top heavy, sort of imbalance there... And I went to a meeting in Cardiff a couple of weeks ago and we were discussing this with regards to this sort of service, and they were saying: Oh well they've been told that they can have up to 5 nurses on their group. So we came back and said: Well where did this magic number come from? Because we assumed, incorrectly, that it had come from the Department of Health, and the government. But nobody knows where these magic figures had come from. Whether or not there was a GP that had said well we only want 1 or 2 nurses, and even the sort of people representing the general public, 1 individual to represent (R6, p.16, paras.51 & 52).

This was confirmed to some extent by the following extract from the HA's Annual Report for1998: *'PCGs in which local GPs will group together to plan, influence and, in time, purchase Health Services for local people'* (my emphasis). This respondent implied that GPs were responsible for the dearth of nursing staff and user representatives. There had also been little effort expended locally to recruit people from the local community to serve on PCGs:

> So you look at people from black and minority ethnic groups. I mean do they know about this? I'll say well how are the public going to know that they can apply to come on these groups? Oh well we will publicise it. I've not seen anything yet, and I've been saying to my clients look this is what's going on, if

> you want patient representation ring up the health authority and say look you want to be included on this. I don't know whether they have or not, but I know that... Because I haven't seen anything in the local press, on the news or anything that says to people we are looking for representatives from the local community to represent the ordinary folk to come on to these groups (R6, p.16, para.54).

In fact she argued that the reluctance to involve users was part of a wider pattern, which appeared to disadvantage minority ethnic communities in particular:

> They're building a new hospital [here]... One of the people who's on the committee for that, rang me up and said, we're doing this and we've actually started the plans, and this is what I was going back to about token sort of ethnic minority on the board. And she said Oh well we've realised that we don't have anyone from an ethnic minority group on our panel, and I said why not? Why have you left it until now to do something about it? So I suggested they contact a couple of people that I work with, a couple of clients who I feel are very articulate and they're very, very strong at getting the patients' voice heard. And I said look contact them. So I rang them up to say look you'll probably be getting a phone call from so and so. Saw them a couple of weeks later to do my usual home visits with them. Oh how did you get on with...? I haven't heard anything. Fine. I went back and they said, Oh well we decided it was too late to actually include anybody on this (R6, p.17, paras.55 & 56).

In short, the influence of GPs on PCGs is likely to be pre-eminent in the local area, and the influence of other groups minimal. This situation was felt to have been manufactured by GPs to fit a consistent local pattern.

The predominance of GPs caused this same respondent further anxiety because she felt that they would work to lower the priority of the service she provides, which mainly caters for minority ethnic communities:

> And I think one of the things that concerns me with regards to the primary care groups now that they're introducing next year is...I provide a service I cover the whole of [the city]. Now you're gonna have different primary groups, what can I do to influence the care of people with sickle cell and thalassaemia when you've got all these different primary care groups you know? Is it that they're going to say, Well actually we don't really want to tap into that service, so people who live in that area are going to miss out? (R6, p.15, para.50).

This she related to the conservative nature of many GPs, who were least willing to challenge the traditional professional/patient relationship, and, the most likely to demonstrate overt racism. These tendencies were discussed in the previous section and have been evidenced most clearly in the role fund holders have played in the recruitment of contracted staff (Cole 1994).

So the power differentials built into the PCG system were already causing anxiety for certain respondents, and part of that was the unwillingness to allow users to make a meaningful contribution. Yet some argued that even if it could be secured and the power differentials negotiated, the opportunity to improve services to minority ethnic communities might be minimal,

> I believe some of the changes in hand could create sort of the patient-led service, but there's still questions about accountability. We have primary health groups which are going to be heavily dominated by doctors, where there's questions about structure and sort of a platform that a single lay member will have for a population of 80 to 100 to 120,000 people. And it may be a locality which will probably contain many different communities with individual needs... And that's a worry because as I said earlier, because if you've got one lay member for a population of 120,000... (R5, pp.6 & 19, paras.18 & 59).

One user representative would be expected to champion the rights and needs of an entire community. This would be difficult enough where communities were ethnically homogeneous (assuming this were possible), but when they are also ethnically diverse, the difficulties multiply.

Another potential problem might be that the user representatives might actively elect to ignore the needs of the local community altogether:

> I think that it's really useful to get user input into your service but I think it has to be very well managed in the sense that typically the users involved in that type of arrangement may not be representative of the whole. They might have a particular axe to grind, and I don't know if you necessarily select users, if you... I'm thinking of patient focus groups or patient committees that sort of thing and you tend to get a particular type of person who attends that and I don't know that that's necessarily representative. But how you get that is very difficult, and also I think that with those types of groups that there's an expectation that whatever

they will say will then change automatically and a) it might not be representative, and b) it may just not be practical (R23, p.6, para.20).

In sympathy with the attitude of the HA representative, this respondent argued that user representatives are individuals and may well elect to pursue their own agendas. Part of the problem is that the type of person attracted to this role is unlikely to be representative of the general public (discussed more fully in chapter 7).

In short, although several respondents acknowledged that PCGs had the potential to improve services, there was substantial suspicion that the potential would remain unrealised. These findings have been substantiated by research involving a nationally representative sample of lay people on PCGs (Foolchand 2000). Although 75% (199) felt that PCGs were already improving service provision, there was a widespread expression of isolation and exclusion. The research indicated that minority ethnic communities are underrepresented (3.9%), that clinical dominance has been strong and unchallenged and that these trends were likely to characterise the development of Primary Care Trusts (effective from April 2000) (Foolchand 2000: 32). However the findings of this research appear to offer some insight into the question raised by Foolchand – is underrepresentation due to non-application or bias? The answer would appear to be that bias may be hampering certain applications, though there does appear to be some more recent improvements in numbers at least (DoH 2001).

Conclusion

Although the internal market was feted by many as a real opportunity to improve equal opportunities, access and service quality (Hopkins & Bahl 1993) the evidence suggests that its potential has not been realised. Although a minority of the trust employees accepted that some changes had been forthcoming, the majority rejected this because they were of the opinion that little change was required. There was however a near consensus about the PC, which was blamed for politicising users and leading to a compensation culture reminiscent of the United States. And yet, as Hari (2005) has pointed out, the compensation culture is at present a myth, and a myth generated by the desire to discourage claimants through guilt. It may be that Health Service employees can call on the additional guilt that complaining about a public service appears to stimulate in the majority. The extra workload in a period of staff shortages was also resented by the trust employees.

The unofficial user representatives felt that the PC had not necessarily produced the effects outlined above, particularly in relation to the minority ethnic communities, because of the general apathy of consumers and the specific disempowerment faced by ethnic minorities. It was viewed as something of a backlash running ahead of schedule. This group of respondents was less knowledgeable about the wider reforms, but there was little acknowledgement of tangible improvements. The head of the local CHC put this down to role confusion and resource constraints, but the unofficial representatives who expressed an opinion consistent with earlier chapters denied that the political will exists to fundamentally improve the lot of minority ethnic communities.

One clear result had been the consultation exercise and the resultant on-going dialogue identified with pride by the HA representative. However, it soon became clear that any nominal involvement that had been achieved might have been less about directly influencing services and more about buying off discontent. Indeed one respondent argued that the main objective of the HA was to obscure problems to ensure a superficial harmony paid for by minority communities. The recurring issues of demography and resource constraint were used to excuse a lack of real commitment to change, underlining the analysis of Carter (2000: 64)

There has been an inevitable tendency among managers within the Health Service to reduce success to equations about time and money. At the same time, 'soft' issues such as equal opportunities have tended to be marginalized precisely because of the lack of quantitative indicators of success or productivity.

As this section progresses it will become apparent that equality issues *per se* have been to some extent demoted or dismissed, and as Carter's analysis indicates also, this is less about appropriate measures for success than a clear unwillingness to respond to the needs of a diverse society.

The work of Jamdagni (1996) and Mwasamdube and Mullen (1998) indicate that community size and funding were central to the level of response by Health Service managers. However, the processes by which certain needs are constructed as peripheral need to be recognised. Jamdagni concluded *'...that a certain type of awareness of racism, and its impact on the health of the black population, is more likely to lead to a level of political commitment which brings about positive change'* (1996: 31). Political will in the region was found to be limited (Mwasamdube & Mullen 1998) and the local HA were only willing to acknowledge racism in the wider society, by implication separating the NHS from the community despite claims about participation and involvement. Therefore, it seems unlikely that the situation will improve in the immediate future.

Indeed, as the interview survey began, the first steps had been taken to set up the first PCGs in the area. Just as with the introduction of the internal market, there had been high hopes that the results would be beneficial for everyone and minority ethnic communities in particular. Yet the power imbalance created by GPs, anticipated and indirectly condoned by the HA, had prevented any attempt to ensure community representation, or at least to minimise any communal influence. Even if a fair representation was to be achieved in the future several respondents were sceptical about the outcomes. How could one or two lay people challenge the clinical pre-eminence and then sensitively represent the needs of such a diverse community? Although there has been an attempt to link generalised health policy with the equality and diversity agenda through initiatives like the

Primary Care Project (DoH 2003a) and the *Race for Health Programme* (Johnson 2004), the Labour government is promoting a formalised specialist agenda for 'racial' equality which will be discussed more fully in chapter 8. Before that we will turn our attention to efforts in Robbinston to address lingual and cultural barriers.

CHAPTER 5:

Minding our language

'I strive to be brief, and I become obscure' – Horace

Introduction

Apparently the potential of the internal market to indirectly benefit minority ethnic communities was not realised, nor was there unqualified support for PCGs, despite widespread recognition of their potential. At the local level the policy issues were much narrower, in line with the central demands of the communities during the consultation exercise the focus was very much on communication. In this chapter we focus on the issue of language barriers and how they have been addressed in Robbinston.

Various commentators have recommended universal interpreting services over the years (Torkington 1991), but this was clearly not a priority in Robbinston. The trust employees were happy to muddle through situations in which language barriers arose and were reputedly happy with a directory of available interpreters compiled by the newly appointed Patient Representative, even though most had never used it. Similarly the representative of the HA was keen to discuss the benefits of Language Line a national telephone interpreting service, which might be considered good practice in less diverse areas (Parekh 2000). The contention that it was in many ways preferable to universal interpretation was not supported by the evidence produced during the consultation process or by this research project.

Link working, a concept which involves bilingual workers forming a link between health workers and patients where communication proves difficult, was popular in theory (with the majority of trust employees) and in practice (with those who had some knowledge or experience of the service). Unfortunately there does seem to be a tendency to prefer the voluntary sector to bear the burden of solving such problems with all the attendant difficulties that this creates (Ahmad 1993b). Here as elsewhere the implicit message appears to be that minority ethnic communities create the problems therefore 'they' bear the responsibility for solving them.

Background

In 1991 Torkington called for the introduction of universal interpreting services in diverse areas. Three years later a national Health Education Authority survey stated that to be universally effective interpreters and advocates must support health services wherever necessary (Rudat 1994; a point raised by Parekh 2000). There was also a need to translate health promotion materials and NHS information into various languages. This was shown to be particularly important for older sections of the community and for women (Gunaratnam 1993; Cohen 1995b; Skellington 1996). Yet as the literature demonstrates (i.e. Donovan 1986a; McIver 1994; Bothamley 1996; Baxter 1997; Fletcher 1997) and as discussed in chapter 3 such support has not been provided on a systematic basis.

Mwasamdube and Mullen (1998) found in the local area that 97% of trusts reported having interpreting services available, but over half (21, 58%) relied on family members for translation and interpretation. The failure of current provision was also highlighted during the local consultation exercise. In particular it was recorded that:

- There are not enough trained interpreters available in doctors' surgeries and hospitals.
- Drug and treatment advice often needs to be translated.
- Leaflets are not effective on their own.

As a result of these issues the HA had resolved to:

- Increase the resources allocated to interpreting and support services.
- Conduct a trial of Language Line – a telephone interpreting service which offers 20 languages and can be available out of hours and for GPs, and Trusts.
- Review, with the help of the NHS Trusts and local people, how Trusts provide interpreting services, in order to identify possible improvements.
- Talk with GPs, Trust and local communities about which material should be translated and whether symbols, tapes etc should be used. This will be a continuing process.

In relation to these issues and policy promises there is once more a clear division of opinion between those who work in and around the NHS and those who unofficially represent minority ethnic communities. While the former consider the current provision of interpreting services to be generally sufficient, this is not a view shared by the latter. Nor are those who work in the NHS entirely convincing on this point. In fact, there appears to be little genuine commitment to improving things allegedly because of the costs involved but more importantly because there is a general feeling, as discussed throughout, that the problem resides in minority ethnic communities and that 'they' must either make do or make their own arrangements.

Language provision: inappropriate or innovative?

There was a distinct difference of opinion about the sensitivity of the local Health Service in meeting the needs of minority ethnic communities, between those working in or in close association with the NHS, and the majority of the unofficial user representatives. One of the central concerns was around language provision. There have been mixed reports about the availability of interpreting provision in the relevant literature. For instance, only 5.7% of the 130 Vietnamese respondents who provided information to Nguyen Van-Tam *et al* (1995) about interpreting provision in Nottingham said that interpreting was not available. Alternatively most research evidence suggests that interpreting services are rarely provided on a systematic basis (Gerrish *et al* 1996).

Torkington (1991) reported that none of the Somali women involved in a discussion about language provision had ever been offered interpreting services, similarly in a small questionnaire survey involving 40 people Leiston & Richardson (1996) found that 65% of those who needed interpreting services when visiting the GP were never offered them. Less than one in ten of the respondents in the fourth PSI survey who reported language problems in consulting GPs had access to an 'official translator', similar inadequacies were reported in relation to in-patient services (though the extent varied by group) (Nazroo 1997). Most of the user representatives, whether official or unofficial, were conscious that the local provision of interpreting services was inadequate and often non-existent. For example,

> It's the same as the whole system, that's supposed to be sensitive to user's needs, and providing a sensitive service to people. But again…that goes back to the fact that they're not providing interpreting facilities for everybody, and they're not always looking at cultural differences, cultural needs (R1, p.10, para.90 & 92).

Even where interpreting services were provided they were often deemed inappropriate. The Chinese respondent argued that the Health Service was frequently unable to provide for different dialects, something the local Housing Department had successfully addressed through consultation, reflecting the truth that social services, particularly social work, have led the way in the public sector (Thompson 1993). She was sceptical about the willingness of the Health Service to do the same.

Seemingly it will be difficult to convince (white) health workers of the need to improve things because, as stated in the previous section, most do not consider language or cultural differences as part of the 'core business'. In any case, they were mostly satisfied with the current level of provision. This had allegedly improved recently with the compilation of an interpreting directory by the newly appointed Patient Representative:

> There are issues that I'm aware of about getting interpreters, but as you probably already know we do have a Patient Representative who compiles the communication directory?... The Patient Representative has quite a unique role. There are others in different parts of the country, but they deal with patients' complaints, concerns and issues. Where people want to talk to more of an independent third party and don't always want to complain to their own doctor or their own nurse because they feel it might affect their own service. And one of the things that's she's done is to compile a communications directory which gives a huge list of names of interpreters who are prepared to work with the trust. And it does include sign language interpreters as well as ethnic minority languages... She's produced this directory which is distributed widely across the trust, and she has a small budget that she uses to finance it (R24, pp.1-3, paras.4 & 11).

Every one of the trust employees made reference to the directory at some point, and several were highly complimentary about it:

> There's a directory, yes, and they can get in touch with them. And our interpreters are paid and they're paid quite well actually, and the majority come from, they are ex-employees, which is quite nice as well... Yes, so we've got a couple of sisters who've retired, ward sisters, and they're on our directory for, I think its Hindi, and some other one. And they can come in and translate for us which is quite good (R13, p.2, paras.4 & 7).

So although two respondents were concerned about the low profile of the services offered and the problems in matching interpreters to patients at pertinent moments, there was a virtual consensus amongst the trust employees about the appropriateness of language provision.

Conversely four argued that they could not evaluate the quality of provision because they had never used the directory compiled by the Patient Representative. Rather than use the directory to identify appropriate interpreters, it seems that the respondents often prefer to muddle through or to allow minority ethnic individuals (whether friends, relatives, community workers or health workers) to overcome language barriers for them.

More than half of the respondents in the study by Nguyen Van-Tam *et al* used a relative (35.7%, 25, called on their children) and another 29% used community workers (Nguyen Van-Tam *et al* 1995: 108). Leiston & Richardson (1996) in a similar study produced strikingly similar results. This was apparently a common experience in Robbinston also, according to one of the working groups invited to comment on the report and action plan of the HA, and in the participating trust. For example:

> To be honest I've never had to use them [interpreters], because if ever, on the few occasions we've come into contact with any non-English speaking people they've normally had family members who've actually acted as interpreters. I've never come across people who couldn't speak English or communicate at all (R26, p.1, para.4).

Where this practice was identified the implication was that minority ethnic patients tend to bring along their own interpreters. The Chinese respondent disputed this:

> And often the hospital expect whenever they phone up, they say can you bring somebody from your family or relatives or friends? And I have women who come to me and say I got women trouble, and when I'm asked, when I'm asked about my relationship with my husband my son is doing the interpreting. I can't answer, I can't, I can't give an answer I would be embarrassed. Traditionally that's the way it is (R4, p.26, para.98).

According to her the service consciously relies on informal interpreting with all its attendant dangers, i.e. the inadequate technical language facility of the interpreter, and possible censorship of sensitive information. There was also a disturbing tendency to employ sign language, which has also been supported by other research evidence (Torkington 1991; Nazroo 1997). In the words of Parekh (2000: 183-184) *'This bad practice places extra stress on patients for whom English is an additional language, as well as on the informal interpreter and health professionals'*.

Another option then has been to use minority ethnic staff members as impromptu interpreters (Donovan 1986a; Torkington 1991; Farooqi 1993). In 1993 the NHSME launched a programme of action to overcome barriers faced by minority ethnic staff members (discussed more fully in chapter 7). One of the recommendations read: *'Regard the variety of languages spoken by staff as a valuable asset'* (1993: 11). However the evidence suggests that this has been ignored. Bagilhole and Stephens (1997) found that minority ethnic health workers, mainly women, were used to plug gaps in language provision without recognition or reward (see also Willmot 1996). This was similarly a common experience in the trust. Minority ethnic staff members were certainly called upon to provide impromptu interpretation.

> So obviously, I mean we have people who speak German and French, we haven't got anybody who speaks Hindi or anything like that... And obviously there are times when we call on these individuals to talk to patients because...mainly to allow some sort of conversation (R15, p.8, para.25).

Admittedly, the minorities in the example cited were likely to be white (though not necessarily), the inference was clear, that were (non-white) minority ethnic staff members available they would be asked to perform similar unofficial duties. A general manager from employment services said:

> Quite often we get calls saying do you know anybody who speaks so and so. You know, and then we've got to try and find somebody who speaks the language because the patient doesn't speak English (R31, p.1, para.5).

This demonstrates that the practices outlined by Baxter, whereby one of her respondents said *'They will come and get you from another ward so you can interpret for them'* (1988: 38) are continuing (see also Gerrish *et al* 1996: 80; Parekh 2000: 176).

Although I was unable to interview any minority ethnic staff members, the Chinese representative confirmed this imposition:

> It still goes on and even local city councils they use their own staff and yet the staff actually told me they don't want to be used, and nurses they told me from health authorities, they don't want to be used. They say very often they are busy, they want one job, and next thing is they were called upon to go to another ward to provide interpreting... It is not what they want to do, no. They don't want to do it, and also they say they feel it's a conflict of interest because when the client questions the facilities, the services and the nurse, and she's in a position feeling... And she'll feel very embarrassed to relay that to the hospital... (R4, p.14, paras.52-54).

So where relatives or friends are not available minority ethnic health workers are used to plug gaps in language provision. They receive, as Bagilhole and Stephens (1997) asserted, no recognition or reward for such efforts. They also found that although this caused work-load problems for the individuals involved, there appeared to be none of the reluctance to provide such services identified by the Chinese respondent. For instance, one said *'I like to translate but the problem is that if I spend too much time with them, I fall behind with my own work and so have to rush really badly sometimes. But I don't like to say 'no' if somebody asks'* (Bagilhole & Stephens 1997: 18). However, she did support her position by referring to divided loyalties. According to her even if these additional skills *were* to be taken into account in terms of employment status and reward, this would not entirely rectify the situation. After all, as the respondent suggests they may still find themselves in the invidious position of having to relay criticisms of the service they are involved in providing to colleagues and superiors.

It is when there are no informal means of interpretation available that the real innovation begins. On a visit to a different hospital in an official capacity the Chinese respondent approached one of the ward managers

> I say to him do you use interpreters if they can't speak English? No problem, we use sign language (R4, p.16, para.60).

This also occurred in the participating trust to some extent. One respondent outlined the steps taken when language barriers did emerge:

> As far as this department is concerned we use interpreters very little. A lot of our investigations are fairly short-lived if you like. The vast majority of our investigations will last no more than 10 minutes max. Some of the more complex ones obviously do. With the shorter investigations it is a case of almost leading anyone through, quite readily, because we can demonstrate to people what we want them to do, and how we want them to do it. For instance, if we want them to hold their breath the usual thing is for us to hold our breath, and show them, because things can be made over-complex. But as I say the vast majority of our work then that's the case. If it is much more complex then as I say patients do tend to come along with relatives or friends who do speak English, and translate for them. If that is a problem then we contact the services that we provide, and they will provide some sort of interpretation for us. And that's basically the 3 sorts of steps that we have depending on the problem's complexity...It's a very sort of practical issue really, it's not like sitting in an office and talking to someone about something specific. It is actually about getting out there and doing things with the patients, so it is much easier (R15, p.2, paras.5 & 6).

So despite the praise heaped upon the directory services, it would appear that for some it is the final resort rather than the first port of call. The dangers of such an approach were ably articulated by the following ward manager (the story bears full repetition):

> Yes we did have I think it was an Indian family, a lady who was actually very, very ill, terminally ill. So she was having a lot done for her, and we did at that time. Her family did ask whether there was any other Indian nurses or I can't think what the other ethnic...But they were specifically saying that because of the

language, because when they went away, went home, she couldn't communicate. Because she'd never, I mean she'd been here for *thirty years*, but she'd never spoken English, and I don't know how they get on, but they obviously do. But I think she said yes and no, but I think that was about it. But I mean we could communicate by gesture and everything, but they were worried that if there was anything serious she couldn't communicate (R13, p.13, para.36).

She was surprised, indeed she seemed during the interview to be actively annoyed, that the family should request an Indian nurse able to speak the appropriate language even though the danger attached to communication by gestures was obvious. She did not regard the much less appropriate requests from white patients for white nurses with the same irritation.

At the level of local hospital and community services the user representatives were highly critical of available language provision. Although the trust employees were generally satisfied with what they could provide, there was substantial evidence that the interpreting service was rarely employed. It would seem that most would rather rely on informal channels or personalised sign language than to ensure the provision of adequate interpretation. The risks associated with this enterprising attitude are all too clear.

The region-wide response

In spite of such criticisms, there was a belief amongst some of the user representatives that things were slowly improving. For example, an ex-member of the CHC said:

The Health Authority have been trying to address that and we have had various reports over the last 10 years about that, and about how effective that policy has been. But the Race Equality Council and the health authority do work together (R8, p.2, para.6).

The current head of the CHC echoed this:

We are aware of course that there are issues in terms of language, interpretation, translation and so on. But having said that the Health Authority who've just completed, well I say just, over a year ago now, a major piece of work consulting black and other minority ethnic communities, put a number of initiatives in place to try and help around those things. Like Language Line, which is translation by phone. There are a whole range of translated leaflets available, or, arrangements can be made to translate them (R12, p.1, para.1).

The representative of the HA was not concerned with the provision of translated materials, as this was not raised to any great extent during the consultation carried out in the region, but she was keen to discuss the telephone initiative.

Language Line is a national initiative in which the health authority had recently invested in order to improve the service provided by GPs to minority ethnic patients unable to speak English:

I only had a little amount of disposable money – about 25,000, 30,000 a year – and we put some of it into general language. I can talk about that, Language Line, which is a support telephone service for GPs... And I think we've done that a bit with GP services and interpreting as an example. When I started this, communities were just saying to us you must provide interpreters. Why don't you provide interpreters? Well over a 2 year period of discussion...which is that GPs see 30 people in a morning, it's not planned, if somebody turns up who can't speak English the chances of ever getting them together in the same GP surgery with an interpreter or an advocate is minute. It would take days of work to arrange it. And so what we've done is join up with this telephone service – Language Line – in London. [It] is rather artificial, it's not perfect, but on the other hand it's very confidential, it's well removed from the local community, and within 90 seconds they will guarantee to connect a GP to any one of 90 language speakers in London, who are trained and who are quality tested. And yes the GP and the patient have to hand the phone backwards and forwards, but it's better than nothing. Now I had a lot of people, the advocates in the community found that very difficult to accept, because it wasn't the perfect solution. The perfect solution to them was the interpreter sitting with the GP or the advocate (R11, p.25, para.92).

She readily acknowledged that Language Line was not perfect but within the context of limited resources it was the best that could be offered. There was some discussion about the development of a universal service jointly funded by the local Unitary Authorities, but it was felt that this would destabilise the link working service (discussed below) and would be prohibitively expensive in relation to the demographic profile of the region. Furthermore, whereas interpreting services had allegedly caused problems for local communities in terms of confidentiality, it ensured a safe distance between interpreter and patient. Although confidentiality would not present a major problem in a significant area of minority ethnic settlement such as London or Birmingham, she felt that it would be harder to ensure in a smaller city with a correspondingly small minority ethnic population.

Parekh (2000) accepts that a telephone service would reflect best practice in areas of low minority ethnic settlement, and although some of the areas for which the HA is responsible would certainly meet that criteria, it does not explain why universal interpreting provision cannot be made across Robbinston. It may be that such a solution would also be culturally inappropriate for certain sections of the community, as identified by the local REC. For example, Bowers (1993: 622) suggests that *'Asian patients are uncomfortable with telephone advice...'* Although the line was acknowledged as a step in the right direction by even the most critical of the user representatives it also came in for some heavy criticism.

Not only was it reputed to be impersonal and insensitive, because of the inability of patients to communicate with GPs, but it also dictated the nature and extent of such communication:

> They got a Language Line now, but it's still not satisfactory because it's still got a lot of teething problems and people did use it and they said it's not satisfactory. It's very insensitive. It's no personal contact and very often you're restricted to what you have to say. It's not as though like face-to-face (R4, p.1, para.2).

The potential for misinterpretation and misdiagnosis must be enormous during this kind of three-way interaction. At times the results were reported to be somewhat impractical

> Sometimes the client actually phone from home to the GP and the GP tap into this line and it's a 3-way thing, it's not satisfactory. No, it's got a lot of teething problems and I think...the [health authority] try very hard to make amends and try to improve the services to the black and ethnic minorities but they still got a long way to go (R4, p.2, para.3).

Without any face-to-face contact at all, the dangers become that much more pronounced. Although the HA representative accepted the imperfections of this system, she considered this to be the most effective method available under existing resource constraints, particularly as the minority ethnic population was relatively small. The level of provision requested by user representatives would be impractical to provide for primary services, so it would be utterly impossible for trusts to entertain such a notion:

> It's a terrible thing for an Asian women perhaps to end up on her own with cancer on a ward in the [nearest hospital], and to feel isolated and not be able to share all the issues that she wants to share and perhaps not to have the language to share it. But equally...one has to recognise it's equally very difficult for that trust to provide expert services, expert Asian interpreting for her. You know because they don't have one, they don't use one often enough to justify it. So any of them they do use will come from some sort of general service who won't have medical training, who won't have relationships with staff on the wards so that they can ask the right questions about patient care. It's just a really difficult thing. It's not that people don't want to do it, it's that they can't see how to (R11, p.11, para.33).

Although she could empathise with those who find themselves in frightening surroundings facing the prospects of a serious illness without the ability to communicate, there just are not enough resources to provide extensive services to such a small proportion of the population.

Actually she often used the issue of population size and the number of people presenting interchangeably. Although this can be done to a certain extent, there is room for slippage. There is a real possibility that inappropriate services may be deterring usage, and that underutilisation may be dictating resource allocation. As Kurtz suggests *'Where there is little take-up of well meaning but unsuitable services, this may be interpreted as a reason for not putting extra resources into services for black and ethnic minorities'* (1993: 82). It would be ironic if inadequate services should be justifying themselves. That they are insensitive and inappropriate enough to deter people from using them, but that this underutilisation is interpreted as a lack of need amongst minority ethnic communities, consequently it is concluded that there is no need to improve provision.

Of course the final point that needs to be reiterated here is that the NHS is funded through taxation, and as taxpayers and citizens everyone is entitled to a satisfactory and appropriate service. An inability to communicate directly with health professionals surely denies people the full rights of citizenship, and whether this can be justified on the grounds set out above is highly questionable.

Whose line is it anyway?

Of course the argument that resources are scarce and that any and every want and need cannot be catered for is frequently used to limit expectations, not only of minority ethnic communities, but also those of the majority population (Lipsky 1980). However, in relation to language provision this explanation was rejected by most of the user representatives. For example, the representative of the REC maintained that:

> The obligation to have the appropriate communication tools still rests with [the] patients (R5. p.22, para.70).

Moreover that,

> ...the expectation's very much...And I think it's fairly typical of the society, where the integration means that people automatically learn English as a language. No matter their age, educational background. You know without providing, often, any clear programme for this to happen (R5, p.1, para.3).

On an institutional level, at least locally, this is largely the case.

In fact the only provision for language tuition has been organised via the voluntary sector through section 11 funding, dedicated funding provided under the provisions of the Local Government Act 1966 to local authorities '...*very much as compensation...having to deal with the 'problems' such as non-English speaking children in schools and immigrants with extra social difficulties'* (Bagilhole 1997: 66-67). The scheme works in conjunction with the link working service, which will be discussed below. Here the co-ordinator explains how it operates:

> I think it is maybe better here than in some cities, but it's moving into looking at those needs and trying to meet those needs. But I think a lot of it is left to the voluntary sector as well... And [this service] comes in by education yeah? And that's trying to meet the need for communities to learn the language so overcoming some of the barriers to ease access to Health Services. So it's trying to get the health or social authority to understand the language and cultural differences and also trying to help the communities [learn the language...]. Meanwhile the link workers are actually doing the interpreting and the tutors are trying to teach the language and give them information about the Health Services (R1, p.2, paras.13-19).

So there is provision made for those who cannot speak English to learn, but this is treated as an educational issue rather than the preserve of the Health Service. Yet the scheme also provides its students with information about the workings of the NHS, making them aware of their entitlements and does so in the security of their own home via one-to-one tuition.

Nevertheless, it does have its limitations. It is a long-term solution to an immediate problem. What happens to people while they are learning the language? Surely the Health Service has an inescapable obligation to ensure that services are adequate and sensitive now? Finally, what about those who are not eligible for such tuition? It only operates on behalf of 'Asian' women, and other sectors of the community with similar needs are excluded (the co-ordinator was only too conscious of this).

This takes us right back to the statement made by the REC representative. It seems likely that it is not only a lack of resources that restricts the quality of language provision, but a general unwillingness to meet what are seen to be illegitimate needs, as the dominant understanding of different needs is constructed via ethnic sensitivity through a biomedical channel. She argued that the obligation to negotiate such difficulties rests with the users and this was most certainly the interpretation of most trust employees.

Link working

An early attempt to deal with both lingual and cultural barriers at once has been the adoption of link working, first identified during the *Asian Mother and Baby Campaign* (AMBC) (DHSS 1987; Johnson 1993). Link workers are similar in some respects to interpreters but are arguably more acceptable to both sides they act as a *link* between patient and professional. It was hoped that their proliferation would follow on from the 1991 reforms (Bahl 1993a), but the evidence as to their efficacy in practical terms is ambiguous. While Bahl (1990) claims notable success in terms of the uptake of antenatal services in the wake of the AMBC (a 50% increase), Hoare *et al* (1994) reported (in a randomized controlled trial of breast screening services in Oldham) that there was no evidence of any positive impact amongst 'Asian' women in the area.

More recent evidence suggests that link working can be effective. For example, due to pressure from a voluntary organisation in Tower Hamlets the NHS set up an audiology clinic at Great Ormond Street Hospital to deal with the disproportionate rate of hearing difficulties amongst Bengali children. They are up to four times more likely to experience such difficulties than their white counterparts (consanguinity has been mentioned as an explanatory factor, despite the criticisms raised by Parsons *et al* (1993) and Ahmad (1994) of the irresponsible use of such factors). Over a third of families missed appointments due to communication barriers many were expected to provide their own interpreting arrangements. Things only improved when a Bengali development worker was employed. One of the audiologists said: *'Before there was a huge communications gap – an invisible screen which fell between doctor and the family. It was incredible how the families opened up in front of her. We can now work with the families to help the children'*. Only 5% of appointments have been missed since that time, although funding was set to run out in 2002 (Cunningham 2000). So it would seem that link workers could be, indeed have been, effective in addressing the problem of communication barriers.

The city in which the research was conducted did have such a service, provided by the voluntary sector through HA funding. It was largely restricted however to maternity issues (although some provision had recently been made for the health problems faced by Somali men). Despite this the central question raised during the interview survey was if the service were to be expanded could link working solve the problem of language barriers? Perhaps predictably, bearing in mind the local concentration on maternity issues, only one of the trust employees had any knowledge of the concept and that was gained through personal experience. She was eager to extol its virtues:

> Well we do have workers in fact we have a Somalian worker, and an organisation [that provides those services]. Well we have a regular worker who's in twice a week and provides interpreting services for us. It's a very well used service, particularly...during antenatal and postnatal periods, with young children, with speech therapy issues. But [they] will also come along with people to the GP if that was what was actually required. (R18, p.2, para.6).

McIver (1994) suggests that link workers might create some tension and even hostility amongst health care workers, with their work dismissed as either special treatment or as an implicit criticism of their own practice. Although most had never used the service, or were even aware of the general concept, once explained the majority of the trust employees thought it a good idea worthy of expansion. This may be due to the fact that it would avoid the need for in-house interpreters and because it is independently provided and might avoid treading on professional toes. (It might also be that it sits well with the view that minority ethnic communities should deal with 'their' own problems.)

The user representatives, both official and unofficial, were also largely supportive of the idea and the actual service:

> Because we have link workers that deal with most languages so if there is a problem, we would actually call upon a link worker whose first language is…And they translate… We have link workers they are specifically for that purpose. There was a problem but I think it was going back quite a few years ago, but there was a need for it, so they incorporated the link workers to work over here. They help out in the NHS health centres and places like that (R3, p.1, paras.2 & 4).

Indeed one of the benefits, contrary to the arguments proposed by the representative of the HA, was that it ensures confidentiality:

> I think in the short-term it's essential really. You can't really expect the patients or clients to rely on family or friends due to the confidential nature of things. They may not want the whole community to know about it, but with a link worker you know that it's going to be confidential (R1, p.4, para.28-30).

It soon became clear that, just as much of the available literature suggests, the role of link workers is ambiguous, in that they tend to do much more than simply interpret, much more than providing a simple link. For one thing, as discussed in the previous chapter, they organised and delivered cultural training for local health workers –

> Oh I think so yeah, oh goodness me, definitely, particularly with the Asian women who don't speak English. I would say that they've made a huge difference without a doubt. And I know that they do sort of like the Asian cultural awareness days. And talking to staff they're just like, because you see it depends on the directorate you work in, whether it's community, surgery, medicine, [gynaecology], obstetrics…and I know that I go in to talk to certain groups as an OT and they have study days. And I always tend to go after the Asian women are talking about Asian culture, and it always ran over because the staff were just fascinated. It's like it's a whole new world, although they've sort of been sort of living in [this city], and looking after patients for many, many years, they've never been comfortable to talk to people about their culture; because they feel it was sensitive and they were being nosy or racist and all the rest of it, and just by saying that they were ordinary people, they would love for you to learn about how they do things and why they do things. So it's just like a whole totally different world, it's like teaching a child something for the first time (R6, p.24, para.77).

According to the co-ordinator of the service this willingness to go beyond its established responsibility was the key to its success. Unlike local Health Services, it was pro-active. Link workers went out into the community, talked to people, and dropped leaflets in accessible places. They sought to take health care into the community and they knew how to do it, because they took the trouble to know the community (R2, p.4, para.5). On the whole then the interview respondents were in favour of the actual service provided and the concept itself. However, both the reality and the potential of link working were questioned.

The weakest link?

Link working has been effective in many cases, both locally and nationally, but it is recognised that communication barriers remain a problem even where services are comprehensive (Alexander 1999). As stressed above the local service was not comprehensive, indeed one of the principal problems associated with the service provided was coverage according to certain respondents. The service is located mainly in the inner city and predominantly caters for the 'Asian' communities:

> There are link workers but they're based in only certain areas. So for example in the inner city here... We have about 3 or 4 link workers based [around this area] and they're mainly here for the Asian languages, but also Somalis. But there are problems for other languages as well. I mean for example, Polish, Vietnamese, all these different communities [in the city] (R1, p.1, paras.4 & 5).

More recently its remit had been expanded to take into account the needs of the newly arrived Somali refugee community, and men in particular, who were persistently failing to register with, much less visit, local GPs. Even the link workers in operation cannot cater satisfactorily for the level of demand due to a shortage of hours:

> I think it should because we have a wide variety of people now from ethnic minorities, and it would help because it would give them more hours. I'm aware

that the hours that are given to link workers are very small. I think that like how they are, you have a clerk, or you have a midwife or people like that, you do have link workers, but I think their hours should be more. 'Cos I think that their job is very important and we have a very large scale of minority people. So I think it should be (R3, p.2, para.8).

The Chinese respondent echoed this:

There is one, and that's only mainly because I've been sitting on the management [committee] for a long time. To start with there was only a 5 hour post and out of 5 hours, 1 and a half hours she had to be involved with staff management meetings, so it was only 3 and a half hours a week. Catering for 7 and a half thousand Chinese, it's just not enough. But at the time she was only her designated post is only for inner city, now it's expanded to the [city]-wide area now... And I was inundated, I had to turn people away, and there were people die unnecessarily, so it was just, upsetting me a lot... We increased that to 25 [hours] but it's still not enough... We're still turning people away, and the health link worker works very closely with me, and she says she's forever having to let people down. And we work very closely together. It's not enough interpreters who are catering for the Chinese community and I think officially 7 and a half thousand has not been recognised. Although in all my reports I always put down 7 and a half thousand or perhaps more because we have got a lot of postgraduate students from China and Taiwan as well, and they need all these services as well. So they are Mandarin speakers you see, and luckily I speak both dialects (R4, pp.9 &10, paras.31-35).

Although she had pitched in to assist the link worker, the level of demand was simply too great to cope with. According to her the consequences of this can be tragic – people die unnecessarily due to the inadequacy of the local provision of interpreting facilities and the inability of the link working service to cope with the level of need.

So coverage is a major issue (Patel 1993). Link working in the city caters mainly for the inner city areas and within those areas mainly for 'South Asian' communities focusing specifically on maternity issues, and these concerns were echoed by one of the working groups formed by the HA to offer comments on its report and action plan. The majority of the user respondents appeared to assume that were link workers more widely available communication would not remain a problem.

According to the representative of the REC this is naïve. She argued that the role ambiguity mentioned above (Bhopal & White 1993; McIver 1994), namely, the tendency to provide advocacy services to patients and to advise health workers, is officially ignored by the NHS:

> It also lays questions because is the link worker just a link? What about their recognised role of advocacy? And I think there's a difference between somebody who may be seen as an acquiescent link rather than somebody who is an advocate... Well the link worker is there to provide a link and to interpret basically, but it depends on the boundary. There are some link workers who only do that as interpreters, but I think people fail to understand the differences between an interpreter and someone who is potentially there to advocate as well (R5, p.8, paras.25 & 28).

Her contention was evidenced by the reaction of the HA representative to this issue. She said:

> Yes they are [effective]... [Do they serve as advocates?] Not here very much. Not officially. In practice I'm sure that some of them do, say where they've got a family who for some reason are suffering from ill health. I think they do probably take up an advocacy role but it's not formalised (R11, p.8, para.24).

According to the REC representative and to a lesser extent the nurse trainer this was because the NHS was not prepared to deal with the needs of minority ethnic communities, to use the current managerial terminology, as part of its 'core business' (Stubbs 1993).

Although she thought that the link working service was invaluable in many ways, she also thought that it was a way of passing on responsibility to minority ethnic communities:

> As I said earlier the [link worker organisation] has been operating for oooh over ten years, it has proved invaluable, and I know that professionals using the service find that. They are much happier with the health care they are able to provide, they feel they're more confident about working with the patients and of understanding their patients more. However, a link worker will often be seen as I also said earlier, that her interpreting skills, or his interpreting skills, are not valued. And given the very Englishness of the NHS, it's incredibly hierarchical

and not, and still not very democratic. And I believe what's been missing has actually been putting value on an attachment worker service. It still remains marginal because it's provided by a black non-professional from a voluntary organisation that's not seen as part of the internal machinery (R5, p.7, para.23).

In a sense then the link working service actually enables the NHS to keep the needs of minority ethnic communities on the margins because they are a marginal entity dealing with marginal concerns (at least as far as the Health Service is concerned) (Bagilhole 1993).

She also argued that locating responsibility within minority ethnic communities allowed the Health Service to encourage divisions within the community, to divide and rule, and deflect any attempt to achieve radical reforms (Ahmad 1993b). Although it would be extremely difficult to evidence the conscious intent she surmises, there was certainly evidence of divisions. In order to provide a more sensitive service to the Somalian refugee community, a male link worker from that community had been employed. This was felt to be necessary for a number of reasons:

We also have a male worker who works from [the organisation] who is specifically there for looking at the health needs of men and also the elderly of the Somali community, and how we can perhaps help address those issues. For example, we've noticed that a lot of men don't register with GPs – the women do for antenatal care or what have you – but the men don't. And so therefore it is difficult if they're either unwell or they're missing out on screening opportunities (R18, p.2, para.6).

According to the HA representative:

I only had a very little amount of disposable money – about £25, £30,000 a year...about £20,000 of it we put into an extra Somali link worker because after much agonising that was perhaps the most consensus you could get around what to spend it on (R11, p.8, para.22).

The consensus was clearly very fragile because the Chinese respondent for one had argued vigorously against this appointment:

I broke in tears when they were going to put up money [the Health Authority] gave the money to the [link working organisation], £40,000. And part of the money should be increasing the Chinese link worker's hours and yet because [that organisation] is also controlled and run by Asians, mainly Asians, and Chinese just very fraction of it right? Therefore, they were going to employ a male link worker by using that money. But I fought, I really fought very hard, I was disgusted...I thought that money was supposed to be designated for increasing the hours. We need it because I myself was working as an interpreter (R4, pp.8-9, para.31).

In concert with the view expressed by the HA representative the majority of the user representatives recognised the gaps in provision – i.e. for the Chinese community – but considered that the resources had been used as effectively as possible under the circumstances. The Chinese respondent argued that this was because the 'South Asian' community had managed to secure most of the funding and controlled most of the voluntary provision in the city.

Whilst it would not be possible to support the view that providing funding for voluntary provision, and link working in particular, is a deliberate means of stimulating divisions between minority ethnic communities it can be argued that this has occurred. The notion that link working locates the problem firmly within the community is much more plausible, particularly in light of the views expressed by those employed in and around the NHS. This may well be why the majority of the trust employees favoured the concept. If this is so then the argument proposed by the respondent from the REC would carry some weight – that link working is a means of preventing a radical restructuring of the Health Service to meet diverse needs. At the very least it is possible to suggest that even if it were expanded link working would be unlikely to solve the communication problems identified in the previous section.

The consultation carried out by the HA across the region underlines the importance of a comprehensive interpreting service to the minority ethnic population. Important though link working has become, it was not seen to be a viable alternative on its own. It was also clear from the consultation, as will be discussed more fully in chapter 7, and highlighted by the representative of the local REC, that interpreting should not be seen as a compromise on matters of ethnic diversity in the workforce.

Conclusion

For the most part the trust employees reported that they were more than satisfied with the trust's provision, emphasising the value of the directory put together by the newly appointed Patient's Representative. However, there was a distinct lack of evidence that it had been used, and it soon became clear that minority ethnic people were often held responsible for their own interpreting needs – either as friends, relatives or as health workers providing *ad hoc* services.

The consultation exercise undertaken by the HA had thrown up these problems and several policy promises had subsequently been made. Just as the majority of the unofficial user representatives feared, and the bulk of the evidence suggests, there was very little commitment to following these promises through. The most that could be done had already been done according to the representative of the HA, and that took the form of the telephone interpretation service – Language Line – based in London. Although she accepted that it was not ideal as far as 'activists' were concerned she felt that it was superior in many ways to their preferred option of universal interpreting services.

The idea that the telephone service was more confidential than face-to-face translation did not outweigh the numerous flaws identified by the unofficial representatives. In fact, there was some dispute about the confidentiality also, with several of the latter suggesting that the best means of ensuring confidentiality, even in the context of a relatively small city with a correspondingly small minority ethnic population, is to provide professional interpreters on a universal basis. This was qualified, as will become clear in chapter 7. Although members of the community were consulted on the composition of the HAs report and action plan they did not want this at the expense of a drive to increase the diversity of the local workforce (see chapter 7).

Ultimately, as stressed throughout, the unofficial user representatives were predominantly sceptical that the political will was present to achieve the range and depth of changes needed to ensure sensitive and appropriate provision. The HA representative was clear that in the context of resource constraints, with such a small community, there was very little more that could be done, and, albeit implicitly, where gaps appeared then the onus fell on the communities themselves to deal with them.

This can be seen most clearly with reference to the approval given in principle at least by the overwhelming majority of trust employees to the notion of link working. Although everyone with any knowledge of or dealings with the local service, funded by the HA, was quick to heap praise upon it and the difference it had made, there were some doubts raised about its long-term potential. The representative of the REC in particular feared that link working was a deliberate means of keeping the needs of minority ethnic communities on the margins by allowing individuals from those communities to take responsibility, whilst at the same time denying them any professional status within the health system. Furthermore, there have been indications contained in the relevant literature that link working is a useful way of creating divisions within and between sections of the minority ethnic community (Ahmad 1993b; Smaje 1995). Although insufficient evidence is provided here to fully support this contention, there was evidence that the way in which funds had been distributed and services organised had caused inter-group tensions.

In the final analysis it seems fairly clear that despite significant lingual barriers identified in the relevant literature and in Robbinston, the policy promises made by the HA are unlikely to be met. Even if they were, the results might not be sufficiently transformative, as the primary goal appears to be to make minority ethnic communities responsible while keeping them on the margins of the Health Service, as argued by the REC representative in particular. Numerous studies have shown that even comprehensive interpreting or link working services on their own are not enough and that more thought and organisation needs to be engaged in clarifying the role of minority ethnic health workers (Gerrish *et al* 1996). We will explore the possibilities of diversifying the workforce as a realistic alternative or supplement to such policies more fully in the third section. First we will set out and evaluate the local plans for filling in the cultural gaps identified earlier.

CHAPTER 6:

The value of Cultural Awareness Training

'Cure the disease, and kill the patient' – Sir Francis Bacon

Introduction

One of the central methods of dealing with cultural misunderstandings between patients and health workers in Robbinston, drawing upon the HAs report and action plan, and, the interview material provided by the organisation's representative was to be cultural awareness training (CAT). Despite the many problems associated with this concept, not least its individualistic, victim-blaming underpinnings (Pearson 1986; Baxter 1988; Culley 1996), there was some support for it from many respondents. The unofficial user representatives were generally keen to stress that such activities ought to be carefully thought out and collectively organised.

However, there was also a great deal of resistance to the notion, particularly amongst the trust employees, who felt that it was both an unfair judgement of their treatment of minority ethnic communities, and because that treatment was perfectly adequate, tantamount to positive discrimination. Any resistance from the unofficial user representatives derived from its tendency to undermine radical change. Perhaps neither camp ought to have worried too much as CAT was only sketchily provided and if the HA representative is to be believed, is unlikely to expand much in the near future. The consistent theme of

168

scarce resources was once again produced to justify any inactivity (McNaught 1988; Smaje 1995).

It was also apparent that where CAT was provided the responsibility lay with minority ethnic communities themselves. Not only were minority ethnic health workers expected to provide *ad hoc* cultural awareness advice to their white colleagues (Baxter 1988, 1997) they are, it seems, sometimes called upon to provide organised training programmes with little or no training or expertise. The role of minority ethnic workers in the provision of services to their own communities has not been openly articulated (Stubbs 1993), but what ethnic diversity means and how it will work in practice forms the heart of chapter 7.

Background

One of the key problems identified by minority ethnic communities during the consultation exercise undertaken by the local HA was located in the insensitivity of white health workers to diverse cultural needs. As a result the HA had made several policy promises. For example, they committed themselves to:

- Arrange training for [HA] staff.
- Develop training for wider groups of staff working in GP practices.
- Work with Trusts to improve awareness in staff.
- Design and issue a "good practice" guide for NHS staff in [the region].

The intention was broadly to encourage as far as possible Health Service employers in the area to introduce CAT. Of course, as one of the working groups maintained in commenting on the HA's report and action plan, it would be wrong to divorce CAT from wider equal opportunities issues. However, this was to some extent the case in the local area, and I have maintained this divide in order to focus on equal opportunities in employment and its service implications in Section 3.

The training of health professionals has been a key issue in the provision of health care to minority ethnic communities for some time (Johnson 1987). There is no doubt that health workers need to be aware of cultural differences, as Jayaratnam states: *'Health care staff need to develop a requisite degree of cultural competence to match their professional skills if they are to give correct information and a good service to people from different cultures'* (1993: 12; see also Baxter 1997; Parekh 2000). Writers such as Leininger (1991) in the United States and Cortis (1993) in the UK have pushed hard to have cultural awareness placed at the heart of professional education, with some success according to Culley (1996). Furthermore, the UKCCs 1984 Code of Practice and the ENBs Equal Opportunities Policy 1993 stressed the importance of providing nurses with the tools to provide appropriate care to minority ethnic communities (Baxter 1997). Yet evidence shows that health professionals generally continue to be poorly prepared for work in multicultural settings (Karmi 1993; Gerrish *et al* 1996; Baxter 1997; Nazroo 1997; Parekh 2000). Too often efforts to improve the quality of professional education and training have been *ad hoc*, patchy and have relied too heavily upon committed individuals (Baxter 1997) - themes which resound throughout the literature on 'race' and health policy (Ahmad 1993b; Johnson 1993; Smaje 1995; Iganski *et al* 2001).

There was a developed awareness of these issues across the region in which this research was carried out. The university responsible for training health professionals in the area was in the process of implementing a policy to diversify student cohorts on health-based programmes *and* to improve the quality of their exposure to diverse needs. This strategy was partly a drive to increase local recruitment but was also informed by the research undertaken by Gerrish *et al* (1996) and Iganski *et al* (1998) on behalf of the ENB.

The problem is, as the nurse trainer responsible for these efforts suggests, that CAT creates as many problems as it solves, and this has been recognised for some considerable time. The report published by Brent CHC in 1981 for example asserted that the actual training of health professionals and the literature involved served to obscure the needs of minority ethnic communities by presenting distorted information on different cultures permeated by negative representations (Brent CHC 1981: 13-14; see also Pearson 1986; NAHA 1988; Hopkins & Bahl 1993; Bowler 1993; Bhopal & White 1993; Bothamley 1996).

The use of CAT suggests that the problem is individualistic and based in false ideas, if only we can enlighten (predominantly white) people they will not discriminate. This can be described diagrammatically as follows:

Ignorance → Prejudice → Intolerance → Insensitive service provision

↑

Educational intervention (breaking this cycle)

In this formulation timely intervention to eradicate ignorance breaks the chain which leads to insensitive treatment. The strategy is counterproductive because it often leads to the reification of ethnic identities and cultures, a cultural and ethnic essentialism, which conveniently ignores the complex, heterogeneous and dynamic nature of culture, including that of the white majority, and the problematic nature of ethnicity (Ahmad & Sheldon 1992). This has been referred to as the Saris, Samosas and Steel bands effect (Penketh & Ali 1997). Thus CAT can serve to propagate the very stereotypes it seeks to challenge (Bowler 1993; Ellis & Sonnenfeld 1994), for instance the passivity of 'Asian' women the generalisability of which is demonstrably inaccurate (Bryan et al 1985), and the tight knit 'Asian' community, the detrimental consequences of which were discussed in chapter 3.

In fact CAT can encourage discrimination by exhorting tolerance, which locates the blame for any perceived difficulties in 'deviant' minority ethnic cultures (Donovan 1986a; Pearson 1986; Bagilhole 1993). This *'health [model sees] many of these [health and health care] problems as internally generated through inappropriate cultures; family and community traditions'* (Stubbs 1993: 40). Further, the individualistic emphasis (relating to the ignorance of white individuals) is highly apolitical, in that it deflects attention away from structural forces and relations, and racism in particular (Jewson & Mason 1993). Embodied in the belief that, as expressed by Henley (1992), and supported by the majority of the trust employees, health professionals never discriminate intentionally.

There is also an implicit instruction for minority ethnic communities in the theoretical foundations of CAT as identified by Culley: *'Appropriate education, coupled with integration on the part of the more 'alien' minority communities becomes the obvious solution to racialized inequalities in both health and access to health care'* (1996: 565). Thus as Baxter (1997) and Mason (2000) have argued assimilationism remains central to the provision of health care to minority ethnic communities.

CAT derives from 'cultural pluralism' or 'ethnic sensitivity' which, as we saw earlier, forms part of the dominant ideological framework informing the practice of those employed in and around the Health Service. It has also been influential in the professional literature (Culley 1996) so despite the fact that the work of Gerrish *et al* (1996) suggests that it has not improved the standard of care provided to minority ethnic communities, one might expect it to resonate strongly with health workers. This did not seem to be the case.

The HAs annual report referred to a number of cultural awareness training events which had recently been sponsored by local trusts, and it identified that in-service training was being provided by certain trusts in the area. However, such training was only provided on a piece-meal and voluntary basis, and attempts to co-ordinate a programme across the public sector had allegedly failed due to a widespread unwillingness to co-operate (one of the unofficial user representatives had been involved in this attempt, R1). Similarly, Mwasamdube and Mullen (1998) found very little evidence of CAT in the region, characterised by an overall lack of training of any kind, other than equal opportunities training in relation to recruitment and selection procedures.

The fact that CAT does not seem to command much support among white health workers has been identified in the relevant literature (Baxter 1988, 1997;

Culley 1996). Apparently concerns have been expressed about the complicated nature of 'cultural awareness', because the scope of information is too large, acting as a further drain on their time (Baxter 1988; Bowler 1993). Some have even argued (and this will be evidenced below) that it is a form of positive discrimination, singling minority ethnic communities out for 'special' treatment (Baxter 1997). Thus it would seem that any attempt to improve the service for minority ethnic communities, even where efforts marry perfectly with dominant ideological constructs promises resistance.

The notion that the training of health professionals at induction and beyond ought to be informed by structural issues and an introduction to the problematic nature of existing research and ethnic categorisation appears a distant prospect (Bhopal & White 1993; Culley 1996). In fact regardless of the demands made by the local communities about the introduction of CAT and the policy promises of the HA, there is little sign that even this arguably flawed remedy will be delivered. The HAs report and action plan asserts that the contracting process should be used to pressurise recalcitrant providers into action, but if the HA representative *was* truly representative, then there appears to be little real commitment to make good on the promises, in the same way that those made in relation to lingual barriers have arguably been neglected. Consistent with the thread running through each chapter, there are also implications for minority ethnic health workers in promoting CAT, which will lead us directly into the third and final section on ethnic diversity in the workforce.

CAT to the rescue

Consistent with the demands of the local communities several respondents expressed the belief that regular in-service CAT courses for professionals are vital if they hope to deliver a sensitive service to minority ethnic communities. As per the material in Section 1 there was a division between trust employees and user representatives but it was less marked than before.

The trust through the Human Resources Directorate provided a half-day voluntary course on cultural awareness. As will become apparent below, it was not well publicised. The Head of Nursing had only discovered it by chance, but she had sent several of her staff along because she wanted to maximise the limited training opportunities offered by the trust (supporting the findings of Mwasamdube & Mullen 1998). Those selected had returned with good feedback and so she now tried to ensure that every staff member attended the course (R27, p.2, para.3).

Several of those that had heard of the concept or knew something about the course argued that CAT was valuable for a number of reasons, primarily in providing sensitive services:

> ...in fact [the co-ordinator of the link working organisation] has certainly in the past offered, and is very willing to provide again, cultural awareness training which I've taken advantage of. And that hasn't just touched on...That's touched on several cultures, just to raise the awareness really that there are different cultural issues for different groups. One group for example that health visitors are involved with would be the travellers, and yet again there are cultural issues there in terms of washing up. You'd have one bowl for washing up your crockery etc. but it wouldn't be acceptable to wash your clothes in, and there are other...Underwear, you wouldn't hang women's underwear on a washing line if you're a travelling family. That would not be...That would be very inappropriate, and it would be utterly taboo. So there are all sorts of things like that. So we need to have an understanding and awareness so that we don't inadvertently cause offence to people and we can tailor where possible our service to meet client needs (R18, p.3, para.8).

It was also argued that a heightened awareness of cultural differences would make life easier altogether because of the diverse nature of the city and the surrounding area, which was ironic as the perceived absence of diversity was so frequently used to justify inadequate services. Nevertheless, it was argued that a wider understanding of cultural difference could only serve to improve relations both inside and outside the Health Service.

For the most part the user representatives agreed that CAT would be useful but were more specific about its ideal shape and nature. The content, design and targeting of CAT were thought to be crucial. Most unofficial user representatives agreed that training would be useful, and two in particular stressed the need for senior managers to receive such training, largely because they are the ones who formulate policy:

> I think in some ways there are officers who have worked closely with grassroots communities, they understand our needs and frustrations, and I think it's the higher hierarchy... That's right and they actually not in touch with the real people, what I call real people we serve everyday. Those are the people who need the services the most and they are not in touch with them. So a lot of things is not reality. Not realistic. To me people like myself fighting trying to bring it to their awareness and this is why when we have consultation meetings we actually insist that like consultants and senior officers should have cultural training (R4, p.11, para.40).

This was only a matter of emphasis however, as it was stressed quite clearly that every health worker ought to receive regular training, which reflected the demands of the communities during the consultation exercise.

The way in which training should be provided was also considered to be important. One respondent argued that it ought to be organised and delivered by a group of people to ensure that it is wide-ranging and relevant, preventing the danger of creating or sustaining stereotypes:

> But then it has to be a partnership for the cultural awareness training, not just one or two people delivering that training. I think it should be maybe a board of people who actually do that and agree the cultural policy... The policy they kind of put forward. The context really of the whole area, because there are so many differences within communities. I mean some people do this and some people do that. It's trying to present a coherent strategy... My colleague does quite a lot actually of multicultural training. And obviously she's, it needs to be done. But that's what I'm saying, it needs to be done in a certain way. We're not perpetuating stereotypes, such as all Asian women wear Yashmaks and veils, which I certainly don't... It's emphasising the differences that are important. Like in presenting, delivering a service and trying to keep away from the stereo...perpetuating the stereotypes. It is a difficult balance to achieve, but I think it's easier to do if there are more people involved in it (R1, pp.6-7, paras.65 & 69).

She also argued that contrary to current practice CAT ought to be provided not as a casual course to established staff only, but that it should form part of the core professional training of health workers:

> I think you need to start when people are being trained. I mean you can do it when they're in post as well, but it shouldn't really start then. I actually think it starts putting it into practice as soon as they get in (R1, p.6, para.65).

Another respondent who called on her own past experiences as a health professional echoed this, although she would prefer a stronger type of training incorporating anti-discriminatory features with more exposure to minority ethnic communities early on (see Gerrish *et al* 1996; Baxter 1997):

> I'd put the base, because I think a lot of what's happening is discriminatory, because basically black patients, Irish patients, Traveller patients. They are not receiving fair treatment. There's a difference of treatment and difference means they're probably getting less favourable treatment. That in a sense in the way that the Race Relations Act operates could possibly be seen to be breaching section 20 because of less favourable treatment. And I think what's needed is an anti-discriminatory racial equality framework where you're getting cultural racism where people choose not to understand, and I think the way to approach it probably, to a degree, would be through core training. Which means getting medical staff, doctors and nurses etc. and all the other fields who don't have that sort of anti-discriminatory practice based within their core three to five year training. I don't believe that they do...I think it's about valuing and appreciating, understanding the other cultures. I don't think negating anything helps. I mean I wouldn't want...I think what is often the case is in terms of training, when I talk to nursing staff, and I've been a nurse myself. I think I've got a day-to-day practice understanding of what was missing in my training, and looking and hearing from patients and staff, twenty years on, I don't think very much has really changed. That organic change hasn't happened (R5, pp.4-5, paras.8 & 12).

Despite the fact that the law is continually breached (Harding 2005), and that the service cannot claim to be sensitive until such training is provided as a component of professional instruction, she feels there has been little in the way of development in two decades. In short, there is support for the notion, particularly amongst unofficial user representatives, depending on its content, design and where it is directed. This supports the conclusions of Batsleer *et al* (2003) who

176

maintained that where training is provided by minority ethnic-led organisations it should be monitored to ensure that a conservative/traditionalist agenda is not being propagated for religious or political reasons.

Policies and plans

There was some disbelief in the commitment of those training health workers, but there are signs that things are changing locally. As mentioned previously there are plans to increase the recruitment of minority ethnic people into nursing and part of this reform will include raising the issue of 'race' inequalities and adding stronger cultural aspects to basic training. The nurse trainer stressed the importance of this:

> We are very conscious in this department of this problem and I think we are taking active steps to improve the basic nursing curriculum... If you look back over the years and you look at nurse education you could have a nurse perhaps who's been informed about different types of diets. Some of these are found in the literature. It depends on the level, knowing about diets and knowing about religion, religious practices and so on is very mechanical perhaps. Whereas I'm interested in having an integrated understanding of culture, and I think there's a need to move away from, these are the procedures, the policies on diet on religion etc., that we all have a good understanding of living and working in a multicultural society. I think that's quite different from the other approaches that have been used in the past (R20, p.2, paras.4 & 5).

However he did argue that CAT is mechanical and that in the longer term the NHS must undergo a radical cultural change if it is to successfully meet the needs of minority ethnic communities (Donovan 1986b; Baxter 1997). Nurses must learn to respond automatically to the diversity they face in the user community. The framework he envisaged to make this possible will be discussed below.

The HA representative also recognised both the demands of the local communities and their validity:

> What we've got to do is find the people, the workers in places like health care, increasingly you've got to be able to look at the person and think what do I see?

Who am I seeing here? This woman's 80, frail, She's Irish, or she's black, she's
Chinese, what does that mean? If she's Chinese, Chinese elders actually are very
unlikely to have good English – at present. They will have led very, very isolated
lives. And it's that ability that to me is the key... And for all health workers to
have an appreciation that you, that that's how they have to work [seeing people as
individuals]. Now, that does mean that they do perhaps need to know more about
some cultures... And good health workers do try and do it. But it's very patchy.
And what black communities say to you is that we ought to be able to depend on
that fact that every health worker: GP, consultant, nurse, physio will understand
enough about what they don't know about our communities to ask the right
questions, you know? And that's why I keep going back to saying the only
answer to this is for a general increase in the NHS staff's awareness of each
person as an individual. So that when they see an Asian woman sitting on a ward
with cancer, breast cancer, they'll have just enough insight to say to themselves
okay, she's elderly, she's Asian, she's got breast cancer, I can ask so and so for
advice about how elderly people cope with this. But I don't know how she feels
about cancer because she's Asian (R11, pp.3-12, paras.8, 16, 17 & 38).

However despite the recommendations contained in the report and action plan she
did not think that any steps would be taken to implement rigorous training
programmes across the region:

Well we try, that's what the communities say to us. First, the first thing is to get
cultural, some sort of cultural awareness, but to do that across [the region] is
huge... (R11, p.12, paras.40 & 41).

She went on to argue, as she did throughout, that apart from the enormity of the
task in geographical terms, the resources required would be disproportionate to
the level of need (see Smaje 1995 for evidence of similar attitudes in the context
of the NHS). In short, the minority ethnic community in the city was deemed –
once again – to be too small to justify such efforts. Obviously needs are calculated
by head of population rather than on any qualitative measurement. Yet, the
voluntary organisation responsible for improving the socio-economic position of
minority ethnic communities were able and willing to provide such training in-
house or at their own training centre at a reasonable rate (according to its
documentation and its representative, R7).

This argument that resources are too scarce to enable the region-wide adoption of CAT had been filtered down to the communities. The Chinese respondent said:

> They said they're beginning to plan it, they're planning it because of the budget, because of the financial reason and they're planning it. It's in their plan. It's in their business plan, whatever you call it, in their strategy to train people (R4, p.11, para.41).

She felt that resources were not really the problem:

> I mean I myself am a cultural trainer anyway, but they haven't approached me. I did train the nurse and the staff at [a local] clinic on one occasion and I train also staff [for various local agencies]. I have trained other people on cultural training, but if they wanted it they could have got hold of me easily... Apart from that one incident I did it for [the local] clinic, and I haven't any follow-ups. But all this about training the doctors and nurses and consultants and senior staff, well they haven't come anywhere near me... Maybe they are in 3 years plan or 5 years plan, I do not know but as far as I'm concerned it's not enough (R4.12, para.45).

If the Health Service was serious about providing CAT there were plenty of local resources – including her own organisation – which could be called upon to provide effective and inexpensive training. Ultimately she blamed a lack of political will, in other words that the NHS chooses to ignore the need however it is calculated. So whilst nurses in the area may receive CAT as part of their basic training they may not be exposed to it during their everyday working lives.

Resistance is not futile

Despite considerable support for the notion of CAT, resistance was one of the strongest themes during the interview survey. However, the notion of 'resistance' was reported to be fairly irrelevant for community-based staff. The very nature of their work, so it was argued, predisposed them towards taking some kind of interest in cultural differences and their implications for health and health care. One of the unofficial user representatives said:

Well I think so yeah. I think what's been done so far [here] they are, that they're very much keen to learn more about and keen to get involved, at least some of them want to learn Asian languages, that's from the majority not the minority community in [the city]. So there is, there are obviously some who wouldn't do that, but the majority I think would want to do as much as they can... We have a number of health visitors who are very keen to learn, for example, Punjabi. Obviously it's not easy to learn but actually the motivation is there to actually help the women that they see. You know they want to be able to understand the women, it's not just that they're going in there just delivering a service, and couldn't care less whether they're understood or not. So they are actually trying to do that. They're trying to do the job the best way they can, and they're trying to involve communities as well (R1, pp8-19, paras.73 & 164).

A health visitor based in the inner city supported this:

People [would] put themselves forward, but very often, more so in this area because it more abuts onto the inner-city and we have a wider cultural and ethnic mix [than in other areas]. People have a raised awareness because this is the people we're working with and so people do actually put themselves forward and say look, I really need some information in order to understand and help this particular group of people I'm trying to do some work with... I certainly haven't been aware of any reluctance for people to actually attend that sort of thing... And you need to understand where people are coming from because if you don't know where people are coming from then you're not going to be able to help them, whatever it is that they need (R18, pp.3-4, paras.9-11).

For health workers based in and around the inner city performing work in the communities in question CAT was seen as vital and there was little resistance. It was seen as part of the job, reflecting the findings of Gerrish *et al* (1996).

However, hospital-based staff were often unaware of the concept, and were certainly ignorant about the availability of the training provided by their employers (despite the eagerness of the Head of Nursing to send as many staff members as possible this included several of her own senior staff). Where they were aware, or made aware, of CAT for the purposes of the research, there was a high level of resistance to it mainly because of the associated implications.

On the one hand, consistent with the material set out in the first section, there was the widespread belief that it was not necessary because current service provision was adequate.

> There are, there are some, but, because it isn't a major issue, or it doesn't appear to be a major issue then I don't think there's many people actually go on that sort of training (R15, p.2, para.7).

A similar attitude was reported amongst GPs in the area. Indeed one respondent argued that when she had tried to organise specific training for health visitors, the move had been blocked:

> A lot of GPs once they're fund-holders they can govern who they employ, they govern what training their staff go on... And when for example we put on training for certain primary health care professionals who work in the community the GPs were saying, No I don't want you to go on that, but the professionals wanted to, because they wanted to learn for their own professional and personal development. And they were told, No you will not go on it, because that isn't an area that affects us. That does not affect us...but it does affect them because the service that they're providing is not a good service is it? So essentially that's rubbish (R6. p15, para.49).

The resistance was based on the notion amongst certain (mainly white) health professionals that the service they provide is already adequate, despite the substantial evidence to the contrary, and, the associated belief that certain needs are illegitimate and therefore should not be met anyway.

CAT also provoked a certain amount of defensiveness, possibly linked once again to the aftermath of the Macpherson Report. Many of the trust employees felt that it was an implicit suggestion that they discriminate against minority ethnic communities. The representative of the HA explained this reaction with reference to past experience:

> There have been bad experiences with training in cultural awareness in the past, when it was very PC stuff. And there was trend in the NHS training anyway, for certain trainers to come in and just berate people for being racist, and tell them

that until they acknowledge their own racism they won't get rid of it. Well that was a complete turn-off... Because racist is such a term of abuse and NHS staff can't cope with seeing themselves in that context... They are caring people. I mean they do a hell of a lot... To be called a racist without further explanation of why. Inevitably we're all racist. I mean black people are racist in certain aspects of the way that they...'cos they don't understand some of where we come from. It's very hard. So there's an awful lot of resistance to it (R11, p.13, paras.42-45).

This simply means that the training provided was not truly about raising awareness of cultural diversity. It would appear that the programme was confused with anti-racist training or had been deliberately hi-jacked for this purpose (Blakemore & Drake 1996). The object of such training is to underline 'racial' inequalities and where necessary to address white perceptions of different cultures and the consequences of those inequalities (Baxter 1988, 1997).

One of the major criticisms about CAT of course – as set out earlier – is that it does not challenge racism. The representative of the REC emphasised this:

All they have is like cultural awareness, which doesn't address those issues about racism (R5, p.5, para.16).

In her view there ought to be an anti-discriminatory aspect to such training anyway, and the disability co-ordinator of the trust agreed. This would certainly fit with the findings of Jay (1992), who discovered that where such training was being carried out across the south west, it often did have a more political feel than traditional pluralistic courses. The disability co-ordinator went on to argue that this would be difficult to implement, due to the insecurity detected by the representative of the HA:

So they either don't think it's a problem, people haven't actually thought about it enough to actually recognise that they do discriminate. They don't realise or they ridicule it. Maybe for all of us it's actually quite painful because we have to confront something in ourselves which perhaps we don't like. I'd hate to think that I'd discriminated but I'm sure I do. I would like to think I don't, racism appals me but I've been brought up in this country, through British institutions, there may be bits there that I'm trying to work out, but it's actually quite a painful process. Certainly having gone through equal opportunities training, that was a painful process. It says a lot. I have to learn a lot about me (R24, p.19, para.78).

However, in her view the insecurities need to be challenged because, as the HA representative accepts, racism is a very real problem. Although minority ethnic people can be racist in their attitudes they often do not have the power to inflict significant damage on the white majority. So whilst CAT is resisted because of its perceived links with anti-racist training, the irony is that the latter, already tried in various places including the research area, might be a better alternative under the circumstances (Baxter 1997).

Another related site of resistance appeared in the idea that CAT would be divisive. On top of the hostile political climate created by the MacPherson Report in which white professionals are perceived by definition to be racist, the majority of the trust employees felt that such training was contrary to the underlying ethic of British society (grounded in individualism) and outside the core business of the NHS:

It's almost the case that on an individual basis, because it's very difficult, though of course it's very easy to generalise, but you can pick any group at all, you know there's a whole range there, and so you can't say because someone comes from the East of Poland then therefore we need to do this that or the other. It is the case that as part of our training we have psychological training as much as anything else, and so it's a case of trying to sense and encourage people to say what they're feeling etc. Because before each investigation we always say what we want to do and what the patient will be expected to do, and you usually find from their reaction just how they feel about that... The difficulty we have is that any patient that comes through the door presents in different ways, if they've got a problem, some people just clam up and say nothing, other people can become aggressive, and, again, as part of our training, we look into that and try not to react as patients react. If they're quiet we try to coax them, if they're aggressive we try to calm them because there's no point in two people shouting at each other, it gets us nowhere, it breaks down totally (R15, pp.3-5, paras.11 & 14).

Yes I think so, I think they have to be careful that we don't make it absolutely a thing on its own. I mean I said to [the co-ordinator] when I was on the sub-group, I'd like to revisit the ethics for all nurses, because they were obviously going to do it from a nursing point of view, and looking at treating disabled people as well as the ethnic minorities. But treating everybody as individuals, and not specifically to pick out things (R13, p.6, para.18).

Indeed the latter respondent argued that CAT could be seen as a form of positive discrimination (discussed as a theoretical concept in all its applicability and complexity in chapter 8):

> Absolutely, absolutely [CAT can be seen as positive discrimination], and I think we have lost a little bit of treating people as individuals because of the turnover now in hospitals is so fast, you are absolutely working very, very busily, and perhaps to get back to actually saying these are patients, treating them individually is no bad thing. So that might be a way forward by doing that (R13, p.6, para.19).

The implication here is that patients ought to be treated as individuals and to provide training for health workers on cultural diversity would be to unfairly advantage minority ethnic communities. That would not be consistent with the core business of the NHS as perceived by the majority of health workers and managers.

This would make some sense in light of the widespread belief that the service is perfectly adequate. However, the adequacy of local health provision is contested and the idea that people should be treated first and foremost as individuals is not reflected in the 'non-attendance' policy administered by this respondent, because individual needs are addressed according to ethnicity. If a white person requests a white health worker, however irrational such a request might be, they are humoured. Should a minority ethnic individual request someone from a similar ethnic background they are not dealt with equally, so, group identity rather than individual need determines policy.

According to the disability co-ordinator equal opportunities more widely, because it is seen to be a group-based, slightly communistic entity, is neglected due to a similar reference to the core business:

> What we've found while I've been working through disability equality issues is that we've had, and if I can just use this example, we've had an access working group on disability access improvements, and we've actually achieved quite a lot of improvements. And one of the things we want to do is try to get staff on disability equality training courses. But we're very aware that although we've been beavering away and we can do a certain amount 'cos we're grass roots and know what the actual practical issues are, unless you've actually got an organisation in which there is senior management commitment to it, how are we ever going to get staff released to go on disability equality training? Unless from the top people are saying that this is important. We'll go. Because people say disability equality, what's that all about? Equal opportunities? No I've got to go and get my updates on this that and the other, I've got to do, I only go on important training. They won't go. We don't have the power to release staff to go (R24, p.16, para.67).

Health is the main preserve of the NHS and there is no time or space for such superfluity; despite the fact that equality of opportunity has far-reaching implications for the successful provision of care. But one of the unofficial user representatives, consistent with the material in chapter 3, argued that it was much deeper even than this and specific to the notion of CAT, she said:

> You're in a Westernised country...The statement has been made that, well if you come to a Westernised country, well then you should be Westernised. But culture, again, we have to know people's culture... It's good to learn about other cultures, but it's like you have to really make them know how important it is, and why it is so important (R3, P.4).

In other words, although the possible failure of services is denied, implicit is the idea that cultural gaps are a problem for the communities not the Health Service. Adopt the culture to which the NHS is designed to respond and things will be fine. Certainly the central point to underline is that problems of this type are perceived not to be the responsibility of the Health Service (see Carter 2000 for a similar analysis).

Whose responsibility?

In the previous chapter one of the ways in which the inadequacy of language provision was addressed was to allow minority ethnic communities to take responsibility for ameliorating or solving any problems. Either patients were expected to bring interpreters of their own, or, minority ethnic health workers were expected to provide *ad hoc* translation – without recognition or reward. In terms of dealing with cultural insensitivities the same process appeared to be in operation.

In a legitimate sense it was argued that minority ethnic people ought to provide CAT as a matter of principle (Jay 1992):

> And it's a very touchy area, and good trainers are very hard to come by, because they should be from a minority ethnic culture (R18, p.12, paras.40 & 41).

In Robbinston this had certainly been the case. The Chinese representative had provided some training in the past so too had the co-ordinator of the link working service. What is more, the link workers themselves continued to provide such training (further evidence of their extended remit),

> Oh I think so yeah, oh goodness me, definitely, particularly with the Asian women who don't speak English. I would say that they've made a huge difference without a doubt. And I know that they do sort of like the Asian cultural awareness days (R6, p.24, para.77).

This would appear to be legitimate because it sits easily with the legal concept of genuine occupational qualifications. Under the Race Relations Act 1976, Section 5., certain types of employment are thought to be performed better by people from particular ethnic backgrounds. This is usually justified on such grounds as cultural competence or authenticity, i.e. Indian waiters for 'authentic' Indian restaurants. Who better to provide tuition on cultural matters than those who are able to bridge the divide? In other words, those who understand something about the culture of the NHS *and* minority ethnic cultures.

However, there is also a sense in which minority ethnic people are being asked to solve the problems of the NHS in a much less legitimate fashion. For example, one respondent said,

> What happened was the training school rang me and said...can you put on some training on the African-Caribbean culture? And I said well because you're black. And I said, yes, but what do I know about African-Caribbean culture? I was born in this country and for me I don't know, I didn't know what a Caucasian saw, I didn't know what they wanted. So I felt it was very difficult for me to say, Oh yes I will put on this training day. So I refused to do it. They found someone else to do it, someone who works in the community (R6, p.2, para.7).

So the fact that she was black was qualification enough, in the eyes of her employers, to provide CAT. There is evidence to suggest that health providers are encouraged to use their employees in this fashion (Henley 1991: 77). This was not the only way in which the respondent was expected to deal with minority ethnic problems in an unofficial capacity, as we shall see below.

Minority ethnic health workers are also expected to deal with cultural issues on a less formalised basis in the course of their day-to-day employment. As mentioned in the previous chapter, Bagilhole and Stephens (1997) found that minority ethnic health workers were called upon to provide informal interpreting services, but they also found evidence of the same workers being asked to dispense cultural advice to their white colleagues. Although there was no significant evidence to suggest that this was the case in the trust, it was more than a strong possibility.

In 1993 the NHSME recommended that '...*managers and staff should view cultural differences positively, as a rich source of ideas and responses*' (1993: 11). However it seems that this also has been ignored and some minority ethnic employees are being exploited. A ward Sister - in response to the question, do you think CAT would be useful? - replied,

> I think because [the city's] quite an ethnic area, it probably would be useful. And obviously we do have one person who is from the ethnic race working in the department (R25, p.2, para.12).

When pressed on the connection between CAT and the presence of a minority ethnic health worker she denied that the worker in question provided *ad hoc* cultural advice. She later confirmed my original interpretation by arguing that it would be an idea to organise minority ethnic health professionals into an informal support network that their white colleagues could draw upon:

> Yes definitely. I think if there is a support network in the hospital where people could go for advice, dealing with issues if they're really not sure about any background knowledge of an Asian's particular way of doing things or about their religion, then I think it would be beneficial to be supportive to those people (R25, p.5, para.39).

As per the language barriers identified earlier, it is, it would seem, down to minority ethnic communities to some extent, to either provide training, or, to dispense the everyday advice to their white colleagues which would make this unnecessary.

It may well be that this type of arrangement will become part of the accepted duties of minority ethnic professionals in future. The HA representative expressed doubts about the use of CAT, as we have already seen, but she also directly connected the recruitment of minority ethnic health professionals with this issue:

> The other thing is about getting more black and ethnic minority staff into the NHS, and that's not so they can act as interpreters and that's not so they can act as advocates. It's so they gradually...that bit of yeast will percolate through the loaf. That when people work day-by-day with somebody who begins to talk openly about their family life or their religious, their thoughts about religion and why they have different attitudes. That subtly informs how everyone works (R11, p.13, para.45).

She denied that they will act directly in this capacity, but that their very presence will improve the quality and sensitivity of services. This connection was also drawn by the nurse trainer (whose responsibility it is to increase the representation of minority ethnic students on nursing programmes locally). He argued that CAT might be good in a limited, mechanical sense but in itself it will not be enough,

> I think they need to be more aware than just having training I think, just training of staff will not do it by itself I think. In the end I think certainly the training with and the more exposure to minority ethnic clients but also to staff, I see those two things going hand-in-hand in supporting development. I think that just having more nurses from minority ethnic groups will make other staff more aware that they need to be more sensitive. That will work I think and make people realise that they need to be much more aware and sensitive (R20, para.25).

So the issue of training and recruiting more minority ethnic staff into the NHS are clearly connected, as suggested by Gerrish *et al* (1996) and Iganksi *et al* (1998). Yet, it is difficult to articulate in concrete terms just what the connection is, unless we accept that they will be given at least some responsibility for sensitising services. This might mean offering advice to their white colleagues, but is just as likely to encourage the latter to wash their hands of these problems and to allow minority ethnic professionals to deal with what are perceived to be community problems. This already happens but will gather speed and legitimacy as those responsible for training and implementing policy and for training and primary recruitment offer their endorsement.

Conclusion

Training must, as Baxter (1997) maintains, be an important ingredient in any coherent challenge to 'race' inequalities in health and health care. However, it seems unlikely, particularly in light of later research (Iganski *et al* 1998, 2001) that the anti-racist curriculum she proposes (building on the work of Larbie *et al* 1988, see also Parekh 2000: 75) will gain much ground in the present climate. Whether the nurse education centre in Robbinston will develop (or has developed in the intervening period) its teaching practices and policies along these lines is unknown. In terms of in-service training the principal means of addressing cultural gaps between professionals and patients from different ethnic backgrounds remains the notion of CAT (Hiscock 2004). Despite severe doubts about its potential to achieve radical reform, due to its founding assumption that problems are based in individual ignorance, and that it implicitly equates difference as deviance, it was one of the key demands of the local communities and one of the subsequent policy promises made by the HA.

There was substantial support for the notion amongst the interview respondents, particularly the unofficial user representatives, who had very definite ideas about how it should be organised and delivered. The Head of Nursing had only found out about the trust's own course by accident and had since tried to get as many of her staff along as possible. Unfortunately she still had some way to go, and there was a distinct lack of awareness amongst the trust's staff about the availability of CAT.

It was widely felt that CAT would be most useful for community-based staff simply by virtue of their work, although it was argued that it would provide all staff members with valuable life skills in the context of a diverse society. Nevertheless resistance was an important theme which emerged and there was evidence of some resistance to the notion amongst hospital staff. Several expressed fears that it would lead to greater hostility and division, and one respondent actually argued that CAT could be viewed as a form of positive discrimination. This has an incredibly ironic twist, because on the understanding that services fail to meet the needs of minority ethnic communities, she is arguing that any attempt to address such failure constitutes positive discrimination. The problem of course is that many do not on the whole accept that the service fails because they regard people as individuals first and foremost, until that becomes unsustainable or inconvenient – i.e. in allocating caring responsibilities for minority ethnic patients to minority ethnic professionals.

As in the previous chapter, we concluded with the idea that the ideal solution appears to be to allow minority ethnic communities to deal with their own problems. This may be due to the idea that the problems are theirs because they refuse to assimilate, and this was recognised by one user representative in particular in relation to the resistance of white employees to CAT.

Where the failings are due to cultural insensitivity the burden has fallen onto the shoulders of minority ethnic health professionals. Although white staff members denied that minority ethnic health professionals were being used in this way, the consistency of the evidence, supported in the literature (Baxter 1988, 1997; Bagilhole & Stephens 1997, 1998, 1999) suggests otherwise. This may actually prevent the development of greater cultural awareness and competence amongst health workers regardless of their ethnicity (Gerrish *et al* 1996; Kandola & Fullerton 1998). Furthermore, it may become accepted practice in the future, for despite vigorous refutations, those responsible for primary recruitment (of nurses) locally, and for implementing health policy, appear to endorse such a development.

It is, it would seem, time to address the appropriate role of minority ethnic health workers, and to consider the possible impact of greater ethnic diversity in the workforce in this context. One demand of the community expressed during the consultation exercise that we have not discussed thus far, though it formed a central concern for the HA, involved the diversification of the workforce as a means of improving services to minority ethnic communities. Stubbs (1993: 39) relates this very nicely to the proposed activity in Robbinston:

> ...in terms of service delivery, there has been much greater attention to link-workers and interpreters, usually low-paid casualized, and exploited, rather than to issues concerning the role of black workers at senior levels of the medical and health professions. Skills such as community languages (a euphemism for undervalued, non-European languages) and 'cultural awareness' are not seen as prerequisites for the recruitment of medical students, GPs, consultants, or administrators.

The assumption here is that with greater ethnic diversity in the workforce and the sensible employment of that diversity services would automatically improve. The third and final section of the book examines this assumption in greater detail, and in particular three important questions. What does ethnic diversity mean? How will it work? And how can it best be achieved?

SECTION THREE:

Ethnic diversity in the NHS

CHAPTER 7:

The meaning of ethnic diversity

'It's just like when you've got some coffee that's too black, which means that it's too strong. What do you do? You integrate it with cream, you make it weak' – Malcolm X.

Introduction

Although the NHS has been ethnically diverse for the bulk of the post-war period the role of minority ethnic workers has been neither fully recognised nor fairly rewarded (Bagilhole & Stephens 1999). As we have seen from previous chapters much is expected of individuals from different communities in both a formal and informal capacity (Thompson 1998). However, there is a formal development in equal opportunities theory which actively links ethnic diversity with improved services and other societal benefits (Bagilhole 1997).

While the trust employees in particular rejected the notion of numerical representation as arbitrary and potentially ineffective there was a consensus amongst the interview respondents that ethnic diversity has numerous benefits for employers and communities alike. This was also reflected by the views of the mail respondents (Human Resource Directors and personnel professionals).

Asked to define and operationalise ethnic diversity, the bulk of the interview respondents moved through various interpretations, from a proportional interpretation, through a structural definition (in which the diversification of managerial positions is emphasised), to rest finally on a model in which minority ethnic individuals are charged with actively representing the needs of their communities (Baxter 1988). This reflects the dominant theme of the research, i.e. the perception that minority ethnic communities must deal with the problems 'their' (deviant) cultures and unreasonable expectations create. As discussed below this may not work, and even if it could, it may prove counterproductive in the longer term.

Background

According to Collier (1998) there has been a disproportionate emphasis on equal opportunities in relation to employment opportunities and policies and too little attention given to equal opportunities in the provision of services. Without unfairly simplifying the basis of her argument it does overlook to some extent the clear connection that has latterly been drawn between employment and service issues (Iganski *et al* 2001). For example, Baxter argues that:

> The two roles [NHS as employer and service provider] are often seen as unrelated. It is as if the nature and standards of health care provided could be divorced from the personnel policies and conditions of employment within which health workers deliver their care (1988: 6).

This same connection was made by the local communities during the consultation carried out by the HA. One of the principal demands alongside better interpreting and cultural provision was greater ethnic diversity in the local NHS workforce. Although no explicit reason was provided for this in the report and action plan we will consider some of the many possibilities in a moment. First we need to consider the issue of ethnic diversity in the post-war period.

As Ward (1993) suggests, the Health Service as one of the biggest employers in Europe has also employed more minority ethnic workers than any other organisation in Britain (see also Doyal *et al* 1981). This remains the case today: although minority ethnic communities accounted for 7.9% of the total population according to the 2001 Census (http://www.statistics.gov.uk/cci/nugget.asp?id=273), collectively they make up 8.4% of the nursing staff of the UK and 28% of clinicians (Stephens 2001: 23; Parekh 2000; Hutton 2003), although recent evidence suggests that 'Asian' groups are actually under-represented in nursing, certainly amongst those applying for and being admitted to Nurse Education Centres (Iganski *et al* 1998, 2001). Nevertheless, the NHS has officially been held up as an example for other public sector employers to follow in terms of ethnic diversity (Straw 1999).

Yet as diversity *per se* has never been a problem, authors such as Law (1996) have argued, consistent with the findings set out in Sections 1 & 2, that *'The NHS provides the strongest case to refute the common argument that opening up an institution to black minority ethnic staff inevitably leads to organisational change in favour of black minority ethnic clients, users, customers, or in this case patients'* (Law 1996: 151-2); Ward (1993) points out that the most insensitive areas of provision for minority ethnic communities have also been the areas in which minority ethnic health workers are disproportionately represented – i.e. psychiatry. Diversity has been used as a defence against challenges to inappropriate services and racism.

There is obviously a serious point here about the practical value of ethnic diversity which needs to be recognised. The location of minority ethnic representation is also important. For example, although minority ethnic groups account for 9.3% of nursing and 28% of clinical staff, around 4% of Nursing Directors are from minority ethnic groups and they make up just 16% of consultants (Stephens 2001; Hutton 2003). This reflects a consistent historical trend in NHS employment.

Several reports and research studies have underlined the fact that minority ethnic individuals are in positions that do not match their abilities and that they have not been adequately recognised or rewarded (Brent CHC 1981; CRE 1983; Anwar & Ali 1987; Baxter 1988; Admani 1993a; Law 1996). They are disproportionately to be found in ancillary and nursing auxiliary grades etc. (Bhavani 1994; Owen 1994) and are barely to be found in middle and senior management (King's Fund 1989; Jewson *et al* 1993; NAHAT and King's Fund Centre 1993; NHSME 1993; Beishon *et al* 1995; Aanchawan 1996; NAHAT 1996/97; Mason 2000; Hiscock 2004). At present only 1% of chief executives are from minority ethnic communities and 3% of executive directors (Hutton 2003).

There is also evidence of significant over-representation in the least attractive specialities – i.e. geriatrics, psychiatry etc. (Ward 1993; Gerrish *et al* 1996) – and in the least prestigious community settings and hospitals (King's Fund 1990). Minority ethnic individuals are also to be disproportionately found on night shifts (Bryan *et al* 1985; Baxter 1988; Cohen 1995a). These patterns were confirmed by the King's Fund in a major report on the plight of minority ethnic workers throughout the NHS (King's Fund 2001; Carvel 2001).

Although discrimination is not entirely responsible for this, it is considered to be centrally important (McNaught 1987, 1988; Baxter 1988; Ward 1993; Gerrish *et al* 1996; Mason 2000). A substantial body of evidence suggests that discrimination occurs at every stage in the employment process, from initial entry, to deployment and promotion, even in the processing of complaints and the distribution of professionals awards (see Smith 1980; Smith 1987; CRE 1988, 1991; McKeigue 1990; Esmail & Everington 1993; Dillner 1995; McManus *et al* 1995; Godlee 1996; Chaudhary 1998; Iganski *et al* 1998; McManus 1998; Alexander 1999; Carter 2000; King's Fund 2001). Nor has there been any real attempt to address and deal with discrimination (Mason 2000, see chapter 3).

It is within this context of stunted careers and aspirations, compounded by the often unchecked racial harassment carried out by white colleagues and patients alike (Baxter 1988; Beishon *et al* 1995; Gerrish *et al* 1996) that Baxter issued her early warning about the 'black' nurse as an endangered species. Minority ethnic numbers continue to decline as existing staff age and are not replaced (reputedly many are either deterred by the experiences of their predecessors or are actively discouraged by them) (Baxter 1988; Brindle 1997a; Carter 2000; King's Fund 2001). As the NHS is experiencing a major labour shortage generally (Browne

2001; Carvel 2001; McGuaran 2001), evidenced by the priorities established in the *NHS Plan*, this trend is even more problematic (Ward 1993).

As Baxter (1988) has pointed out, it is not merely to solve a staffing crisis that ethnic diversity is required there are allegedly many practical benefits (see chapter 9 for a fuller discussion). Historically these assumptions about the practical benefits emerged from the United States and particularly the higher education system (Dworkin 1981) with the initial momentum provided by the Bakke case in 1978[1] (Nickel 1990; Edmonds 1994). Aside from the loss of staff and the associated waste of talent, low morale will undoubtedly impact upon the productivity and effectiveness of those who remain (DoH 2003b). Furthermore, greater ethnic diversity could have real implications for the sensitivity of the services provided, a diverse workforce is more likely to understand and react appropriately to diverse needs (Anionwu 1996; Gerrish *et al* 1996; DoH 2003b; Weston & Walsh 2003). Baxter (1997: 96) argues that a diverse workforce can improve institutional/communal relations and identify gaps in service provision *'...in a way that is impossible for any white person to do'*. There may even be negative implications for wider 'race relations' if diversity is not actively pursued.

In actuality the Health Service has recognised the value of ethnic diversity since the 1970s, targeting the membership of HAs in particular. Smaje (1995) argues that this and related measures such as the employment of ethnic advisers at the local level and the establishment of the Ethnic Health Unit were 'pluralist' in tone and assimilationist in intention. He also makes reference to the NAHA report *Action Not Words*, which maintained that:

> An effective way of making Health Services responsive to the needs of a multi-racial and multi-cultural population is to ensure that members of minority ethnic

---

[1] Alan Bakke applied for admission to the Medical School at the University of California but was refused because a quota system was in place reserving 16 out of 100 places for minority ethnic students. The Supreme Court ruled that although quotas were unconstitutional, ethnicity could be used as one aspect in the admissions process. Justice Powell said: *'The diversity that furthers a compelling state interest encompasses a far broader array of qualifications and characteristics of which racial or ethnic origin is but a single though important element'* (Nickel 1990: 54).

200

groups are employed at all levels in the Health Service and thus involved automatically in the planning, management and delivery of those services (1988: 10).

Similar proposals were made in the report of a 1987 management seminar on the health needs of minority ethnic communities, during which Tony Newton (then Minister for Health) claimed: '...*an NHS where there is a better ethnic mix across the hierarchy will be better equipped to identify and remove obstacles to equal access*' (DHSS 1988: 2, my emphasis).

This was also a key theme in the subsequent action programme on minority ethnic staff launched in 1993 (see Alexander 1999: 7). The benefits of a diverse workforce have been recognised in a number of policy arenas, from policing (Etzioni 1997), through the criminal justice system (Rose 1997) and the military (Joyce 1997), to the business sector (Ross & Schneider 1992; Pandya 1997). In the context of the latter a business case for diversity has emerged emphasising the pragmatic rather than moral justifications for engaging in equal opportunities activities (Torkington 1991; Jewson & Mason 1993; CRE 1995a; Hiscock 2004), and this has been supplemented by the CRE with a quality case for the public sector (1995b; see also Thompson 1998: 196).

To be effective it has been argued that it is at the higher and highest levels that diversity must be achieved (Baxter 1988, 1997; Johnson 1993; Smaje 1995; Dreachslin *et al* 2004). In discussing the under-representation of minority ethnic groups on Health Service boards, Mason (2000: 203) said that:

It is difficult...to see how these functions can be effectively and credibly discharged unless members are drawn from a broad cross section of the population served. The presence of minority ethnic members would seem to be a key element in the successful placing of ethnically different needs on the local health agenda.

Similarly, Bagilhole has argued that *'The lack of ethnic minority staff in decision making and powerful positions in the NHS has important consequences for the type of service provided'* (1997: 152). The government shares this emphasis, evidenced by the Prime Minister's first speech to the Labour Party conference after their 1997-election victory:

> We cannot be a beacon to the world unless the talents of all the people shine through. Not one black high court judge; not one black Chief Constable or permanent secretary; not one black army officer above the rank of colonel. Not one Asian either. Not a record of pride for the British establishment. And not a record of pride for Parliament that there are so few black and Asian MPs (Travis & Rowan 1997: 17).

Furthermore, the recommendations of the MacPherson Report (1999) lent added moral and practical weight to the pursuit of ethnic diversity. Although there has been some progress in terms of diversifying senior and managerial levels of the NHS, as evidenced by Alexander (1999), there remains much to do (Parekh 2000).

These arguments have certainly been widely disseminated not least through the operational management structures of the NHS (Iganski *et al* 1998). It would be wrong to dismiss the importance of ethnic diversity *per se*. However, as will become clear the practical value of *ethnic* diversity has not really been satisfactorily identified (Iganski & Johns 1998). For example, diversity forms a major theme throughout the Parekh Report (2000), in chapter 13 it is argued that *'Black, Asian and Irish representation could help to ensure that the impact of racism on health is properly researched and recognised and appropriate action taken'* (2000: 181).This suggestion is quickly qualified thus, *'This is not...to say that the burden of race equality action should fall on black, Asian and Irish people, but rather to affirm the crucial importance of direct experience'* (Parekh 2000: 181).

Unfortunately, as much of the relevant literature confirms, supported by the previous chapters, the burden has and does rest on the shoulders of minority ethnic individuals. Furthermore, this will continue unless the assumptions set out here are supported by a rigorous debate and convincing evidence. Ethnic diversity incautiously invoked may further illustrate the 'otherness' of minority ethnic communities and further underline 'their' responsibility for solving 'their' own problems. The central function of this chapter is to provide an insight into popular perceptions of ethnic diversity and its value.

Diversity and representation

One of the key concepts in any discussion of 'diversity' whichever groups are involved is numerical representation, and it is not an entirely clear-cut issue. As Bagilhole (1997) suggests it depends very much on the local area, and the availability of suitable individuals (see also Edwards 1995). In terms of the interview survey the question of representation in the local NHS produced some very interesting contrasts. The overwhelming response from the user representatives both official and unofficial was that minority ethnic groups were under-represented in the local workforce. Reflecting the demands of the local community the representative of the HA said:

> The other thing is about getting more black and minority ethnic staff into the NHS (R11, pp.1 & 13, paras.2 & 45).

There was, however, some qualification of this in relation to horizontal and vertical considerations. The problem was thought to be more extreme in certain areas and at certain levels:

> ...also the issue of - which has been raised and brought to our attention again through public meetings - employment in the NHS. How when people from the black and other minority ethnic communities are in the NHS they tend to be at the lower levels for want of a better phrase. They don't seem to be able to progress in terms of the proportion in the NHS, in relation to the community isn't right. I mean it's lower in the NHS at higher levels (R12, pp.1-2, para.2).

Among the user representatives the HA representative was alone in thinking that things were slowly improving, particularly in relation to the boards of local trusts. One other respondent accepted that boards had changed but only with regards to non-executive positions (Smaje 1995) and even the representative of the HA accepted their limited potential.

In relation to the trust employees opinions were divided. Several accepted that *their* organisation did not reflect the diversity of the surrounding area:

> No, I would say from my own experience that there's not a large, I don't come across a large population of ethnic minorities within the trust, no...I wouldn't say that I'd come across them at any level. I'm just trying to think. I wouldn't say they're very evident...That's based on my general perception of my day-to-day visiting of the hospital, I wouldn't say that I see large proportions of ethnic minorities in the domestic side, certainly not in the management side, on the wards, the nursing side. Not on the wards no... I mean for example I don't think I ever remember seeing a Sikh with a turban on, just as a minor example (R26, pp.2 & 3, paras.12-16 & 18).

In sympathy with the views expressed above, where under-representation was identified it was seen as a feature of certain areas and levels:

> I think they're well represented in certain groups of the trust's workforce, but I wouldn't say that they are as a whole. I certainly don't think they are in management grades. I certainly don't think they are in professions allied to medicine, like all the paramedical type services. But they probably are in the sort of nursing and ancillary staff groups. There is certainly a high percentage in the sort of ancillary staff groups (R17, p.1, para.1).

A similar number thought that the trust was broadly representative of the local area:

> My perception is that the hospital does represent the community, but that's more by luck than judgement. We don't particularly go out to say well we must get our numbers up. I think it's just kind of happened (R28, p.6, para.21).

> There's no barrier obviously we have got people from minority ethnic groups in senior posts but not, not the same proportion as in the population as a whole (R31, pp.1 & 2, paras.1, 2 & 13).

204

There was some residual concern about the numbers of minority ethnic individuals at the higher and highest levels but it was assumed that natural evolution would rectify this.

Representation *per se* is a highly problematic concept. As both Flew (1986) and Sowell (1994) argue, it assumes that interests, skills and abilities are randomly distributed and that were discrimination to be eradicated a near perfect representation of groups in all areas and at all levels would result. This may not be the case. Can discrimination be blamed for the preponderance of African-Americans in professional basketball or Jewish intellectuals among Nobel Prize winners? Sowell argues that this explanation is related to biological racism because both have dogmatic views about under-representation, due either to genetic inferiority or discrimination. They ignore human agency and societal complexity.

Whether such arguments influenced the respondents is difficult to establish, but there was certainly a consensus amongst the trust employees about the arbitrary nature of numerical representation,

> I wouldn't have thought so there are ethnic minorities as there are everywhere. But I'm not sure what the level has to be, or what is seen as a reasonable level. I mean there are quite a number but whether it's the right amount? Or if it's too low or too high, I'm not sure... ...and in fact we do have a number of what you might call minority representatives at the higher levels here, again, as I say whether it's the right number or not I don't know (R15, pp.7 & 12, paras.22 & 35).

Who has the responsibility to determine adequate or inadequate levels of representation? For the majority of these respondents this was an impossible question to answer. One person was concerned that the very notion implied failure on the part of the trust:

> You could say that it's under-represented, but if you look at who's applying then maybe it's a fair representation...It's just one of those that it could look unfairly represented, but I don't know without knowing facts and figures of who actually applies for jobs and things. It might be proportionate to the number of people that apply, with the number of people who get jobs (R19, p.1, paras.3 & 4).

She immediately linked the notion of representation with blame - that the trust might be failing. In her view it might simply relate to the preference of minority ethnic individuals to work elsewhere.

So while the user representatives were convinced that minority ethnic communities are under-represented in the local Health Service, the trust employees were divided on the issue. They did agree on one thing, that the notion of representation is problematic. So if ethnic diversity is to be more than a numerical question, there needs to be some discussion about its practical benefits. Despite divisions on the concept of numerical representation, there was a virtual consensus from all of the respondents about the multi-dimensional value of ethnic diversity.

Benefits of ethnic diversity

The benefits of ethnic diversity for individuals, organisations and for society have been rehearsed since the early 1970s at least. One of the earliest claims was that it was simply a matter of justice, it *'...should decrease the difference in wealth and power that now exists between different racial groups, and so make the community more equal overall'* (Dworkin 1981: 229). Thinking about diversity has moved on and justice appeals are thought to be insufficiently persuasive in the context of a capitalist labour market. Actual benefits for the organisation and the service population must be evidenced (Ross & Schneider 1992; Schneider & Ross 2002).

In fact some evidence exists that increasing workforce diversity can be *detrimental* to firms and organisations. It can generate conflict and lead to breakdowns in communication, increasing both employee dissatisfaction and staff turnover (Jain & Verma 1996: 28). Ethnic diversity may be most unworkable, due to racism and incongruent communication styles (Fine 1995; Kandola & Fullerton 1998). This was certainly the interpretation of the ward managers who participated in Carter's (2000) study. They worked hard to achieve homogeneity in ward teams. However, the mail and interview respondents were largely enthusiastic about ethnic diversity, rehearsing many of the benefits identified in the relevant literature.

For instance, one suggestion, a utilitarian argument, has been that greater ethnic diversity would reduce social tensions (Dworkin 1981; Baxter 1988; NAHAT 1996/97). The mail respondents were not entirely clear about the value of diversity in this respect, see Chart 1.

Chart 1
Diversity would ease social tensions

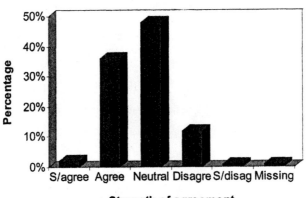

Faced with the statement: *'Diversifying the workforce would ease social tensions'*, 48% (125) remained neutral, while 38% (99) agreed that it would have this effect. The response might have been more definite had 'workplace' been used rather than 'social' tensions.

The interview respondents were much clearer, arguing that it would send out an important message to minority ethnic communities, that the service belongs to everyone, and, it might help to promote a greater understanding and lead to the erosion of prejudice,

> We have the benefit of different attitudes and cultures, and hopefully we can, in terms of learning to live in an harmonious world and environment, then hopefully that could be mirrored at the hospital. If we're going to live and work alongside one another (R28, p.2, paras.5 & 7).

The implication here is that ethnic diversity, by virtue of proximity, creates a better understanding between people of different cultures challenging stereotypes and reducing discrimination. Although evidence suggests that conditions need to be right for this to occur (Cook 1978; Dreachslin *et al* 2004), several respondents had seen the process at work:

> I mean you see it, because people who are totally prejudiced and then you give them a working colleague and suddenly they become best of mates and realise that there's no difference whatsoever. I see that all the time (R17, p12, para.42).

Trust employees provided several such examples though there was a minority view that prejudice is impenetrable and diversity would only heighten division (see chapter 3). Although the data provided by the interview respondents were much clearer on this particular issue it must be recognised that the method does provide the opportunity to seek clarification, whereas self-completed questionnaires provide data that are *'necessarily, superficial'* (Robson 1993: 243). On the other hand it is possible that interviewers produce 'public' and 'private' accounts with the former tending towards a more 'politically correct' account (Robson 1993: 230). This must not be ruled out in interpreting the findings.

An associated benefit was the enhanced trust a diverse workforce might engender in the wider community (IPD 1996; Walker *et al* 1996). For example, a publication by the National Association of Care and Resettlement of Offenders (NACRO) (1992: 7) suggested that:

> The presence of black staff in numbers proportionate to their representation in the community would help to dispel the perception of an all-white system which deals harshly with black offenders, and would go some way to restore confidence in the fairness of the process.

Similarly the Nolan Committee argued that every Quango ought to reflect its service population because '...it...may also enjoy greater public confidence, thereby making the implementation of its work more effective' (cited in Sperling 1997: 119). This argument has also made ground in the NHS (Anionwu 1996). For example, Chevannes (1991:17) argues that 'One aspect of Asians' and Afro-Caribbean's perception of 'fairness' of the service may be their observation of the presence or absence of black nurses and doctors. This has both a symbolic and a real importance'. This same point has been raised in relation to disciplinary processes (King's Fund 1990: 5) and the revision of the merit award system for consultants (Moore 1998: 3). Locally the action programme designed to encourage more students on to health-based programmes emphasised the need to have more minority ethnic staff members because their dearth can 'be an obstacle to winning the confidence of potential students from these communities'.

There is some evidence that a diverse workforce would promote greater trust and confidence within minority ethnic communities also (McFarland et al 1989; EOR No.84, 1999). The majority of respondents supported this argument, as Chart 2 illustrates the mail respondents in particular.

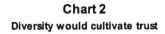

Chart 2
Diversity would cultivate trust

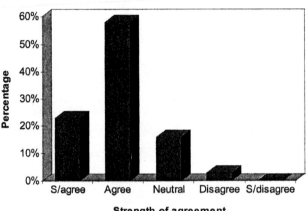

Strength of agreement

Eighty one per cent agreed that diversity would cultivate trust between providers and communities. The interview respondents provided some background into the processes involved.

> I mean patients are a diverse group and it's therefore only right that our staff should be as big a diverse group as possible. You associate particularly with race, sex, creed anything out of it one associates yeah? And I think that for ethnic groups it's important that they see ethnic groups in the workplace. That's my personal view... I think human nature suggests that you have faith in those you know (R21, p.3, paras.11 & 12).

This might serve to increase rates of utilisation and compliance, indeed the respondent responsible for running a sickle cell clinic actually identified this process at work:

> The consultant has said to me that it's been so much easier since I've been in post because they've found that patients haven't been taking medication, they haven't been complying with treatment, they haven't been coming to clinic (R6, p.4, para.11).

She used the experience of a white colleague in London to form a meaningful comparison. He had found it very difficult to develop a working relationship with the local community because they were unhappy about his ethnicity.

It has also been argued that ethnic diversity once achieved would become self-perpetuating and inherently quality enhancing. Although Dworkin (1981: 229) was evaluating the justice of preferential treatment in higher education the parallel is evident: *'If blacks are seen as successful law students, then other blacks who do meet the usual intellectual standards might be encouraged to apply'*; diversity ensuring greater diversity in a virtuous cycle. This would come about as a result of role modelling, and as Chart 3 Illustrates, this appealed to the mail respondents, when asked about their agreement with the statement 'Minority ethnic groups need more role models', four out of five (84%, 221) either agreed or strongly agreed.

Chart 3
The need for more role models

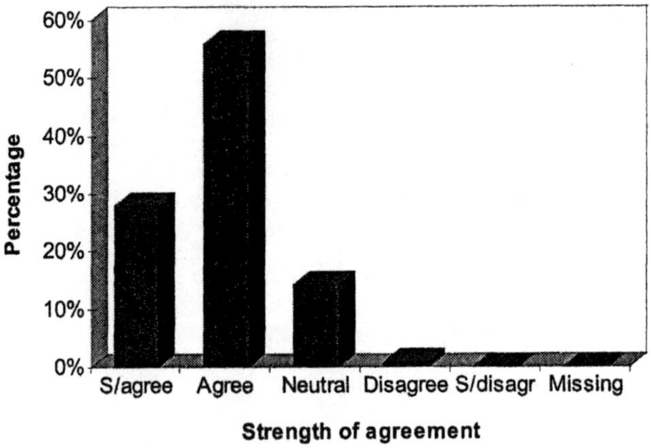

This was described by one of the interview respondents as the 'visibility' factor, and was similarly resonant:

> Yes that one person's just as good as the next person and providing that you have the relevant attitude or qualification or whatever then there's no reason why you couldn't also do or achieve a job or role that appeals to you. So yeah it is about opening up opportunities to people, opening up ideas to people (R18, p.9, para.30).

According to much of the relevant literature providing role models would not only get people into the NHS, it would encourage them to stay there, if they were diffuse throughout the organisation (Nickel 1990; Cortis & Rinomhota 1996; Iganski *et al* 2001):

> I think they would be good role models. He was probably discriminated against too, as a child, and look where he is now. You can beat the system. It would be encouraging (R9, p.16, para.49).

> Oh it is a key issue [role modelling] there's no doubt about it. It is a general perception that nurses don't get far and it is recognised that black nurses get an even worse deal in terms of career progression (R20, p.7, para.19).

Several respondents argued that role modelling had influenced them in their careers and one in particular identified it in practice:

> We actually promoted an individual from an ethnic minority background to the role of supervisor. And that's actually had a really positive effect on lots of the other staff in there. And people who would never really have aspired to be a supervisor are now sort of thinking well if she can be a supervisor perhaps we could do that in the future (R17, p.8, para.25).

So the achievement of ethnic diversity would have a number of benefits according to the respondents, not least in perpetuating itself in a virtuous cycle. Getting people into the NHS and keeping them there, infusing them with new aspirations.

One of the most popular arguments for the pursuit of greater ethnic diversity has been the belief that it will open up an untapped labour resource to employers (IPD 1996). This has slightly less relevance to the NHS than to other organisations, because it has relied so heavily on minority ethnic communities in the past, although as we have seen this has been contained within certain areas and at certain levels. It may be more accurate to suggest that the NHS needs to retain and develop the employees that it has as well as to convince younger generations to enlist (Bagilhole & Stephens 1999). The King's Fund (1990) underlined the work of Baxter (1988) by arguing that the talent of minority ethnic nurses in particular has been wasted. Where it clearly can exploit untapped labour is at the higher and highest levels of the service.

The sophisticated nature of the historic relationship between minority ethnic communities and the Health Service was not recognised by many of the interview respondents, particularly the trust employees. Focusing strictly within the confines of the city it was commonly argued that pursuing greater ethnic diversity - in the context of a severe labour shortage - would enable the Health Service to tap into a wider pool of labour (Hutton 2003):

> I think we've always got to say that there is this wider pool of labour available, a lot of it possibly currently untapped, let's make sure we actually have mechanisms to access that complete pool of labour to get the best person for the job. I think that's the only way it can work (R17, pp.5 & 7, paras.17, 18 & 22).

There is, as one of the respondents recognised, a cynical motive to this argument, in that minority ethnic communities (and others) become a valuable reserve army of labour in the context of the present labour shortage. Local trusts, in line with national trends (Brindle 1999), had been recruiting foreign nurses for some time, much to the consternation of one of the unofficial user representatives:

> Well I think I remember Diane Abbott making some comments about this in terms of the shortage of nurses that we've got. And it is quite interesting that we have a significant number of people unemployed here in Britain, particularly those from minority ethnic groups who are not being encouraged to train in this particular area where there is a severe shortage. And they are going to the expense of recruiting people from other countries (R7, p.17, para.35).

Alongside the reduction in opportunities for British people from minority ethnic backgrounds there has been concern about stealing the human resources of 'developing' countries. Some countries have been ruled off limits for active NHS recruitment, but large numbers of individuals are still recruited through voluntary action and the work of independent agencies (Carlisle 2004, 2005; Laurance 2005).

Should the well of foreign workers dry up the reserve army of minority ethnic nationals will become much more valuable, though how enduring those advances might be should the environment change is debatable. The Training and Development Officer for the trust felt that once the value of diversity had been recognised it would endure, and part of this was due to the distinct skills that minority ethnic communities can offer.

This reflects the most common argument in the literature, that greater ethnic diversity will actively improve the quality of services (King's Fund 1987; Baxter 1988; CRE 1995b; Anionwu 1996; NAHAT 1996/97; Bagilhole & Stephens 1999). The general idea has been labelled 'multicultural competency' by Coker (1997: 30), it is reputedly *'...when both the organisation and the people entering it respect each other's cultural identities and values, and are interested in learning from each other's differences'*.

The document setting out the action programme of the local university argued ethnic diversity in the workforce was vital *'to understanding how best to develop recruitment and marketing strategies'*. A diverse society needs diverse public services. While many of the mail respondents accepted this, an equal number were uncertain, see Chart 4

214

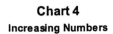

Chart 4
Increasing Numbers

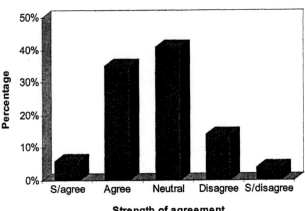

Strength of agreement

Forty one per cent of the mail respondents (105) agreed that an ethnically diverse workforce would improve service quality, while 41% (108) remained neutral. Again the different methods employed may have influenced the responses (see above discussion), but it would seem likely that either the framing of the question, or, as some of the respondents commented on the questionnaires, their lack of experience with diversity, influenced their responses. Once the shape of ethnic diversity is made clearer the level of support apparently increases (see below).

The interview respondents on the other hand were overwhelmingly convinced about the practical benefits of an ethnically diverse workforce.

Oooh yes, I'm sure there are [benefits], I mean especially in a hospital from a patient's point of view if we've got diversity. So probably to have a diverse workforce as well would be helpful. And obviously in terms of culture, drawing on as many views as possible (R31, p.1, paras.4 & 5).

Well yes, because we're providing a service to a population and the workforce comes from the population and so we're not different animals, we're the same people. And I think if you're looking at providing to a certain mix of the population, then I think it's quite helpful if you have representatives within the workforce that might be more able to understand the wants and needs of the members of that mix really... Your decisions about what's appropriate come from your basic values, and if it's a completely different culture that's making those value judgements how do they know if it's right or not? (R30, pp.7 & 14, paras.29 & 52).

So ethnic diversity, it was argued, actually enhances the cultural sensitivity of the service. Indeed the head of a voluntary mental health organisation even argued that without internal diversity a diversity of provision would be impossible:

I would be really delighted if we could attract some black people in, but we've got one Asian woman here on the [phone] lines... From a purely selfish point of view it would impress the funders. But we do have an equal opportunities policy here, and we do think that it's right that we should provide a service to all sections of the population. And in order to do that we need to attract the staff and the volunteers to go with that policy (R8, p.4, para.15).

Seemingly ethnic diversity would be a positive development for individuals, communities and organisations. It could be self-replicating, might create the basis for a harmonious society, improve the range of talent available, and, expand our understanding of merit in the interests of society.

However, in terms of the argument that a diverse NHS would better meet the needs of a diverse society, there is an implicit assumption that diversity will benefit *everyone*. This has been questioned by white supremacists in particular (Taylor 1997: 3),

Today, one of the favorite slogans that defines the asymmetric quality of American racism is 'celebration of diversity'. It has begun to dawn on a few people that 'diversity' is always achieved at the expense of whites (and sometimes men), and never the other way around.

The author argues that white people are not allowed to maintain separate institutions because that is racist, but for minority groups it is seen to be affirming. There is some merit to such claims, in as far as the claim does open up the possibility for white racists to claim that an entirely white staff is vital for the

sensitivity of services in a predominantly white area. This will become clearer as
we proceed. Having discussed the prospective benefits of ethnic diversity we now
need to clarify what the concept means – what is ethnic diversity?

Modelling ethnic diversity

Although a great deal has been written about ethnic diversity and its
prospective benefits very little energy has been devoted to defining it. Of course
the governmental preference for goals and targets provides some shape, discussed
more fully in the following chapter but the concept itself is rarely discussed
explicitly. Almost every respondent had a view about the shape and nature of
ethnic diversity. For many respondents simply reflecting the diversity of the local
area was considered the clearest starting point. As we can see from Chart 5, 84%
(221) of the mail respondents agreed that *'A workforce that reflects the community
would be better equipped to meet its needs.'*

Chart 5
Reflecting the community

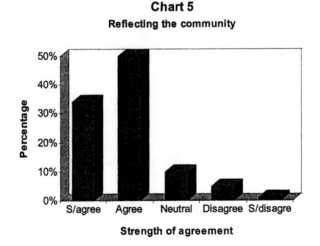

Strength of agreement

Yet, as will become clear in the following chapter the mail respondents were generally unhappy about conflating diversity with ethnic diversity. Similarly the interview respondents accepted reflecting the local community as something of a theoretical starting point,

> Well I think the bottom line would be that it would have to reflect the local population, definitely. If you could go further then and try to reflect the national picture that would be better. But I think the essential thing is that you should reflect your local population (R24, p.14, para.59).

Perhaps the most straightforward notion, drawing from the conceptual framework produced in an exploratory paper (Iganski & Johns 1998), was *proportional diversity*; that the proportion of minority ethnic members of staff ought to match those in the user community (EOR No.84, 1999). This can be the local or national community and often involves availability data[2]. This has been advocated by Etzioni (1997) in relation to community policing, and corresponds with the idea of establishing goals and targets.

It has also been criticised, for instance Nelson (1990) refers to this as the 'Noah's Ark Syndrome'. Here numbers are muddled up with effective action. This was recognised by the majority of the interview respondents. It was pointed out that proportional diversity equated numbers with need:

> It's not going to be an easy way, you can't just say well there are more Indians, sorry but we need to put more funding into that area. It's going to be...Diverse communities mean that you're going to be looking at diverse needs as well (R1, p.12, para.102).

It was argued that often the smallest communities need most assistance. Another problem was that it would be impossible to achieve a perfect reflection:

---

[2] Rather than a simple numerical target, it is usually necessary as per the practice adopted in the US, of establishing how many suitable individuals are available in the local workforce, see Edwards (1995). Similarly for a discussion on the statistical processes involved in establishing indirect discrimination in the UK see Kandola and Fullerton (1998: 113).

You're not going to get one Somali person, one Asian person. So I think it's a step towards raising awareness and looking at different needs, but it's a big responsibility to place on one or two people isn't it? (R1, p.14, para.112).

Some communities will never be accommodated either because of their size or the scarcity of posts available (Walker *et al* 1996). Finally there was the question of appropriate measures, which should be used local or national figures? Although a national target would force areas such as the south west to increase the numbers of minority ethnic staff, it would lead to massive under-representation elsewhere.

The weakest point about proportional diversity for the user representatives in particular was that it had already been tried:

In the same way let's not forget that the NHS was built on black communities being employed, that immigration policies have been sort of very flexible to allow black people from the Caribbean, Irish people, South Asian doctors to save the NHS thousands in not having to train them, and that diversity hasn't made a good deal for black patients. I think what's needed is a diverse and not discriminatory NHS so that black staff are valued, and that there will be, they are able to influence the sort of service that we have. But if we look at service areas such as psychiatry and learning difficulties they are often very heavily staffed with black nurses. If we look at the Cinderellas of the medical profession, such as again psychiatry, again we've had many more black doctors there as well. And I think it's seeing black people throughout the professions and at all levels of the professions. So I want to see more black people get to be chief executive officers (R5, p.9, para.29).

The key is not simply to reflect the population it is more complicated than that.

If you had to employ 8%, if your workforce has to be black and providing that 8% at each level. I mean 8% of your workforce is black and they're all porters. Fucking awful innit? Worse than useless in my view (R12, p.21, paras.58-60).

So it is important, as set out in earlier in the chapter, not only to achieve proportionality because that can be contained, but also to achieve diversity at the higher and highest levels. It is possible to achieve proportionality without touching managerial or policy-making positions (Bryan *et al* 1985; Baxter 1988; Karmi 1993).

This slightly different interpretation, defined by hierarchical concerns rather than simply numerical representation, was by far the most popular definition of ethnic diversity for the interview respondents (though the least popular notion for the mail respondents, see chapter 9) -

> I think it's also at the kind of policy level, that there are people there who can actually make a difference there... So if they can actually provide that then that's good, but there needs to be structural change at the top (R1, p.12, para.106).

> I think it [increasing the number of minority ethnic people in senior positions] would be important, because often the culture of the organisation is set by the senior members in that organisation. And I think that's important. And our trust board has members from the ethnic minorities on it for that reason, but as far as I'm aware none of the clinical directors are from the ethnic minorities (R30, p.9, para.34).

Whilst many respondents had set out their initial definition of ethnic diversity in proportional terms, they appeared to feel very strongly that unless minority ethnic people managed to gain a foothold in the higher echelons of the NHS, proportionality would be irrelevant.

This equates to the notion of *structural diversity* identified by Iganski and Johns (1998). Just as proportionality without structural change can be tokenistic and ineffective so too can structural diversity if it is the *only* aim. For example, Richard Nixon allegedly used affirmative action programmes to prevent radical reform. By targeting the most 'able' and/or vociferous sections of minority ethnic communities he was able to 'decapitate' them, and he also boosted the electoral prospects of the Republican Party by creating a new black middle class (Cockburn 1995). There is some suspicion amongst sections of minority ethnic communities here that a similar phenomenon is occurring. Gary Younge picking up on the long-term fears of Sivanandan warns that, *'The advancement of a few makes others feel that progress is possible. The denial of the many suggests that faith might be misplaced'* (2000: 19). This suggests not only that structural diversity alone will be insufficient, but also stresses the limitations of role modelling.

Perhaps this was implicitly recognised by the interview respondents because they unerringly went on to articulate what minority ethnic people at all levels ought to be doing:

> But I think it's important to make those changes at the policy level to let it filter through, because you could be doing things at the grassroots level which may not actually be recognised by the people at the higher level who deal with funding. So it needs to be at the policy-making level as well, and I think that is good that they've actually started to recruit more ethnic communities into the NHS (R1, p.13, para.110).

There is an expectation of agency here, an unspoken awareness about how diversity will operate. This has its antecedents in the earliest articulations of ethnic diversity (Dworkin 1981). The King's Fund (1990) having argued that the talent of minority ethnic nurses had been wasted then claimed that this had lowered the quality of care and adversely affected accessibility.

Iganski and Johns (1998) relate such expectations to the notion of *needs-led diversity*. This essentially means that diversity will be shaped according to the needs of target communities. What was not as clear then, but which this research has underlined, is that needs-led diversity comes in different strengths. At the most extreme end there lies what might be known as *segregational needs-led diversity*, a reflection of apartheid in South Africa and the Southern states of North America (Taylor 1999). This requires complete segregation in terms of service provision. The Chinese user representative maintained that the Chinese population had persistently demanded a separate service:

> Now that was a very good consultation meeting, the Chinese actually say we want a Chinese clinic with Chinese doctors, with Chinese nurses, with professionals speaking mother tongues all centralised in one area. But up to today it hasn't been addressed because we were told because a lack of resources we can't do it. And they do it in Birmingham they do it in Manchester, they do it in Leeds, they do it in Sheffield, they do it in London but they can't do it [here]...

That is what we want, we want all the Chinese speakers, professionals like nurses all in one place...That was what they wanted most but it's not been provided. Not even been addressed so far (R4, pp.17 & 18, paras.64, & 66-68).

The HA had dismissed these demands on the grounds of resources, and the representative confirmed that there would be no such concession. Not only would it be prohibitively expensive, according to the HA representative in particular, it would also be divisive (interestingly questions about distinct services provided according to gender are now subject to debate, Moore 2003). Yet in the UK, unlike the US, segregation only seems to be dangerous where minority ethnic communities seek it. The furore about state funding for Muslim secondary schools is a prime illustration (Smithers 2001). The Chinese respondent did ultimately recognise the futility of the claims, but suggested a compromise of making Chinese professionals available to deal with specific problems. This suggests another form of diversity, what might be termed *specific needs-led diversity*.

This is actually legal under the existing equal opportunities legislation. Under the Race Relations Act 1976, (section 5(2)(d)), the ethnic group, or the cultural characteristics of the health care worker become a key criterion of merit in relation to other qualifications and attributes, a genuine occupational qualification (GOQ) (Iganski & Johns 1998). There is, however, some confusion about the accurate identification of specific cultural needs and even if this were straightforward, it would only amount to a small fraction of health care *per se*. Nevertheless, several of the interview respondents were aware of it, and the trust had recruited such staff when necessary.

During the 1970s in response to community pressure black health advisers were appointed (Bryan *et al* 1985), and there have been subsequent calls for a natural extension of specific needs-led diversity. Anionwu (1996) during a survey designed to identify personal and professional profiles of Sickle Cell and Thalasaemia Counsellors, found an overwhelming majority of her respondents argued that matched ethnicity was important for effective counselling (80%, 27). To some extent this would appear to be happening already.

However, the model of diversity articulated by the majority of respondents required a massive expansion of needs-led diversity. They wanted to see minority ethnic health workers and managers working specifically on behalf of 'their' communities in a generalised way. We might refer to this as *general needs-lead diversity*[3] because it has the effect of expanding those areas to which ethnicity is seen to be relevant. As commentators like Edwards (1995) have argued, ethnicity may have more relevance to the merit principle (i.e. apportioning employment opportunities using criteria such as ability plus effort, Saunders 1996) than previously acknowledged. It seems that ethnicity might have a large impact upon the way in which services are provided. In a sense general needs-led diversity would turn minority ethnic individuals into community representatives (Iganski *et al* 1998, 2001).

Thinking back to the benefits of ethnic diversity anticipated by the respondents we can see that this is indeed how ethnic diversity is expected to work. The clearest example of this is the argument that black and minority ethnic staff members will sensitise the service to the diverse needs. How is this possible?

> But it is very important to have assertive black, and I don't like using that term generally, assertive black people working in the NHS, because they will have to be assertive in the right way, which is difficult. They'll have to say I know you're delivering a really good service on that ward, but you just perhaps, could I suggest that if a black person with very little English came here they would have a difficult time for these reasons. That has to be part of a general debate about how care is improved... One Asian person can't speak for the Somali people, black people and Chinese people. But what they do bring is the perspective of somebody who's experienced the difficulties of relating to the NHS, because they've got different... And I mean they may well be a financial expert or they may be a personnel expert but in all the broad debates that perspective will inform...it's about transmission (R11, pp.12, 14 & 19, paras.38, 46 & 67).

---

[3] It should be noted that the exploratory article by Iganski and Johns (1998) included the notion of team-based diversity, but this did not appear to have any resonance with the interview respondents. Furthermore, according to Kandola and Fullerton (1998 102-103) the concept is organically related (although they obviously do not put it in quite these terms) to general needs-led diversity with all that that implies.

It works on the basis that they will actively represent those needs. Even where they do not take on an active role the idea is that they will transmit their knowledge to their white colleagues by association (Gerrish *et al* (1996). There is some evidence to support this (Batsleer *et al* 2003) so it is not wholly surprising that this was a resonant concept:

> The other thing is about getting more black and ethnic minority staff into the NHS, and that's not so they can act as interpreters and that's not so they can act as advocates. It's so they gradually...that bit of yeast will percolate through the loaf (R11, p.13, para.45).

The idea of representation moves away from 'numbers' towards 'agency'. Minority ethnic individuals will improve the service provided to minority ethnic communities by directly or indirectly representing the interests of 'their' communities.

Here we can see that the arguments raised by Taylor (1997) are to some extent justified, ethnic diversity defined in this way is really designed (or at least the appear to be designed) to benefit minority ethnic communities. When faced with the argument that predominantly white areas ought to be entitled to a white workforce there was consternation amongst the interview respondents:

> No [we can't have a white workforce in a white area] because you've got to represent everybody (R9, p.9, para.29).

Straw (1999) has argued that even where areas are homogeneously white, some ethnic diversity will be required in the workforce of the public sector, to allow for geographic and demographic change. This is entirely inconsistent, because on the strength of what has been said before we each act as representatives for our communities. If this is the case then a white community should be entitled to a white work force, not as some commentators suggest (Weale 1983) as a matter of simply 'fitting-in', but to provide sensitive and appropriate services. Consequently it is fair to say that ethnic diversity, as defined by the interview respondents at

224

least is mainly about improving services to minority ethnic communities. Is this what people want, as they are likely to bear full responsibility for the needs of 'their' own communities?

There is evidence to suggest that minority ethnic groups want to consult with doctors from their own ethnic background, although this appears to vary by ethnicity and gender, men being less concerned than women (Gerrish *et al* 1996; Nazroo 1997). The key issue was lingual but mention was also made of cultural and religious reasons and a minority would just feel more comfortable. This was not recognised by the majority who work for the NHS. The mail respondents appeared largely unaware of patients' demands for workers of a similar background, 24% disagreed with the statement, *'Patients prefer workers from their own ethnic group'* and 55% (142) remained neutral (see Chart 6)

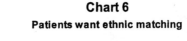

Chart 6
Patients want ethnic matching

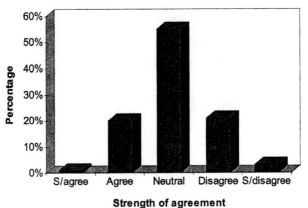

Similarly the trust employees were largely unaware of any such demands but there was some recognition of the issue:

Another side of it may be that people from ethnic minorities may prefer to be cared for by a member of their own culture, I mean that may not always be the case (R30, p.8, para.30).

My mother has been with her GP for years. I said mum why don't you go to that practice it's nice, and she said Oh no, they won't understand. Oh yeah, because they feel that they understand the culture more, and I mean from the patients point of view we've got a doctor at the moment and he is superb. He's from Trinidad, and this girl, this patient, she is very difficult to treat because her veins are quite poor, but this doctor he is so wonderful. He's very sort of calm and confident and he gets in there, and she has built up such trust with him, and she said to me: Do you know why? Because he's from the Caribbean. And when he had a couple of days off she refused to be treated unless he came back. And I said if there was another sort of African-Caribbean or Asian doctor would you allow them...? And she said, Oh yeah. She'd be happy for them to treat her, and I think people they feel comfortable with their own, you know? Because I'd be exactly the same (R6, p.25, paras.81 & 83).

The demand for greater diversity from the community has already been identified. If they were adopting the same model as the respondents then representation was the key issue.

Furthermore, this is already occurring to some extent, though it would appear to be forced upon individuals (see Gerrish *et al* 1996; chapters 2 & 5). Minority health workers are routinely used to provide interpreting services and cultural advice. One respondent said:

And also I find that doctors if they're faced with a problem with a patient of African-Caribbean descent they will call me, and it's not necessarily directly linked with my work, they will call me because I am a black health professional. And I say well what do you expect me to do in this situation? Well we thought that you'd be able to intervene and I say well this isn't my area, I'm not employed to do that. You need to seek help from another source (R6, p.3, para.9).

She had also found herself caring disproportionately for minority ethnic patients due to the neglect of her white colleagues, and when expressing her guilt to colleagues discovered this was a common experience (see Baxter 1988 and George 1994 for similar accounts):

> I know a couple of the doctors and nurses and I've sort of said to them, God isn't this awful and I feel so guilty for doing it, but they say well we're the same (R6, p.26, paras.84-86).

This substantiates the claim by Baxter (1998: 38) that *'There is a general feeling among black nurses that in many instances they are only encouraged to look after black and ethnic minority patients at the convenience of their white colleagues and not at their own professional discretion'*. The respondent, as discussed above, had even been asked to run CAT courses without adequate expertise. It is commonly assumed that minority ethnic individuals will be able and willing to deal with the needs and interests of 'their' communities:

> Our equal opportunities unit is made up of people from ethnic minority backgrounds which is very important because of course they know the issues. You couldn't have an equal opportunities unit full of white men. Yeah, I mean they might be very enlightened white men, but there's no substitute for life experience (R9, p.21, para.68).

Indeed one potential respondent declined to participate in this research because, in her words, she was *'always being volunteered'* for things related to equal opportunities or 'race' issues.

Having underlined the evidence that it is already happening in the NHS, we must now consider in more detail the concept of needs-led diversity, more specifically general needs-led diversity. All the benefits associated with ethnic diversity appear to depend upon minority ethnic individuals representing the interests of 'their' communities at every level, by directly providing services or by influencing policy decisions. As the reluctance of the potential respondent illustrates, the concept is dubious.

Who wants to be a representative?

This assumption that minority ethnic individuals, with their greater awareness of the needs of 'their' communities, and a shared history of oppression, will be ready and willing to take on this role has been around for some time (Baxter 1988). For example, Johnson (1987: 131) argued that:

> For such a perspective, and for a growth in training materials which have sought to assist in the fight against discrimination rather than simply to describe the culturally specific features of minorities, we have by and large had to await the arrival in positions of authority (i.e. the obtaining of power) of ethnic minority professionals who find it easier to relate to minority community demands – and the disturbances caused by young people intolerant of delay and taking their own form of 'community action'.

It is a commonly held belief then that minority ethnic individuals will have a better understanding of the real health priorities of 'their' communities and will be prepared to meet them. Undoubtedly some individuals may accept, even relish the opportunity (Baxter 1997). For instance, in response to the survey carried out by Anionwu, 50% (17) reported that helping clients was the best part of the job. A typical response read, *'I like helping my own community and being there for them'* (1996: 178).

What the respondents said about the benefits of ethnic diversity would suggest strong support for this, and yet when faced with the implications of their suggestions, few were willing to accept them. When presented with the statement, *'Minority ethnic workers should act as representatives for their respective groups'*, 35% (92) of mail respondents disagreed and 41% (108) remained neutral (see Chart 7)

228

Chart 7
Workers should act as representatives

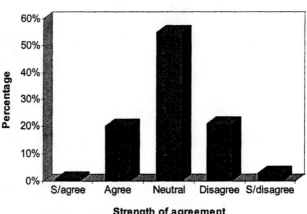

Strength of agreement

From the interview survey only three respondents believed that minority ethnic individuals would want to represent 'their' communities in this way:

> I think in some cases that inevitably happens because there are people who go in who are from ethnic minorities who have a particular concern for their particular community, and therefore strive to improve services (R14, p.4, para.16).

One had actively done so throughout her career, particularly since she'd been appointed to run the local sickle cell clinic.

However, the notion of active representation is highly problematic (Aanchawan 1996). For one thing, there is evidence to suggest that the notion of ethnic or 'racial' allegiances is a myth. In discussing the value of the Asian Women of Achievement Awards in 2005 Chowdery said:

> I do not automatically feel a close affinity with anther woman simply because she happens to be Asian. I make no apologies for it and I resent that this stance is

sometimes taken to be a deliberate act on my part of distancing myself from my heritage (2005: 35).

The idea of active representation outlined above subsumes individuality beneath group-based characteristics. This tendency was identified by several of the interview respondents. For example:

> So we'll know because of them what that community needs. Well I would say that's crap because those Somali people know what those Somali people want, what they: I'm a Somali person, I might know what I want, I might know what my immediate family want. But why in the hell would I know what the wider Somali community want? Why should I? I'm just one person. I'm a doctor, I'm a nurse, I'm a porter. How do I know? (R12, p.14, para.37).

The idea of representation overlooks the complexity of identity, privileging ethnicity over other characteristics (Ahmad 1993a; Culley 1996):

> Another thing is if you do recruit black people they might actually be so well integrated into the white community that they've taken on the white cultural values, and then not be in touch. So you can make assumptions... I mean when I was on the Mental Health Act Tribunals we had a black woman, and she had originally come from the Caribbean and her mother still lived there. And she'd come over as a child and she'd worked in the NHS as a psychiatric nurse, and she'd become a manager and I think her partner was white and she lived out in a white area and... She might have been in touch with her own community back home, she used to go home quite a lot, but not [the community here] (R8, pp.7 & 10, paras.27, 43 & 44).

It was felt that other facets of identity, such as class, nationality or even regional background might serve to prevent minority ethnic individuals from understanding, therefore representing the needs of 'their' communities (Torkington 1991; Fine 1995; Gerrish et al 1996; Law 1996; Batsleer et al 2003; Dreachslin et al 2004).

There is empirical evidence from the United States to suggest that the assumption of active representation is flawed. During the 1980s and early 1990s several police departments deliberately assigned minority ethnic officers to patrol 'their' own communities. This was partly about conforming to legal requirements and about good public relations. It was also argued that they would provide a qualitatively better service. In reality the officers acted in virtually the same way as their white colleagues (Walker *et al* 1996: 109). Why? Because '...*most experts on the police argue that situational and departmental factors, not race or gender influence police officer behaviour*' (Walker *et al* 1996: 109). In short, professional allegiances often outweigh presumed cultural allegiances (Ahmad 1993c; McLaughlin & Murji 1999).

There is evidence that minority ethnic health workers in the NHS might feel exactly the same way (Ahmad *et al* 1991). In fact the Chinese respondent argued that in the course of her work she had been given the opportunity to gauge the feelings of local nurses in this respect and they did not want to act as representatives, their main allegiance was to their employers. According to the HA representative non-executive directors actively reject the role:

> It's very interesting they reject it [representation] strongly... They're, from bitter experience, people from minority communities are very reluctant to be forced into the 1-dimensional role (R11, p.19, para.67).

Therefore, there is significant evidence that representation might run aground on the rock of individualism (Baxter 1988, 1997).

Even if people accepted the role of representative there is no guarantee that they will improve the quality of service provided to minority ethnic communities. They may use their position to pursue their own interests rather than that of the community (Ward 1993):

> Hopefully they'd be championing the right cause it wouldn't just be somebody who's on a hobbyhorse. And that's the other thing, that it should be somebody from the same ethnic group, but if they've got their own hobbyhorse, it doesn't necessarily fit with what the rest of the community want (R26, p.6, para.37).

The HA representative and the trust employees were particularly worried about this, and stressed very strongly the importance of professional neutrality:

I think it's about getting an equal balance of communities, which is not just getting someone who has black issues, because otherwise it's making us the ones who are going to be discriminated against as well isn't it? White, Caucasians, other ethnic minorities. So everyone should have a broad understanding I feel (R25, p.6, paras.47 & 48).

There was a very real fear that some individuals might abuse their role as representatives to pursue their own ends, or, worse still, to reverse past injustices. Ironically, injustices the majority of trust employees had persistently refused to acknowledge.

Conversely, it was argued that using individuals as representatives could prevent significant reform of the Health Service (Ward 1993). This would be about tokenism, a means of demonstrating that action is being taken without any real changes being made to service provision (Smaje 1995; Gerrish et al 1996). In proposing the introduction of specialist teachers to strengthen the quality of 'race' equality aspects in nurse education, Baxter notes that every effort must be taken to avoid marginalisation (1997: 95, see Bryan et al 1985 for a similar discussion about ethnic health advisers). Many of the respondents felt that this would be easier to propose than achieve:

There's going to be a temptation, conscious or unconscious, to say: well we've cracked the Somali problem. Not only in terms of employment, but also in terms of service provision and access because we've got Somali people working for us... Well at the moment there's a recognition that the Somali community because it's a refugee community, fundamentally, it's marginalised and it's got particular problems that relate with having refugee status. You've been kicked out of your country concerned about what's going... I mean there's a lot of stress on a community like that. So a lot of work's been done with that community to understand its needs. Would that stop if there were sufficient Somali people working in the NHS? I'm only using the Somali community as an example...Yeah well we've cracked it because look we've got open access support, equal opportunities employment policies. We've got that profile now in the workforce, we must be doing alright. Well you know, no you're not doing alright because you're not actually involving the wider population in decision-making about your services (R12, p.14, para.37).

It could lead, as stressed throughout, to the abdication of responsibility to communities themselves:

> We've got this employee who is black and there have been issues in the past about performance, and I know of instances where those have not been taken up because of the potential of being accused as being racist. But in our, from our recruitment we've actually got another black supervisor and that person is from another cultural background, and they have dealt with that person in a different way, and a most refreshing way. Because they haven't had perhaps some of the hang-ups that we've got. I mean we as a white person. They've just gone in and dealt with it. And that's been really good in some ways. (R23, p.12, para.37).

This would certainly be consistent with the findings of this research, whereby any problems are located in the community rather than the service. The inevitable outcome of ethnic diversity as it is currently conceived, it seems, will be to ghettoise minority ethnic individuals in a much more pronounced way than that already in operation in the NHS (Baxter 1988; EOC 1991; Carter 2000; Batsleer *et al* 2003).

Conclusion

Diversity as a concept, particularly ethnic diversity has been around, in the US at least, since the late-1970s early-1980s. It has been incorporated into equalities theory in the shape of the business case for equal opportunities and more recently the quality case (see CRE 1995b). Ethnic diversity is a major policy priority for the Labour government and the reasons for this are varied, though the justice-based arguments articulated early on by Tony Blair may be less influential than functional realities – i.e. a labour shortage and the everyday problems of disadvantage and discrimination experienced by minority ethnic communities in Britain. The aftermath of the MacPherson Report has arguably lent more urgency to these issues than ever before (Parekh 2000).

However, very little energy has been devoted to defining the concept of ethnic diversity, and even less to articulating its practical application. Although the NHS has been the most ethnically diverse employer in the UK since the post-war period, there have been distinct patterns of under and over-representation of minority ethnic groups almost unerringly to their detriment. This was recognised in Robbinston by many of the interview respondents, although several of the trust employees were happy with the diversity of their trust. There was a consensus amongst trust employees however about the arbitrary nature of numerical representation. They preferred to see people as individuals, despite the contradictory evidence presented throughout.

Despite this uncertainty, the vast majority of both mail and interview respondents thought that the attainment of ethnic diversity would be beneficial for a number of reasons, primarily because it would lead to an improvement of services. In defining the concept the interview respondents began with proportionality, drifted through structural diversity before settling on a model labelled here as general needs-led diversity. Minority ethnic individuals were charged with actively representing their communities throughout the Health Service. When this was fed back to the respondents, making the maximum usage of the possibilities presented by active interviewing (Holstein & Gubrium 1997), most rejected it, especially the trust employees, again because they favoured individualism. There was also a range of problems identified with active representation, just as with the numerical interpretation.

The central problem appeared to be that it would not work, and this has been supported by research evidence from the United States (Walker *et al* 1996). Many people tend to offer their allegiances to organisations rather than 'their' communities. Perhaps the best means of achieving adequate representation is to encourage mass participation as per the proposals that formed part of the internal market, except that this has not really been achieved, and at the local level at least has been misused to buy off discontent. Indeed Law has argued that the overemphasis of ethnic diversity in the workforce has partially been done to prevent user participation, by sidelining black-led health forums, which could from a position of strength articulate demands, lobby for sensitive policy change and promote innovative projects. *'In many local areas these forums and groups can provide a focus for the establishment of key alliances and networks between black and minority ethnic communities and health care providers'* (1996: 155; see also Jay 1992: 44; Ahmad 1993b; McIver 1994).

Even in the context of sensitive provision many feel that ethnic diversity is overplayed. For example, according to Proctor and Davis (1994) *'racial similarity between helper and client may be less important than the worker's level of skill in using culturally appropriate communicative and trustworthy behaviours'* (1994: 318; see also Kandola & Fullerton 1998: 103). Similarly, commentators in the UK have warned that ethnic diversity should not be used to allow white health professionals to wipe their hands of diversity issues, leaving minority ethnic patients to their colleagues (Gerrish *et al* 1996). This would certainly be consistent with the central theme of this book which is that white policy-makers and providers seem intent on placing the onus for change on minority ethnic communities.

The message appears to be 'accept the service as it is or do something about it'. However when this fails, because of marginalisation and ghettoisation, it will allow policy-makers to further underline the deviance of minority ethnic cultures and communities. Even 'they' cannot solve the problems 'they' present. This suggests that the 'New Racism' first articulated by Enoch Powell in the mid-1960s, whereby biological difference is displaced by cultural incongruence, remains potent (Barker 1981; Gordon & Klug 1986). The inevitable segregation reflects the foundations of apartheid in South Africa (Taylor 1999).

I do not wish to dismiss the value of ethnic diversity, for the structural representation of politicized minority ethnic individuals would, along with greater community involvement, contain genuinely transformative elements (Ahmad 1993b, 1993c). However, the material presented here suggests that without careful articulation and debate the pursuit of ethnic diversity could be counterproductive, it could be used (as at present) to deflect attention away from inappropriate services and the need to challenge racism and shift responsibility onto minority ethnic communities to an even greater degree (Ward 1993; Marable 1995). In the next chapter we will set out the development of equal opportunities policies in the NHS, focusing on the use of positive action, and pre-emptively set out the current strategy of the Labour government. However, as will become clear, there are numerous counter forces at work which may ultimately thwart any radical attempt to achieve greater ethnic diversity.

CHAPTER 8

Taking Positive action

'In England, Justice is open to all, like the Ritz hotel' – Sir James Matthew

Introduction

The achievement of ethnic diversity has become a policy priority and we have explored some of the ways in which it can be manifest and flagged up some of the implicit dangers of the concept. The object of this chapter is to consider ways in which diversity might be achieved. In theory at least this has involved improving and extending equal opportunities policies, and the strong traditional connection between equal opportunities and ethnic diversity was a feature of the HAs report and action plan.

The development of equal opportunities, however, has not been entirely satisfactory as we will see, and there has been little attempt to engage in positive action measures[1] (Iganski *et al* 2001). This may now be changing, as the Labour government seek to gain greater central control after a period of decentralisation and devolution (Carter 2000; DoH 2003a). Nevertheless, the climate as tested by a series of mail surveys (see below) including the one which informs this book suggests that a more radical approach will face strong opposition from within the

---

[1] Positive action requires a limited amount of differential treatment – though not at the point of selection – which is lawful under sections 35, 37 & 38 of the Race Relations Act 1976. Possibilities range from adding a welcoming statement to target groups at the base of job vacancies, to the establishment of goals and targets. The rationale for PA is that disadvantaged groups require assistance to reach the starting line, it is an attempt to level the playing field, not to provide those groups with unfair advantages.

Health Service. Furthermore, those responsible for making day-to-day employment decisions may have very little sympathy for any measure which strays from the concept of equal treatment. Ironically, the interview respondents, who provided the material for this assumption, are much more radical in their attitudes towards ethnic diversity than the government but are not prepared to follow their beliefs through to their logical conclusion.

Background

Although equal opportunities policies and diversity have traditionally been organically linked within the NHS as elsewhere, the progress achieved in this direction has arguably been negligible. For example, the final report of the King's Fund Equal Opportunities Task Force (1990) asserted that equal opportunities had not been a priority for the NHS and until it became part and parcel of the management function little progress would be achieved.

Since then there has been a growth in the profile of equal opportunities within the Health Service. The NHS became involved in the Opportunity 2000 Campaign (subsequently Opportunity Now) and on the recommendations of the Equal Opportunities Commission (EOC) a Women's Unit was established in 1991 to improve the position of women, but was replaced in 1996 by an Equal Opportunities Unit. More specifically a programme of action was launched in 1993 to overcome some of the many barriers faced by minority ethnic groups. HAs and trusts were charged with

- Adopting equal opportunities policies and action plans.
- Collecting and analysing ethnic monitoring data, establishing corrective action where necessary.
- Monitoring personnel procedures.
- Training staff in recruitment and selection procedures (NHSME 1993).

Despite the high profile, and recent endorsements of the action programme (Mason 2000), there has been limited consistent progress (Jamdagni 1996). In fact Mwasamdube and Mullen (1998) found that less than half of the 12 HAs in the region (45%) had implemented the programme.

There *was* a strong positive action element to the programme, and according to many commentators (Baxter 1988; Iganski *et al* 1998, 2001; Mason 2000; Parekh 2000), this is crucial if greater ethnic diversity in the NHS is to be achieved. There was some recognition of the importance of positive action in the research area. For example, the HAs consultation report and action plan promised to:

- Develop a positive action recruitment and training programme for [the HA] in partnership with the [participating voluntary organisation, as discussed below].
- Encourage local NHS Trusts to join this partnership and talk to them about the possibility of targeting positive careers guidance in schools with large numbers of black students.
- Discuss with the [local university] any action which may be possible in relation to recruitment to specific health training courses.

Judging by the commitment demonstrated in relation to improving service delivery there is no reason to believe that significant progress will be made in this direction.

However, there is a raft of measures designed to improve the service provision to minority ethnic communities and in particular to create and sustain a diverse workforce at all levels and across all areas of the NHS. The HR in the *NHS Plan* stressed the importance of equality and diversity and series of policy papers have been produced to support that direction. For the first time the Health Service has a co-ordinated human resources framework. *Vital Connections*, published in 2000, provides the outline of what the government expects of the

NHS in terms of equal opportunities over the next ten years. This is supported by the framework strategy detailing the operational aspects, supported by national development programmes such as Positively Diverse (DoH 2004b) and the partnership on *Tackling Racial Harassment in the NHS* (EOR No.76, 1998), and the *Improving Working Lives* standard, to which all NHS employers had to be accredited by 2003. In support of these measures the Chief Executive of the NHS Sir Nigel Crisp has developed a 10-point Race Equality Plan (DoH 2004c) and a Equality and Human Rights Director, Surinder Sharma, was appointed in 2004 (DoH 2004a).

The head of the CRE Sir Trevor Phillips has expressed his cautious optimism about these developments (Phillips 2004), and there is evidence of progress at both a national and local level. In terms of the former the National Recruitment Campaign launched in 2003 produced a large increase of minority ethnic applications, with 21% of applicants identifying themselves as such. The Ambulance Service Race Equality Programme of 2001 saw numbers of minority ethnic staff members double to form 3.5% of the workforce. By 2003 90% of NHS employers were accredited under the *Improving Working Lives* standard, and the Positively Diverse programme had seen the involvement of 1,170 NHS organisations, with 12 lead sites providing advice and support (DoH 2003b). From a local point of view it is clear that the *Improving Working Lives* standard is having some impact, particularly with regards activities in the north west of England (Weston & Walsh 2003).

Independent assessors of the achievements in relation to these initiatives and policies have been less satisfied with the overall progress. A recruitment agency found that only 30% of trusts reported no designated person leading efforts towards equality and diversity. The impact of the *Improving Working Lives* standard has been questioned nationally, and while the growth of Positively Diverse is accepted, the number of organisations fully on-board numbered only around 200 by 2004 (HSJ 2004).

Much of the impetus, however the progress is evaluated, for these divers measures emerged from the passage of the Race Relations (Amendment) Act (2000) which placed general and specific duties upon designated public sector employers (EOR No.96, 2001). For the first time public authorities, including the NHS were required to:

- Ensure non-discrimination in relation to its primary functions.
- Promote equality of opportunity.
- Promote good race relations (CRE 2001).

The amendment therefore requires employers to be pro-active and to take proportionate measures according to specific functions (CRE 2001). Furthermore, alongside these obligations the NHS along with other public authorities has been provided with its own framework for action. It is hoped that the amendment will make radical changes in service delivery and employment policies, however, doubts have already been expressed (Parekh 2000, who favours along with others (see Lester 1998) a new comprehensive Equality Act). Of course there has also been activity at the EU level which has been acknowledged in Department of Health planning (DoH 2003a; DoH 2003b).

Within a year of the legislation being passed the CRE had produced a report (2002) evaluating the achievements of public sector bodies in relation to the duties set out in the amendment. It found that NHS organisations were less advanced than comparable public sector employers, and the Race Equality Schemes introduced were patchy and where present not always very robust (CRE 2002). Moreover 108 warnings have been issued against NHS employers by the CRE with regards 'racial' discrimination, and there have been 12 interventions since January 2004 (Harding 2005).

While it would be possible to question the efficacy of the legislation from the perspective of the Health Service, it is too early to say that it will not have a significant impact of direct discrimination. Indeed steps have been set out in the latest Race Equality Scheme to make genuine improvements in this area (DoH 2005) and the CRE are working with the Health Service to this end (Harding 2005). Nevertheless, there remains strong scepticism that any genuine commitment exists in the NHS to take *positive action* to improve the service delivery for or employment prospects of minority ethnic communities (Mason 2000; Iganksi *et al* 2001). Commitment to equal opportunities, as will be demonstrated below, is far from strong even taking the recent policy measures into account, and developments such as 'New Public Management' have provided Health Service Management with room to manoeuvre to marginalise equal opportunities in the same way that minority ethnic health needs appear to have been marginalised (Mason 2000).

However, it seems that the poor understanding of positive action and lack of commitment highlighted by Gerrish *et al* (1996) and Iganski *et al* (2001) in nurse education centres may not be reflected in those making day-to-day employment decisions in the NHS. Rather it seems that positive action is adjudged to be both unnecessary and unfair, and taken to its legal limits, tantamount to positive discrimination. Thus there is '...*a genuine difference of view about the nature of equality, and the measures by which it may legitimately be pursued, which has a long intellectual history'* (Iganski *et al* 2001: 313). Ironically, although in many ways the interview respondents are more radical in their attitudes than even positive discrimination demands, they remain firmly attached to the status quo.

Equal Opportunities in the NHS

The head of the Equal Opportunities Unit Elisabeth Al-Khalifa has argued that the Human Resources Framework Strategy would achieve radical change because although the collective will in the NHS is strong, practical know-how has been generally weak. It will work '*by making it a fact of daily business for trust managers'* (Agnew 1998b: 14). However, early reports suggested that the response thus far has been patchy (McGauran 2001) and the notion that the collective will is strong is questionable.

A number of surveys conducted from 1993 onwards to chart the commitment and progress of NHS trusts have revealed remarkably consistent themes. The first was carried out by the *Equal Opportunities Review* (EOR No.53, 1994) in the early days of trust formation, but since then similar surveys have been conducted by (or for) the NHSEs Equal Opportunities Unit (Hurstfield 1998), the CRE (2000), albeit 'race' oriented and limited to England, the *Health Service Journal* (HSJ) and the study which informed this book. The findings promise significant difficulties for the government in the attainment of their objectives.

The first feature of the surveys is low response. The EOR survey mailed to the extant 292 trusts received a response rate of just 32% (92), similarly the response to the CREs survey was 51% (128 from 250 mailings) and that of the author 58% (266 from 461 mailings). Although it must be stressed that the response rate of 58% for this research project was creditable, the general trend would appear to illustrate almost as clearly as the actual findings that equal opportunities is peripheral for many NHS employers. The principal exception to this trend was the NHSE survey which achieved a response rate of 98%, but this simply suggests a greater incentive to respond to a centrally co-ordinated research programme.

Perhaps the central theme of the surveys is a paper commitment to equal opportunities. The EOR survey found that virtually every trust had a written policy statement, as did the other surveys (Hurstfield 98% (412), CRE 98% (245), and 98% (258) in the present survey). However, there was less evidence of palpable action from the majority of trusts. For example, less than two-thirds of the EOR respondents had established any kind of action plan to support their policies, and this was reflected in the survey for this research. Only 61% (156) reported having an action plan in place, and 81% (126) of those said that it included ethnicity. Similarly a mere 5% of the CREs respondents had designated 'race' equality programmes or action plans in place, with another 45% planning or about to implement them. The majority of trusts appear to monitor their workforces. For instance, Hurstfield's (1998) survey demonstrated that 90% of trusts gathered information on ethnicity, gender and disability, though very few actually evaluate that data or use it to inform or develop policy-making (see also Carter 2000: 69; Iganski *et al* 2001: 306). Similarly the CRE found that 88% carried out ethnic monitoring but only 65% actually use the data.

The survey for this research supports this general trend. For example, 95% (250) of respondents reported that recruitment and selection procedures are regularly reviewed. 85% (224) said that they always drew up person specifications for employment vacancies, 86% (226) kept records of the reasons for short listing or otherwise and another 81% (214) for reasons of appointment or non-appointment. In terms of detailed monitoring however the picture is less impressive. Asked whether equality audits are conducted 61% (157) said that they were not, and of those less than half, or 47% (74), were planning to conduct an audit in the future. This demonstrates virtually no improvement since the EOR survey was conducted in 1993.

The relative inactivity as a result of monitoring reported in other surveys was also identified. Just over two-thirds of respondents (64%, 166) regularly analysed records for equal opportunities purposes. Echoing the CREs survey, 95% (246) collected data on the ethnicity of job applicants, but only 69% (167) regularly analysed this information. Although 80% (77) of the respondents for this survey reported that their trusts conducted equality audits and had provided a subsequent report of the findings the overall picture of equality activity is disappointing.

Perhaps most worrying of all has been the rate of adoption of positive action measures (see Iganski *et al* 2001 for an account of its early development). Even a recent Department of Health strategy document has highlighted this as an issue *'There are a limited number of Positive Action programmes within the NHS'* (DoH 2003a), and this is borne out by the evidence. For example, the EOR survey revealed that only 8 (9%) had set goals and targets for minority ethnic communities, 23 (25%) on the basis of disability and 49 (53%) for women. Only 21% reported future plans to introduce targets. The emphasis on gender was attributed to the Opportunity Now campaign and was, according to the EOR, in need of urgent attention (see also Sharda 1993).

Although more trusts reported the use of goals and targets in the NHSE survey, the trend continues. 33% had goals and targets for women, 25% for minority ethnic communities and 13% for disabled people. Only 10% (44) reported that their most successful initiatives involved assisting minority ethnic communities. The CRE found that 13% of their respondents had taken any positive action measures and that 11% had set goals and targets for minority ethnic communities.

The majority of the mail respondents for this survey were in favour of positive action as a means of achieving diversity. Seventy three per cent (194) reported that they approved of its use for this purpose. However, there was a distinct deficit between attitude and action. Asked to specify their trust's activities via a range of options the results can be seen in Table 1.

Table 1. Positive action measures permissible under the RRA 1976

Measures taken	Yes	No
Additional training	13% (34)	87% (223)
Setting of goals and/or timetables	19% (49)	81% (209)
Out-reach recruitment efforts	39% (101)	61% (158)
Targeted advertising	38% (98)	62% (161)

Twenty one respondents reported 'other' positive action measures but none were relevant for the purposes of this study. Furthermore, 4 (25%) listed activities which would not be classed as positive action, demonstrating a limited understanding of the issues at hand. A survey conducted by the *Health Service Journal* (HSJ) confirmed that 45% of trusts and 27% of HAs actively recruit from minority ethnic communities (Agnew 2000: 12). Therefore, while there is support for the use of positive action in principle in practice it is less often employed (Iganski *et al* 2001).

Furthermore, a consistent trend appears to be that those taking most action, setting aside for the moment its efficacy, tend to be most critical of themselves and to be located in ethnically diverse areas (see also Gerrish *et al* 1996; Jamdagni 1996; Baxter 1997; Iganski *et al* 2001). One respondent from the HSJ survey wrote, *'This area has NO ethnic minorities'* (Agnew 2000: 12), and Jay (1992: 30) found that statutory agencies, particularly in the south west, did not take equal opportunities seriously for the same reasons. Only two respondents from 49 provided documentary evidence of a rigorous policy. Mwasamdube and Mullen (1998) revealed highly consistent themes in relation to the 36 participatory trusts in the region. As discussed in the previous chapter the government requires every NHS employer to be prepared for geographic and demographic change, and a sensitive service and equality of opportunity are seen to be fundamental citizenship rights (Straw 1999). So why do the majority of trusts, indeed Health Service employers, fail to recognise this?

The Sanctity of equal treatment

Numerous studies have demonstrated the inadequate nature of equal opportunities implementation in the NHS. Beishon *et al* (1995) and more recently Bagilhole and Stephens (1997, 1998, 1999) found that policies were poorly communicated and understood, that different people have different ideas about equal opportunities and its value, and that there is a general unwillingness to take responsibility for their implementation. Carter (2000) has since argued that the decentralisation identified in chapter 4 has enabled equal opportunities to be demoted and even dismissed in the face of competing priorities. Ward managers see equal opportunities as a burden rather than an opportunity and use resource constraints etc. to conceal the stereotypical – or racist - use of informal employment procedures (see also Baxter 1988; Bagilhole 1993; Jewson & Mason 1993; Ward 1993; Carter 2000; Iganski *et al* 2001). The common factor however appears to be a straightforward unwillingness to accept any disruption of the status quo.

This is confirmed to some extent by the material obtained via the interview survey. However, its purpose was slightly different, in that it was designed to explore the views of respondents about the best means of achieving ethnic diversity. The trust employees very much reflect those in Carter's study in that they were all responsible in one form or another for day-to-day employment decision-making. The concern of the majority was that diversity should not jeopardise equal treatment:

> I think that is what we should aim for treating everyone equally, not going either one way or the other 'cos I mean it can work both ways (R31, p.5, para.29).

This was very much in tune with the ethos of the trust, as set out by one of the personnel advisers:

> I mean the general way we work at the hospital is we look at things like qualifications, experience, and we have a person specification that someone might meet, they might have experience with computers or a particular computer system. Or they might need to have experience of writing reports or presenting training courses, but it depends on the individual job. It's different for each job, the person specification or the individual for each job (R28, p.13, para.50).

The trust was in the process of reinforcing its equal opportunities framework with the establishment of an equal opportunities committee and associated working groups. There had been a lull in activity since 1991 due to the loss of HA influence according to several respondents. Even so, most were satisfied with the performance of their trust in this respect, although a small minority wanted better dissemination of monitoring information and greater training opportunities, reflecting the findings of Bagilhole and Stephens (1999: 242).

There was little support for anything that remotely resembled differential treatment (reflecting the findings of Carter 2000: 69; and Iganksi *et al* 2001) particularly in the interests of ethnic diversity. For one thing, as stressed in the previous chapter, where it was relevant at all the trust was perceived by most to be adequately diverse. The primary reason was that it simply was not necessary; if there are any barriers to ethnic diversity they are not attributable to the NHS, either locally or nationally. The actual barriers are demographic, relate to specific professions and recent reforms, and/or have been raised by minority ethnic communities themselves.

The trust would find increasing its diversity difficult due to the ethnic profile of the immediate area; the main hospital site was located in the suburbs in a predominantly white area. (Although even in the inner-city clinic there were very few minority ethnic staff members.) The main site was reported to be beyond the reach of the local communities, due to an inadequate bus service. Not only was there an assumption that other modes of transport were unavailable but the basic argument was flawed, the bus service was reasonably reliable.

A related argument was that it was also a problem of availability. Trusts should not be held responsible for the failings of other institutions:

> 'Cos I mean really the trust is picking up, although we're almost like a second round of recruitment if you like. I mean it's like nurse education. Nurse education are really doing the recruiting for us but 3 years previously, so if they're not taking in a diversity of people onto nurse training, we cannot then recruit a diverse population of people (R17, pp.1, 2 & 19, paras.2-5, 71 & 72).

It was common to argue that if the education system failed minority ethnic communities (Stone 1981; Kurtz 1993) and those institutions responsible for training health workers do not select a diverse student body then the trust cannot achieve greater diversity. Although the local university was in the process of implementing a new policy framework, and so this might become less of an issue over time, although as several of the respondents acknowledged this would not solve the problem of discrimination and disadvantage in the school system (Blackstone 1998; Mason 2000; Parekh 2000).

Perhaps fittingly then the respondents felt that nursing was a priority. Despite the disproportionate numbers of minority ethnic nurses in the past numbers have steadily fallen since the mid-1990s (DoH 1997). This was felt to be due to Project 2000, the promotion of a single registered nurse qualification and the accompanying community care programme, because it was perceived to have pushed minority ethnic people out of nursing (Baxter 1988; Ward 1993; Law 1996, for a detailed discussion on the transformation of nurse education see Baxter 1997: Ch.4). State Enrolled Nursing (SEN) had disproportionately appealed to minority ethnic groups. There was some hope that these trends would be reversed though none of the respondents considered the possibility that people were deliberately channelled into SEN courses (Bryan *et al* 1985; Baxter 1988; Carter 2000; Mason 2000).

This may be due to the majority belief that diversity is problematic because minority ethnic individuals are simply choosing not to enter the NHS. Alternatively it might be due to a range of factors. For example, certain authors have noted much higher ambitions on the part of second and third generation settlers (Bryan *et al* 1985). Several respondents also recognised this process at work:

> But I do not know whether there are that many ethnic people going into nursing, of course there's not that many British people going into nursing either... ...just going into other areas of work altogether. Whereas probably they go into the private sector where they get more money...When you think that some of these girls have A levels and O levels and things like that. Well they can go off and do a computer course or something else, where they start off on 25,000 or 30,000 a year, instead of 12,000... And I know a lot of people say, Oh money's not everything, but you ask most kids today, money is what they're looking for, a job with money and prospects (R16, p.12 & 12a, paras.40, 42b & c).

There might also be a cultural element to this, as several authors have suggested (Baxter 1988; Ward 1993). Again this was acknowledged by certain interview respondents:

> Why are you not? Well, we all work in my dad's shop, well okay, fine. That's the reason is it? I mean some groups, they're very family orientated and they work within their family, that could be a reason. But I think we need to examine, we need to ask the groups what is the problem? Is there a problem? I still think it's the religious and the family orientation that prevents them from coming forward for whatever reason, from coming into this kind of area (R21, p.17, para.57).

> Because back at home you've got this whole raft of stuff about what your status is in your group, and how you're leaving that group, you know, perhaps to do work which is seen as not culturally acceptable (R11, p.14, para.47).

On the other hand it might be due to popular misconceptions about racism in the NHS and other institutions (they were apparently oblivious to the work of Beishon *et al* 1995 and Gerrish *et al* 1996 etc.). The majority of the trust employees were clear that the major barriers are located in the communities themselves.

Although institutional discrimination as defined by the MacPherson Report was recognised by one respondent, there was a very strong denial, in line with the earlier discussion about discrimination that (white) individuals discriminate. This was partly due to increased tolerance in a multi-ethnic society, but more about labour shortages:

> So we've moved away from discrimination, we're just, we're actually saying now, dear God if you can do the job, we have to be sure that you can do the job, because we do not want to put our patients at risk, you've got the job. So that's where we're at (R21, p.21, para.73).

This is not entirely reassuring, because to rely on changing circumstances to in turn change attitudes and discriminatory practices is to invite disaster. Hancock (1992) and Butler and Landells (1994) illustrate this same problem with reference to the relative position of women during and after two world wars. Furthermore, discrimination persists in spite of labour shortages (Carter 2000).

The terminology used by the respondents illustrates the presence of prejudicial attitudes – i.e. that 'ethnic' people cannot be British and the argument that Bangladeshi people work in family shops. Furthermore, there was an enormous premium on 'fitting in'. For example:

> I mean partly in an interview you do think if that person will mix with the people out there as well because we've got a funny old band. But colour is not one thing that would ever come into it. It would be more of their personality. If it was someone who was a bit...I mean I've interviewed before for jobs and someone was, he'd been in the army before and you could tell he was going to be quite regimental about things and that won't work out there, they would rebel against that. I mean there were other things as well, that was not the only reason he didn't get the job... You have to think of that person as well. 'Cos at the end of the day you do not want to waste their time, when you know that they probably won't last two weeks out with my lot. So you've got to look at both sides. What's right for that person as well as what is right for the job. But that's a minor thing, the main thing is the experience thing (R19, pp.5 & 18, paras.19 & 57).

One respondent argued that a Palestinian nurse had experienced problems in her ward because she did not understand the dominant sense of humour (see Carter 2000 for evidence of similar processes at work). Yet Employment Tribunals have for some time interpreted 'not fitting in' as *prima facie* evidence of direct discrimination (Bagilhole 1997: 22), officially acceptability criteria ought not to displace suitability criteria (Jewson & Mason 1993; Carter 2000).

Ultimately, the majority of trust employees, those who make the day-to-day employment decisions, emphasised the importance of equal treatment because ethnic diversity depends upon factors largely beyond the control of trusts in particular and the NHS in general. It was asserted that people are treated as individuals (although much of the evidence suggests otherwise) and minority ethnic individuals are electing for whatever reason to work elsewhere.

Different can be equal

The remaining interview respondents were not as rigidly committed to equal treatment as the best means of achieving ethnic diversity. There was some recognition that barriers are not altogether structural. For example, the head of the CHC and the REC representative argued that minority ethnic communities are perhaps more ambitious:

> I mean a lot of people do not wanna do shit work. Their parents came over... In the fifties people came over to do the manual labour that white people...were able to move out because the economy was growing. And they came over from the Caribbean to work as nurses and manual labourers. Their sons and daughters do not want to do that kind of work necessarily and why the hell should they either? (R12, p.17a-18, paras.49a & 50).

There may be a perception that the NHS is or has been guilty of racism.

> Because this is seen to be a racist organisation might be one. It's because somebody's heard that, Oh my mate went and worked there and this, that and the other happened to them. I'm damned if I'm going to. And that kind of thing gets around very quickly. It's about the wider cultural and political framework people are in. The NHS is a public service if you're in a community that experiences institutional racism on a regular basis you will identify a public, any public organisation, as part of that wider framework (R12, p.17a-18, paras.49a & 50).

The unofficial user representatives in particular, as set out in chapter 3, blamed direct institutional discrimination for the lack of ethnic diversity in the NHS and the lack of an effective policy response to rectify the problem.

For this reason equal treatment would not be enough to achieve greater ethnic diversity:

> I think [a diversity policy] would go hand-in-hand with an equal opportunity policy, in the sense that we have an equal opportunity policy, which is a statement that clearly indicates that this organisation not only supports, but is also actively involved in being an equal opportunity employer. And as part of that it needs to have an action plan. I've seen too many companies with very glossy equal opportunities policies but no action plans to implement those policies (R7, p.2, para.4).

One respondent underlined the marginality of equal opportunities policies with an instance from her own experience:

Oh my goodness me. It is just there and it's rubbish. I tell you when I first started they give you all these documents about the trust that you're working for, and you have to go on this orientation thing. And I didn't receive an equal opps policy, and I think it was the Chaplain approached me and said that he was asked to revamp the equal opps policy. I do not know why they asked him but they did... So he contacted me and said, Oh do you fancy, 'cos I know him anyway, and he said do you fancy helping us out, and he said Who else do you think we should invite, and together we came up with a few people. So we started working on this equal opps policy and I thought we did a really, really good job. Anyway, we took it to the person who had requested it be revamped, and it was very much Oh (and we spent ages working on it and getting it right) and they said You've done a really, really good job here. Unfortunately we cannot use it (R6, p.35, para.119).

The belief that the NHS does not take equal opportunities seriously enough was partly confirmed by certain trust employees who stressed that it was not part of the 'core business' (for similar sentiments in the relevant literature see Baxter 1988; Jewson *et al* 1990; Carter 2000).

Unsurprisingly, then, there was a high degree of generalised support for the notion of positive action amongst these respondents. Yet only one was prepared to provide a blueprint for this. He was the head of a voluntary organisation established to increase the professional, managerial and entrepreneurial prospects of minority ethnic individuals. Part of this work involved the organisation of placements with employers to provide qualified candidates with badly needed experience. Although the programme had been highly successful, NHS employers had shown little interest, only the HA had agreed to take part.

More surprising was the fact that a small minority of the trust employees would favour certain activities associated with positive action (as Gerrish *et al* 1996; Bagilhole & Stephens 1999 and Iganski *et al* 2001 also found), i.e. outreach recruitment activities,

But on the other hand it might well swing it. That people say Yes okay, and also I think if you had somebody whom was very, very enthusiastic...I think maybe a double act probably between my Jamaican colleague and myself we might sort of do quite well. Yes I think probably thinking about it now it would probably be a good idea. I'm on the recruitment bus at the moment (R13, p.15, paras.40 & 42).

User representatives were generally supportive of the notion of positive action, although few entered into specifics, and, despite a strong belief in equal treatment several trust employees would support certain activities. However, this is not entirely inconsistent because out-reach methods would make sense in the current labour shortage, and allowing minority ethnic individuals to bear the responsibility has been one of the central themes of this research.

Goals and timetables

Although the government is using a range of measures to mainstream 'race' equality the most radical would seem to be the use of goals and targets for the recruitment, retention and promotion of minority ethnic individuals (HO 1999; Alexander 1999). This has been recommended for some time (Gunaratnam 1993), but as set out earlier there has been very little activity in this direction in the NHS. Although the *Race Equality Agenda* promised that *'By March 2000 we will set challenging targets for all levels of the Department'* (DoH 2000: 6). The targets for board level representation set out under *Vital Connections*, however, had been met by 2004 (DoH 2004a; though the means by which this was measured have been questioned, see HSJ 2004).

Although these targets were not on the agenda for the respondents at the time of the interviews, they were aware of those established by the Home Office and were also aware that a similar development might reach the NHS. When faced with the prospect of such measures there was virtually a consensus amongst the respondents. Although a small minority initially felt that they would *'concentrate minds'*, fit well with the goal-oriented culture of most organisations (Kandola & Fullerton 1998), and reinforce the need for ethnic diversity, there was very little actual support. The problems associated with goals and targets reflected those identified in relation to proportional diversity. They are artificial and arbitrary:

> It's not even in my head that I think I've only got x origin, I need some more of those because I do not seem to be employing enough. That does not even enter my head. I'm not trying to strike a balance here of white, yellow, red, pink, blue, not at all. I want a member of staff who will do a job and do it satisfactorily (R21, p.16, para.53).

They rarely reflect reality and will therefore be difficult to meet:

> I think it's a bit like everything with the government targets for the NHS, they never actually relate to the sort of community you recruit from. If you take a hospital [like this one], there are not that many pockets of ethnic minority groups that are within a sort of travelling to work distance of it. So to suddenly expect a whole group of one community that lives over the other side of [the city] to travel all the way over here to sort of meet our target statistics seems a little bit strange. Whereas if you were somewhere like Aston in Birmingham they'd achieve their targets tomorrow. But there's no sort of recognition about the locality of where people are; they just sort of set blanket targets which is not terribly logical to be honest (R17, p.14, para.49).

Consistent with the views about representation the feeling was that goals and targets work on this basis, and there is no shared understanding of what representation means. Representation and proportionality are inherently arbitrary, and questions about what is desirable and possible are conveniently ignored.

There is also a feeling amongst those already required to meet local targets that they are a knee jerk reaction to a minor problem. For example, a spokesperson for the Devon and Cornwall Constabulary – required to meet a 1% target by 2009 – argued that it would not only be difficult to meet but that it was heavy handed. For demographic reasons racism is a minor issue in the south west (Mitchell 2000). Although this position was attacked by the Exeter REC and leading academics, it echoed many of the trust's employees

> If I was to look at this organisation, there is an overt, an overtly, well like in terms of recruitment obviously there was a particular incident of a consultant and

> I think there may be pockets of it. But in my experience of my colleagues and me I would hope it wouldn't arise, but if I was told you have to recruit this person, that person, it would seem to be wrong to me (R23, p.20, para.62).

Nothing justifies such draconian measures, which imply that individualised racism is rife (argued also by writers such as Kandola & Fullerton 1998):

> It's not that managers are not employing – I'm not saying none – there are some – so I'm not saying none. Some managers may have a problem, but I think the majority, certainly the people I've ever come across shows any outward signs of being discriminatory. I suppose someone will say you've got to look at why they are not applying, but at the end of the day we all know how to go about getting a job wherever you're from...There's Job Centres, there's papers, there's ringing up employers and things. So we're all human beings at the end of the day. We've all got common sense, so really I think it's up to each of us as individuals to go out and look to get a job. It should not be that you put more emphasis on one group, and say come on we're trying to support you to get some jobs because...They could go out the same as everybody else. At the end of the day we're all human beings and we can all work out how to get a job (R19, pp.12 & 17, paras.37, 38 & 55).

Goals and targets smooth over the complex reality that ethnic diversity is restricted by various factors, including choice, educational achievement etc., which even the most critical user representative could appreciate.

In fact it was felt that goals and targets could serve to increase complacency amongst those responsible for day-to-day employment decisions:

> Because there may be more than 2% of the Chinese community that actually get to do the job. The Chinese community may be highly educated and may have greater skills than the white community in proportion, and therefore, you might say we've got the 2% we'll sit back now so we do not have to worry about it... So it may be that the Chinese community, kids in school, and the Chinese community actually their A level results are much higher than, in proportion to white kids. And therefore it may be more appropriate that we have 3 or 4% of the Chinese community (R14, p.16, paras.59 & 60).

Once they'd been achieved managers might decide to look no further. As the respondent cited points out, in some areas numerical over-representation might be appropriate. This chimes with the criticisms of Kandola *et al* (1995: 32) that targets lead to tokenism, the assumption that once the target is met managers will not extend themselves. In fact they argue that they can actually be used to control the numbers of target groups as has happened in universities in the United States (Dworkin 1981) and allegedly in the UK also (Esmail *et al* 1995). The respondents consistently argued that to be successful they would have to be sophisticated enough to take into account every relevant factor and that would be virtually impossible.

Shifting the goal posts: the drift towards positive discrimination

There is a widespread belief abroad that goals and timetables simply do not work (Kandola & Fullerton 1998). For example, those established by the Home Office are yielding mixed and sometimes disappointing results, particularly at the managerial level (http://www.homeoffice.gov.uk; Dodd 2004). Several of the interview respondents agreed that goals and timetables would fail but for different reasons, mainly by drawing upon examples from the United States,

> I do not think we're really into quotas. I do not think they work. I mean we've got examples from the States where they haven't really worked (R5, p.9, para.30).

The reason for the alleged failure of goals and timetables in the US[2] is that they have tended towards quotas (Sowell 1996a), that goals and timetables lead inevitably to positive discrimination (Weale 1983; Kirton & Greene 2002):

> I think it promotes positive discrimination. We'd better get our statistics up on disabled people or whatever... It's the same with disability. That became the same a couple of years ago we had so many disabled people it almost went the

[2] 'Alleged' failure because the evidence about the efficacy of goals and timetables is mixed. On the one hand white conservatives have argued that since the onset of affirmative action measures there has been higher unemployment, higher levels of poverty, and no reduction in pay between minority ethnic groups and white men (Glazer 1983). Furthermore, it has been accused of exclusively helping middle-class individuals and ghettoising minorities in the public sector (Edmonds 1994). On the other hand there is evidence that women and the black community have reaped many economic benefits (Agocs & Burr 1996; Walker 1997) and since the removal of affirmative action programmes in higher education the University of Texas has seen the numbers of minority ethnic admissions fall drastically (The Economist 1997; Lewis 1997).

other way. So if someone is disabled when they apply for the job, have them (R17, p.14, paras.50 & 51).

When goals and timetables are built into the management function individuals will feel pressured to meet them, particularly where performance indicators are attached to their achievement. The respondents did not mistake this form of positive action for positive discrimination, as has been detected elsewhere (Jewson *et al* 1990; Iganski *et al* 2001) they felt that it would inevitably lead to positive discrimination.

Apart from a brief period in the 1960s and 1970s when positive discrimination was poorly understood in the UK (Edwards & Batley 1978, Iganski 1995) there has been widespread disapproval of the concept in Britain (Lipsey 1987; Linton 1995) and the results of this mail survey confirm this. Ninety three per cent (247) of the mail respondents disapproved of engaging in positive discrimination in the pursuit of diversity. Yet there have been calls from unexpected quarters recently for positive discrimination to improve the position of minority ethnic groups. Roy Hattersley (1997) has persistently argued that the position of many minority ethnic people is invidious enough to justify such measures; though it is clear that the government will not consider such a strategy (Brown 1996; Wooley 2005).

In fact only one of the interview respondents felt that positive discrimination was acceptable, indeed unavoidable. It would seem that there would be support for this within certain sections of the community:

> And I know that a lot of my friends say that's the way to go, it's the way to go... They feel that's the only way to get people in... I mean a few of my friends have said Oh god here she goes again, and that's why I say I'm so different. That's why they say I'm not black enough (R6, pp.39, para.132).

Otherwise there was no active support for quotas, despite the fact that they would undoubtedly be the quickest and most effective means of achieving ethnic diversity.

The respondents of both surveys raised a number of seemingly insurmountable obstacles to their use, essentially raising and rejecting many of the traditional arguments. In essence these can be divided into utilitarian and justice-based categories (Nickel 1990; Edwards 1994). In relation to the former, the principal argument has been that without some assistance for disadvantaged minorities' civil unrest, or at least social discord, will result. As this is not in the interests of society as a whole, i.e. the happiness of the greatest number will be adversely affected, a remedy is required and that might include positive discrimination (Nickel 1990; Hattersley 1997; Meikle 1997a).

This argument did not convince either set of informants. The mail respondents were asked the extent of their agreement with the statement, *'positive discrimination is necessary to avoid civil unrest'*. 82% (215) disagreed with that statement. Although the interview respondents were not presented with these arguments directly, they were aware of them.

> A backlash if you have a surfeit of the majority and not many of the minority. It seems that they're being given status purely on the basis of ethnicity. I think that could be counterproductive. I think we would all criticise somebody for not doing their job very well, but if they got the job because of a certain reason...then they're open to more hostility (R15, p.24, para.70).

The general feeling was that it would create more tensions than it would release, partly due to the perception of unfairness by white employees but heightened by the presumption that the individuals selected would be unable to perform. The divisiveness of positive discrimination was one of the primary reasons for the assault on affirmative action in the United States during the mid-to-late 1990s (Glazer 1983; Cockburn 1991; Edmonds 1994; Sowell 1997). Furthermore, Edwards (1988) has argued that justice rather than expediency ought to direct important social policy decisions.

Several claims for the use of positive discrimination have been based in a sense of justice, more particularly distributive justice, that aspect of justice by which the allocation of social goods, such as employment is legitimately made. In the United States one of the initial arguments for the use of positive discrimination was that it ought to be adopted as a means of compensating minority communities for the effects of past injustices (Nickel 1990). *'The essential idea is that people who have hitherto been discomfited and disadvantaged in some way should now, in justice be correspondingly advantaged'* (Barrow 1982: 77).

Asked whether *'positive discrimination is required to compensate minority ethnic groups for past disadvantage'*, 65% (169) disagreed, while 20% (52) were not prepared to comment. There might be a number of reasons why people felt this way. In addition to the geo-historical objections to adopting a North American solution to a British problem (Edwards 1988), there are a number of inherent problems with this argument. In practical terms it would be difficult to establish which groups deserve compensation and which do not, and making a decision would require establishing a date from which compensation would be appropriate (Bowers & Franks 1980). There would inevitably be a degree of arbitrariness to this and achieving a consensus might be impossible. Further, it has been argued that using positive discrimination as a means of compensation is in itself unjust. On the one hand it is unfair to place the burden of past discrimination upon the present generation reversing the patterns of unjustified discrimination (Weissberg 1993), and the interview respondents readily acknowledged this:

> But I'm not going to take people just because it's like Oh right you're black so you've got the job, because that's then discriminatory against the white person (R19, p.18, para.58).

In effect those responsible for the disadvantage of minority communities are not being asked to make amends, and therefore a central component of compensatory justice is lost.

The flip side of this is that it is also thought to be unfair on those who benefit because their ability and achievements will be constantly questioned, possibly to the detriment of their self-esteem (Sowell 1997). Heilman (1994, cited in Kandola *et al* 1995) labelled this as *'the stigma of incompetence'*. Bagilhole & Stephens (1999) revealed a similar attitude amongst the managers involved in their research and this was resonant with the majority of the interview respondents,

> It's not fair on the person who comes in from say ethnic minorities, because I think they could always be viewed that they're there because they're the token goal... And that's not fair to anybody (R23, p.20, paras.58, 59 & 60).

There are as Richards (1994) suggests better ways of offering the genuinely deserving compensation. Rather than gift them occupational opportunities they are not qualified to take, which would, if it were undertaken on a national scale, reduce the gross domestic product, it would be better to maximise that product by allowing those able and qualified to do the most demanding work to do it, and then to distribute the resources generated more fairly. According to Richards it makes little sense to reduce gross domestic product, giving those worthy of compensation a larger share of a smaller whole. It would make more sense and would therefore be fairer to give them a larger share of a larger whole, that way everyone would be happy because the best qualified would also retain a sense of occupational fulfilment.

Although there was concern about the individuals involved and any contravention of procedural justice (that procedure should always be followed where established) the central concern seemed to be that it would lead to a direct contravention of the merit principle. Indeed 91% (238) of the mail informants agreed that *'Appointments should only be made on the basis of merit'*. This reflects the major criticism of positive discrimination over the years, as this principle is a facet of distributive justice and is of central importance to the allocation of such societal goods as employment opportunities (Nickel 1990). Ordinarily the merit claim can be articulated thus: *'A, deserves some good X, in virtue of some personal characteristic, C'* (Weale 1983: 160). In common parlance it simply means appointing the best person for the job – *'Aristotle's remark that we give the best flutes to the best flute-players captures this idea perfectly'* (Weale 1983: 160).

The majority of the interview respondents were less concerned about the injustice of thwarted expectations, those expectations created by the established pattern of attainment and reward (referred to as procedural justice) (Weale 1983) than about implications for service quality of employing less qualified or unqualified people (Stephens 2001). For example,

> In my profession anyway, I wouldn't be wanting to be looking at a social need and compromise in order to achieve that, because if you compromise on competencies you're coming into the areas of segregating people. Not just effectiveness, but potential safety issues (R30, p.20, para.76).

The trust employees were coming from the perspective that service provision for minority ethnic communities was largely adequate. Furthermore, few recognised that positive discrimination need not imply inability (Sher 1979; Nickel 1990).

Ultimately, goals and timetables were viewed with intense suspicion by the majority of interview respondents because of the implicit danger that they might slip into quotas:

> I mean we've tried saying to trusts you must make sure that x percent of your workforce is...but there's always a reason why not... Because it feels artificial... It feels like quotas (R11, p.18, paras.62-64).

One respondent even suggested that she would resist goals and timetables:

> At the end of the day, and I probably should not say this, but I probably won't take any notice of them. Because at the end of the day, personally, for here, it's the people, the application forms I get. And if this person looks as if they're right because they've got the appropriate experience then yes they're coming for an interview and then we take it from the interview regardless of where they're from (R19, p.16, para.53).

So there was very little support for the use of goals and targets amongst the interview respondents predominantly because they tend towards quotas. The mail informants were also very clear about the invalidity of positive discrimination. Throughout the research there was an overwhelming disapproval of this concept. The resistance to goals and timetables went beyond the hypothetical, and the government must recognise that there may well be active contravention of their wishes by those who make day-to-day employment decisions (Bagilhole 1993).

The elasticity of merit

Perhaps the most fascinating feature of the idea that goals and timetables will naturally lead to quotas is the implication that ethnicity has no relevance for the merit principle. Other than a few exceptions under the Race Relations Act 1976, GOQs, this is widely held to be the case. The common assumption is that merit is a universal concept with prior claims on morality, and that it must generally be confined to criteria, such as formal qualifications and experience. However, as Weale argues the use of merit in allocating employment opportunities and associated inequalities is not about morality at all. First, there is no universal agreement about how different skills and abilities should be rewarded. Second, there is no universal agreement about the extent of resultant material inequalities (Weale 1983: 165).

However, the assumed morality of the merit principle remains inviolable even when it is habitually, even systemically, ignored. In the early part of the twentieth century Harvard University set quotas to limit Jewish enrolments, on the grounds that Jews were too intellectual and Harvard wanted to produce 'well-rounded' individuals (Dworkin 1981; see also Kandola & Fullerton 1998: 142). In fact, merit has been regularly cast aside by North American universities to reserve places for legacy students (the offspring of alumni) and children of the rich and famous (Reed 1996). Closer to home, the 11-plus results of boys were boosted to ensure that they obtained the greater (unearned) share of Grammar school places

(Deem 1996). There is also evidence to suggest that acceptability criteria often outweigh suitability criteria in the allocation of employment opportunities. In other words 'fitting in' is sometimes more important than ability (Jewson & Mason 1993; Carter 2000).

One common reaction to the false attribution of morality to merit has been to challenge, using philosophical arguments, the justification of the existing merit system (Sher 1979; Weale 1983). However, the nature of the debate appears to have changed. As Parekh (1992: 276) has asserted *'...what constitutes merit is a social decision and a matter of social policy'*. He argues that merit has traditionally been defined in order to maintain the status quo by rewarding the qualities of the powerful. Therefore, it needs to be revised to take into account different qualities and skills associated with identity, or facets of identity, such as ethnicity (Coussey & Jackson 1991; Robinson *et al* 1994; Fine 1995).

In fact we can take this argument further, as has been done recently, and use it to inform international policy making. Fisk (2005) asks the following question: *'Do nations which we once called "Third World" make better peacekeepers? Would it not be more appropriate – if this is not already happening – to have soldiers who understand poverty to keep the peace in lands of poverty?'* He suggests that soldiers from poorer countries not only have a greater understanding, but that they are actually more useful in practical terms than their Western contemporaries.

This underlines the point that merit is much more complicated than we have previously thought. Richards provides the following justification for amending the notion of merit in just the way set out above:

> ...this does not offend against the principle that there should be no discrimination in the selection procedures, because we are still concerned to choose the best people for the work which needs doing. It is just that the nature of the work to be done has changed, so that different people become suitable for it (1994: 151).

She maintains that this revision should be motivated by a sense of justice (to make society fairer to women) and that it will therefore be a transitionary measure. This reflects something of what we have been arguing, except that we are suggesting that ethnicity may be relevant to the merit principle in its own right and that this will be a permanent revision (Edwards 1995: Glazer 1998). As Dworkin (1981) maintained, merit should be used to secure the best results for society (a contractarian argument, Weale 1983), rather than to reward individuals, and he recognises the implications of ethnic diversity for merit.

The mail respondents were seemingly aware of this contention. For instance, 39% (101) agreed that *'In certain circumstances ethnicity can be classed as an element of merit'*. In fact only 34% (88) actively disagreed, although it might be that they were influenced by the existence of GOQs. Of course the interview respondents had already implicitly acknowledged this in supporting the notion of general needs-led diversity, by arguing that minority ethnic people should act as representatives for 'their' communities. Even if this does not require greater empathy there may be a greater determination to change services for the better.

The confusion surrounding this issue was immense. Aside from the fear that quotas would emerge, the irrelevance of ethnicity was continually underlined by most but not all of the interview respondents. For example, two argued that they would take ethnicity into account in the event of a tiebreak:

No I haven't a problem with that I've done it in fact, when I've had two candidates of equal status, providing I'm very clear they are equal and I have to make a choice. I feel reasonably comfortable in making the choice, in terms of the organisational needs there. If my organisation is under-represented in terms of women I do not feel uncomfortable with that. I'd never do it officially though. I do not know how comfortable I'd feel doing that. I'd certainly feel extremely uncomfortable if I had to say to a man, or a white woman you didn't get the job because you drew with somebody and the successful candidate's black or the successful candidate's a woman (R12, p.22, para.62).

The respondent went on to argue that any such action would require clear under-representation and procedural transparency, but under-representation is a moral not a practical consideration and the implication remains that ethnicity is otherwise largely irrelevant. This interpretation was lent further weight by another respondent who advocated positive action placements. Though he pressed the business case for diversity, this was not the primary concern:

> [The local] health authority in particular has taken on positive action training and is in constant discussion with us and others, around ways and means of improving the end service delivery aspects. So there is consultation taking place, but certainly my, and this organisations' prime area of concern is to address the under-representation in employment. That is not to say that we are not concerned about the service delivery side, but our task is to recognise that there are high levels of unemployment, higher levels of unemployment amongst minority ethnic groups which are not explained by differences in academic or other characteristics. And there is under-representation in most of these companies and our job is to address that. So we focus on that. We do not necessarily focus on the service delivery side of it. I'm sure that there are other organisations that are more attuned into that area. Our focus is on employment and addressing the under-representation in and at levels of employment within these organisations (R7, p.14, para.31).

Although there is a functional question here about wasting talent (conventionally defined), the idea that services will improve is abandoned. Ethnicity cannot be used to expand the merit principle. His primary concern is morality and not necessarily the business case, because the main objective is to improve the position of minority ethnic communities rather than benefit employers. This would support the contention of Rubenstein (1986) that a business case for diversity is actually a myth, or at least that it remains speculative (Blakemore & Drake 1996).

Yet in the previous chapter we saw from the benefits associated with ethnic diversity, and the general needs-led model of diversity articulated by the majority of the interview respondents, that ethnicity *is* relevant to merit. Effectively it was argued that services would only improve where minority ethnic individuals actively represent the interests of 'their' communities, whether in service delivery or in developing policy. Surely then quotas would be the most efficient way to achieve ethnic diversity?

When the paradoxical nature of their opinions were reflected back to them, in accordance with the tenets of active interviewing (Holstein & Gubrium 1997), the confusion grew. For example,

> I think first and foremost if I was appointing someone for a job I would be looking for the best person for the job and I would have to set my criteria out on that basis. The fact that somebody is disabled or black, although that may benefit the organisation in a way, and I believe that it would. Because it would increase people's understanding, it may increase that service, it may increase the quality of service etc. that would not be my criteria in choosing them. My criteria would be would they be suitable candidates for this job? (R14, p.11, para.43).

There was some acknowledgement of the paradox, i.e. that ethnicity is both relevant and irrelevant, but a great deal of resistance to redefining the principle of merit. This also extended to the mail survey respondents in their views about the place of ethnicity in relation to merit (see above).

The general resistance to this redefinition of the merit principle was founded on various grounds. For example, the argument that it would still be widely viewed as positive discrimination by the general public:

> Social validity might also be an issue because we would advertise all our positions in a certain way, and then all of a sudden we decide to throw out a job description and person spec which is nothing like anything that we've thrown out before. And it would be seen probably by all the workforce here as positive discrimination. And that we're not legitimately being good employers by recognising the skills that someone from ethnic minority backgrounds would bring. 'Cos if it went to an industrial tribunal it probably wouldn't stand up in court either. Especially by a white man saying look I've been racially discriminated against because how could I possibly have these things which you're asking for which a white person would have difficulty in bringing? And we'd probably lose the case, and we'd probably be blasted all over the [local paper] saying the NHS has racially discriminated against a white man. And we'd say no that's not what we were trying to do at all. So the system would be against us too (R9, p.21, para.65).

Even if public perception were to play no part, it would still be difficult to put it into practice:

> Obviously there are some jobs where it is more important. Admin and secretarial jobs it's not really an issue, but certainly in terms of drafting up policies which a lot of those are drafted, then that would be an obvious area where that could work. But it would have to be done in such a way that we wouldn't be seen as just targeting people from ethnic minority backgrounds. But I have contradicted myself because I originally said that we should short-list people from minority ethnic backgrounds just to try and boost our representation in the regional office and I just do not think there is anything inherently bad about that... They bring in different skills to those you've already asked for and we haven't recognised because we're so entrenched in formal qualifications, and right from the word go, as a personnel person, we are told to draft and to look for these qualities. And this is how you draft a job description, and this is how you draft a person spec. And they're all very tailored as to how they've been traditionally done. And a lot of that is very good. But it does ignore what you're saying that we've been so focused on what the norm is, we're not actually, we're blind to the positive things that someone who hasn't got all the experience and skills that we've asked for. They haven't go those, but they've got a wealth of other experience, a background and knowledge, an understanding, an awareness which was not in the person spec, and which we overlooked because we've never drawn up a job description and person specs to take account of those things. So yes it's a good point but I'm not entirely sure how I would take that forward (R9, p.20, paras.63 & 64).

Although the point was generally conceded, and the paradox recognised, there was no way in which the majority of the respondents could see how to legitimately take ethnicity into account without having their efforts labelled as positive discrimination.

Even in the ranks of the unofficial user representatives there was some resistance to the idea. Most were happy to accept that ethnicity has relevance for merit in a much broader range of activities than has theoretically or legally been acknowledged:

> Would you say that's positive discrimination? I mean that's employing somebody because they have those skills, not discriminating against somebody on their colour... So that's different. It's like you said actually recognising people's skills that they already have. I do not think that would cause resentment because it shows that the appointment is based on achievement (R1, p.17, paras.138 & 144).

Many rejected the idea in relation to their own positions. For example, one respondent recalled her experience of applying for her current job. She had been working in a different part of the country and felt that her career was being retarded by direct institutional discrimination:

> I applied for this job and I was not qualified for it. And I knew that I was not, but I knew I wanted it. So on my application form I really sort of went to town on it. I really did and I thought I can do this job, although I'm not qualified but I know I can do it. So at interview I just sold myself I really did and it came up between, it was a choice between me and another person and it was split. And they said we'll let you know our decision by whatever time on that day. And they rang up and they said we're really finding it very difficult and I think there were 8 people on the interview panel and 4 of them wanted me and the other four wanted the other person. And the other person I think she really, really wanted the job, and in the end they decided on me having it. And I spoke to them afterwards and said Well why did you choose me? And it was they didn't tell me honestly, they said it was very, very hard, they said it was very close, and I was aware that there were two people in particular who were not happy that I was employed. I handed my notice in from where I was working before, and the woman who was preventing me from moving forward said You know why you got the job don't you? I said well because I was the best person for it. She said No, because you're black. And I was appalled by that, that really hurt me, it really did... I sold myself because I read through the job description, the person specification and I thought right, this is what they'll be asking me, and I did my research round the topic. What could I do? Looked at what was going on in [the city], this is what is needed and I presented it to them and said look, this is what needs to be done, this is what I can do. But I will need help. So I really had thought it through, and so the person who didn't get the job, I met up with her. She's working in [the city], and I said to her, in hindsight do you think you'd have wanted it? And she said Well no, she said when I think about it now it's just too much. I couldn't do it. I wouldn't be able to. Yet she was qualified to do it (R6, pp.41-42, paras.141 & 142).

She recognised that ethnicity was often relevant and that it played a part in her appointment, but she also refused to believe this and so re-created a conventional notion of merit. She succeeded solely on the basis of formal skills and experience.

Some resistance to the idea was grounded in the belief that if ethnicity were to be taken into account in the generalised way suggested above, that it would be ultimately self-defeating and detrimental:

It's got to be the skills that are needed, and I cannot see that the necessity for including cultural factors unless you were going specifically into an ethnic minority area. Perhaps that's just because I'm so used to the way that we work at the moment I do not know? But it always has been the criteria for the post and nothing else (R31, p.6, para.30).

Because there's still a lot of mess and a lack of clarity about what's happening now. We've seen evidence in situations where positive action measures have been used under the legislation where staff have got jobs under section 5.2 (d) which, as I've said, are the GOQs. But perhaps where it hasn't been thought through properly, you then have a service which is operating where you have, for example, five white staff providing a service to their white patients (R5, p.12, para.35).

She felt that where ethnicity is taken into account there is perceived to be a real danger that it will lead to segregation. Minority ethnic individuals writing policies and delivering services predominantly if not explicitly for minority ethnic communities, and white individuals similarly employed (Weale 1983). Only one respondent, speaking on behalf of her community, favoured this kind of segregation.

Another difficulty with amending merit in this fashion is that – consistent with attempts at justifying positive discrimination – it will only really help the most privileged members of minority ethnic communities (Weale 1983; Nickel 1990). Employment opportunities will still require competence using fairly traditional criteria and middle class individuals will be better placed to obtain those qualifications. In a sense taking ethnicity into account could create a minority ethnic middle class professional ghetto, while the masses remain wholly marginalised.

Conclusion

We have seen throughout this section that the achievement of ethnic diversity has become a policy priority for the Labour government, yet it has been a major policy priority for some time. However, the prospects for success in the NHS are not very encouraging. The postal surveys carried out over the last eight years have shown that trusts are committed on paper to equal opportunities but very rarely convert that commitment into practice. Furthermore, positive action has barely made any impact at all. Recent research indicates that HAs are also failing to deliver, and have made very little progress since the King's Fund reported in 1990 (Agnew 2000). There is a strong feeling articulated here and elsewhere (Bagilhole & Stephens 1999; Carter 2000) that such matters are not part of the core business of the NHS.

The interview survey provides an insight into the processes involved. The trust employees, who were all responsible to some extent for day-to-day employment decisions felt that positive action was too group-oriented and they preferred to treat people as individuals (despite the overwhelming evidence to the contrary, i.e. see chapter 3). Although the user representatives were keen on the notion, the only activity the trust employees would sanction was out-reach recruitment methods. This appeared to be because it put the onus on minority ethnic professionals and would be helpful in the context of a labour shortage.

In terms of goals and targets, towards the more extreme end of the positive action continuum (what Nickel 1990 has referred to as an element of strong affirmative action) there was a near consensus that they should not be used. It was argued that they had not worked in practice and would inevitably slip into quotas. Positive discrimination was as unpopular with this cohort as it has consistently been demonstrated to be since the 1960s and 1970s.

The ironic thing about all this is that the interview respondents were actually more radical in their way than goals or targets, or even positive discrimination, albeit by separating out recruitment from issues of service delivery. In supporting the general needs-led model of ethnic diversity they had argued for minority ethnic individuals to act as representatives for their communities to improve the quality of service provided. In effect they had redefined the notion of merit to show that ethnicity has much more relevance than has traditionally been acknowledged. However, while they accepted this position in principle they were much more conservative in practice fearing the attribution of positive discrimination and/or the professional apartheid that might emerge. The business case for equal opportunities has implicitly relied upon this redefinition in trying to sell diversity as a bottom-line issue to employers and managers (Ross & Schneider 1992, 2005; CRE 1995a).

It will be interesting to see how this plays out in practice; the Metropolitan Police Service has recently introduced just such an amendment to recruitment strategies, largely because they are not going to meet their 2009 target of 25% minority ethnic staff without radical action (Smith 2005). This will really test Rubenstein's (1986) argument that no such case exists, but however it operates the injection of moral justifications for equal opportunities and positive action is long overdue (Iganski et al 2001). We have seen from the material presented above that functional arguments may fail in the wake of unfriendly or inconvenient circumstances.

One of the central problems is the fractured structure of the NHS (Carter 2000; Iganski et al 2001) which will require greater leadership from the centre. This may not be forthcoming as,

> ...the translation of national level commitments into effective local policy would appear to require a pattern of central target setting and monitoring, and a range of potential sanctions, which there is, as yet, little evidence to suggest is high on the agenda (Iganski et al 2001: 314).

Whether the equalities framework recently established by the government will achieve the radical change necessary it is too early to say. It should be recognised that if the government wish to pursue a programme driven by strong positive action measures in the NHS there may be little support even from what have been considered natural allies (Carter 2000).

Interestingly, as will be demonstrated in the penultimate chapter, now that policy-makers have seemingly accepted the need for strong positive action measures (i.e. to establish goals and targets for minority ethnic communities, DoH 2000), then the personnel professionals and Human Resource Directors, marginalised to some extent by 'New Public Management' (Carter 2000), who might be considered natural champions of such a project, may also prove hard to convince.

CHAPTER 9:

The management of diversity

'He led a double life...He was a man of two truths' – Iris Murdoch.

Introduction

In the previous chapter it was argued that the government is seeking to take back some measure of central control over equal opportunities after a period of decentralisation and devolution. It has been argued that personnel and human resource professionals might be a natural ally as they have lost a certain amount of influence over line management as a consequence (Carter 2000). However, as discussed earlier, there has been very little sympathy from within the NHS for positive action measures in particular.

One possible reason for this lack of support would seem to be the rise of a theoretical development in the equalities tradition known as managing diversity. More particularly the model set out by Kandola *et al* (1995) has made a distinct impression on the personnel function of the NHS. The authors have argued that its inclusive, individualistic emphasis and its cultural implications for organisations make it an evolutionary step beyond conventional equal opportunities.

Although it promises to muster more widespread support than the traditional notion, there is evidence that it has yet to be widely adopted and that significant confusion abounds in the available literature about the distinction between positive action measures and managing diversity. Furthermore, where managing diversity has been adopted research evidence suggests that organisations are not significantly more diverse than those who claim to be equal opportunities employers (EOR No.87, 1998). This may be intrinsically linked to the individualistic emphasis already mentioned, because this arguably makes it very difficult to judge when greater diversity has actually been achieved.

Ultimately a paradox exists at the heart of managing diversity, whereby individualistic or group-based elements can be referred to where convenient. It is distinctly possible that managing diversity amounts to a process of self-justification for its architects and for those engaged in its implementation on the ground. Although there have been calls for managing diversity to be seriously considered for adoption by NHS employers more widely (Bagilhole & Stephens 1999), there may be detrimental consequences for diversity as a wider theoretical concept and policy objective.

Background

In the previous chapter it was clear that, although equal opportunities policies at least as a paper commitment have become central to the personnel function of the NHS, certainly within the framework of NHS trusts, there has been much resistance to influencing outcomes via differential treatment. Any attempt to impose differential treatment in the form of goals and timetables, for example, is likely to be met with hostility and may even be actively resisted in some quarters (Cameron 1993; Blakemore & Drake 1996).

However, with the government's attempts to re-establish greater central control over equal opportunities issues, it might be that personnel directors and human resources professionals become useful channels or natural allies. Having apparently lost a substantial amount of influence in the wake of the internal market, they would appear to have most to gain (Carter 2000). Yet it would appear that personnel managers are as committed as other NHS staff to the sanctity of equal treatment set out in the previous chapter and it would seem that they have sought another route out of their relative marginalisation.

From the early 1990s, according to Bagilhole (1997), equal opportunities became bound up with organisational change theory, and one manifestation of this has been managing diversity. It appeared during the mid-to-late 1980s in the corporate sector of the United States, and Kandola and Fullerton (1998) cite a publication for the Hudson Institute, *Workforce 2000*, in 1987 as the beginning of its widespread dissemination. The central message was that employers needed to look beyond white males as demography was changing rapidly. According to Jain and Verma (1996) it also emerged out of the development of diversity as a socio-political issue and the march of globalisation across world markets. Fine (1995: 32) and Teicher and Spearitt (1996: 109) add that it grew from the growing importance of human resources management and quality concerns and a backlash to affirmative action. Wrench (2005) also adds post-industrial migration and the virtual displacement of manufacturing by service economies as other significant drivers.

Although it is not purely about responding to legal requirements the impetus achieved both domestically and across the EU has also increased the momentum of managing diversity (IPD 1996; Kandola & Fullerton 1998; Wrench 2005). It fit well with employer-led initiatives of the time such as *Investors in People, Total Quality Management, Race for Opportunity*, and, the CREs *Racial Equality Standard*. It also dovetailed with a perceived growth in business ethics (IPD 1996). As far as its proponents are concerned it is the best means of securing workforce diversity (Thompson 1998).

However, we will not be discussing the concept, or related concepts, in the widest possible sense (Caudron 1994; Ellis & Sonnenfeld 1994; Robinson *et al* 1994; Fine 1995; IPD 1996; Kossek & Lobel 1996; Coker 1997 etc.). Rather the model, albeit welded together using elements of other models, developed by Kandola *et al*. The reasons are two-fold. Firstly because they have been largely responsible for bringing the idea to the UK, as evidenced by their dominance in the relevant literature (Blakemore & Drake 1996; IPD 1996; Bagilhole 1997; Thompson 1998; Wrench 2005), and secondly, and most importantly, because their interpretation has already made some impact upon the personnel function of the Health Service. The devolved, decentralised management structure which formed part of the New Public Management developments from the 1980s onwards have apparently provided managing diversity with fertile ground (Carter 2000).

Although the questionnaire survey was not designed to explore the existence and progress of managing diversity within the NHS it soon became clear that when the majority of those involved in personnel matters thought about diversity at all they were framing their ideas in the language of Kandola *et al*. Although the actual take-up of managing diversity has been slow in the UK thus far, as the authors themselves have discovered, and despite the apparent lack of success attributed to it in attaining a diverse workforce, the ground would appear to be very fertile in the NHS. Whether or not managing diversity is already dated, as Blakemore and Drake (1996) suggest, because it aims to influence workforce decisions rather than shape the work process, is therefore arguably irrelevant in this context.

However, there is a danger that the essential nature of their model might be lost because of misinterpretation and misapplication, but more serious perhaps is its reliance on the business case for diversity. Blakemore and Drake (1996) and others (see Rubenstein 1986) remain unconvinced that a business case actually exists and this is difficult to dispute despite the claims of Kandola *et al*. The real problem it would seem is that if the business case is taken seriously it can lead to general needs-led diversity as discussed in Chapter 7. The proponents of managing diversity are as guilty of this as anyone, as will become clear. Although they emphasise the individualistic nature of the concept when it suits them they are also able to emphasise its group-based elements when necessary. Playing with the merit principle in this way provides employers with the opportunity to discriminate or to ghettoise minority ethnic individuals, as needs dictate. It also provides personnel professionals and consultants with an important weapon in the fight for self-justification.

The Kandolian model

The Kandolian model works on the principle that diversity is broadly based, being virtually individualistic, and that it has positive benefits for adoptive organisations. The definition of diversity they provide accepts:

> ...that the workforce consists of a diverse population of people. The diversity consists of visible and non-visible differences which will include factors such as sex, age, background, race, disability, personality and work style (Kandola *et al* 1995: 31; 1998: 8).

The successful organisation will take on the attributes of a mosaic, where the differences come together to form a coherent pattern, in which *'Each piece is acknowledged, accepted and has a place in the whole structure'* (Kandola *et al* 1995: 31). They argue that managing diversity constitutes the next step in equal opportunities implementation.

According to the authors (and most other commentators, e.g. Teicher & Spearitt 1996) it is an evolutionary step beyond equal opportunities for several reasons. The latter is limited because it is a defensive measure designed to protect organisations against legal challenges, and is therefore exclusive because it concentrates on ethnicity, gender and disability (Cameron 1993). Because of its legalistic emphasis it is peripheral, the exclusive preserve of human resources professionals. Its final limitation relates to implementation, because equal opportunities relies on positive action to be effective. However, as discussed in the previous section there is no vital or immediate link between equal opportunities policies and positive action (Jewson & Mason 1986, 1993; Blakemore & Drake 1996). In fact they recognise this in arguing that positive action *'forms an important ingredient of **many** equal opportunities strategies...'* (Kandola & Fullerton 1998: 125, emphases added).

Conversely, managing diversity is inclusive as it embraces everyone and aims to maximise each individual's potential. This is more positive than simply reacting to possible legal threats. It is also cultural, because it focuses on the movement of people within the organisation and fits well with business objectives, thus diversity programmes are essentially organisationally specific (EOR No.78 1998), although Liff (1989) has shown that conventional equal opportunities policies can be flexible and meet organisational objectives if implemented imaginatively. In order to justify itself managing diversity must show genuine improvements, which it does, as discussed below. Because it is cultural and inclusive it is the responsibility of every member of an organisation and not the exclusive preserve of human resource professionals. Finally, it does not rely on positive action, which is held to be counterproductive because it is based in group-based characteristics. Managing diversity is inclusive because it is individualistic, although certain measures recommended by Kandola and Fullerton (1998) do bear a striking resemblance to positive action by stealth (see pp.112-114 and p.135).

The benefits of undertaking managing diversity fall into three categories proven, debatable and indirect because,

> Our review of the diversity literature has led us to the conclusion that some of the benefits claimed for managing diversity have been exaggerated. We hope that by removing some of the more extravagant claims and promises that have been made for diversity we can identify the real and actual benefits that will accrue to an organisation by adopting the approaches we are putting forward (Kandola & Fullerton 1998: 2).

The full range of benefits is presented in Table 2.

Table 2: Categorisation of the perceived benefits

<table>
<tr><td colspan="2">

Categorisation of the perceived benefits

</td></tr>
<tr><td>

Proven benefits

Access to talent:

• making it easier to recruit scarce labour

• reducing costs associated with excessive turnover and absenteeism

Flexibility:

• enhancing organisational flexibility

Debatable benefits

Teams:

• promoting team creativity and innovation

• improving problem-solving

• better decision-making

</td><td>

Customers:

• improving customer service

• increasing sales to members of minority culture groups

Quality:

• improving quality

Indirect benefits

• satisfying work environments

• improving morale and job satisfaction

• improving relations between different groups of workers

• greater productivity

• competitive edge

• better public image

</td></tr>
</table>

Source: Kandola et al (1995: 33; 1998: 35)

The benefits set out in Table 2. involve a fairly common set of claims, many of which are supported by illustrative examples, although other authors (Jain & Verma 1996) also identify the improved distribution of economic opportunities between different sections of the community. However, despite the grand claims as to the distinctiveness of managing diversity, symbolised in specialist language like MOSAIC[1], an acronym designed to capture the essential features of a diversity oriented organisation (Kandola & Fullerton 1994), there are a number of difficulties with their claims.

For example, the proven benefits associated with the practice generally relate to traditional minority groups. Staff turnover problems are illustrated using gender and ethnicity, and flexibility, though stressing the need to cater for the needs of individuals, mainly refers to maternity leave arrangements (Kandola & Fullerton 1998). Therefore, its individualistic emphasis can be questioned.

In terms of implementation the authors developed a model through evaluation of the relevant literature and tested it empirically via two large mail surveys as detailed below. The model has eight components listed as:

- Organisational vision.
- Auditing.
- Top management support.
- Planning/objectives.
- Clear communication.
- Clear accountability.
- Co-ordination of activity.
- Evaluation.

They claim that their model is the first to be properly validated empirically via survey evidence (Kandola & Fullerton 1998: Ch.6). However, none of the components listed here would be out of place within a rigorous equal opportunities policy (Coussey & Jackson 1991); as the authors more or less accept: *'Although the breadth and focus of managing diversity is quite different from that of equal opportunities, they do in fact have many initiatives in common'* (Kandola *et al* 1995: 34).

---

[1] MOSAIC: Mission and values; objective and fair processes; skilled workforce: aware and fair; active flexibility; individual focus; culture that empowers (Kandola & Fullerton 1998: 147).

The main difference in terms of implementation involves the level of cultural renewal required, because managing diversity must be placed at the heart of the organisation's activities if it is to be relevant and effective. Conventional equal opportunities has arguably failed because it has been marginal and marginalised. So the evolutionary nature of managing diversity depends upon its individualistic emphasis and its implications for cultural renewal (IPD 1996). We have already raised some questions about its ability to deliver on both dimensions, but each will receive more rigorous attention below. Before we attempt to evaluate the potential of managing diversity in any depth it is worth considering the ground upon which it is likely to fall in the NHS. In other words will managing diversity appeal to those overseeing and taking part in the day-to-day decision-making process?

The value of managing diversity for the NHS

Despite the case presented by authors like Kandola *et al* for shifting the focus of equality theory and practice, the possibility of doing so in the NHS would appear to be limited, primarily because the Health Service has only just begun to grapple with conventional equal opportunities policies (see chapter 8). Even the more centralised components are only just beginning to come to terms with equal opportunities, so how much more difficult will it be to encourage the adoption of a whole new raft of policies and procedures, particularly something as all pervasive as managing diversity? Yet it may be that it can expect to secure much greater support than equal opportunities.

Managing diversity has seemingly already taken root within the human resources function of the NHS (Carter 2000; Foster & James 2001; DoH 2003a). Although the questionnaire was not specifically shaped to explore the notion, it is possible to make an educated guess about the progress of the Kandolian model. Initially the respondents were asked to prioritise different definitions of diversity from a set list as follows, in order to identify their interpretation of the concept:

- Diversity means allowing health care to be delivered in the context of a free market (natural).
- Diversity means designing services in accordance with the expressed needs of users (user-led).
- Diversity means increasing the number of health professionals from minority ethnic groups (reflective, or proportional).
- Diversity means increasing the number of people from minority ethnic groups in managerial positions (structural).
- Diversity means ethnically matching professionals and patients to deal with specific cultural needs (needs-led).
- Diversity means changing the culture of important institutions such as the Health Service (cultural).

The results which emerged from reversing the numbers and totalling the scores, i.e. a highest priority was counted as six rather than one (and which derive from 81% of the sample – 50 respondents did not answer as required) can be seen in Table 3.

Table. 3: Notions of diversity in order of priority

Diversity type	N	Highest priority	Second priority	Third priority	Fourth priority	Fifth priority	Least priority	Total score
Cultural	216	492	260	140	39	58	5	994
User-led	216	498	230	132	60	60	4	984
Reflective	216	162	205	224	159	68	5	823
Needs-led	216	102	240	188	135	88	15	768
Structural	216	24	105	108	231	144	15	627
Natural	216	24	35	71	24	14	172	341

Interestingly, other than the question about the free market, those definitions that explicitly refer to ethnicity are the least popular (and structural diversity, the most popular interpretation of the interview respondents, fared worst of all). This would suggest a strong desire to move away from group-based identities. Furthermore, if we consider that one of the principal elements of the Kandolian model is cultural renewal, we can assume (if cautiously) that this influenced their prioritisation of 'cultural' diversity.

Fortunately we do not have to rely too heavily on such assumptions, because several respondents felt compelled to add at times fairly lengthy comments about diversity issues. From these comments it became clear that many trusts have begun to implement programmes in the name of managing diversity.

> Having just completed The Trust's 'Diversity Strategy' and implementation plan, I have found this questionnaire difficult to complete. You appear to only be asking about ethnic diversity, where as we see diversity covering visible and non-visible differences such as sex, age, background, race, disability, personality + workstyle ie all ways in which people are different.
> We also see diversity as being different from equal opportunities and this questionnaire [seems] to view them as one concept.
> * Diversity is about staff maximising their potential —it is not about concentrating on issues of discrimination
> * It embraces everyone – it should not exclude anyone
> * It concentrates on the culture of the organisation and meeting of business objectives – it is not about looking at numbers employed in different groups.
>
> Implementation will not rely on 'Equal Opps' Policy or positive action, as equal opportunities does. Diversity needs to become inherent in the organisation. Like quality, it should not stand alone.
>
> For me diversity is about more than race, gender or disability issues – it is about respecting and valuing every individual and the differences which make them special.
> Managing diversity means that managers should ensure all their staff are treated fairly (which does not mean treating everyone the same).

What is more, it seems evident that the work of Kandola *et al* is being used to guide the efforts of trusts in this direction.

We can further evidence the impact that Kandola *et al* have made with reference to the interview survey. The Training and Development Officer for the trust was in the process of organising a training programme for management taken entirely from the work of Kandola *et al*. He was working in conjunction with the personnel office of a neighbouring trust:

> We have been developing both [this trust] and [another trust] who are going to merge on April the first, the two training departments have been working together in developing a training programme for managers entitled, *Valuing Difference*. And the actual format of that isn't completely formalised yet, because as you said earlier, your project is growing and so is mine. Mine was a little new project to start with, now we have moved to a much larger project. Partly because the government brought out its human resources strategy, and therefore put equal opportunities at the top of the trust's agenda's. And therefore made Chief Executives responsible for it. And if you make CE's responsible for anything it will get to the top of the agenda. So steering groups were set up in both trusts and we'd started developing a training programme (R14, p.18, para.64).

The document presented to the management boards underlines this influence. For example, though the emphasis was health provision, it listed the key features of managing diversity thus:

- Diversity has as its primary concern organisational culture and the working environment.
- Diversity and differences between people can, and should, if managed effectively, add value to the organisation.
- Diversity includes virtually all ways in which people differ, not just the more obvious ones of gender, age, profession, ethnicity or disability (see Kandola & Fullerton 1998: 8).

It also referred to the benefits in proven, debatable and indirect terms, selling it mainly on the grounds of wider recruitment in the context of a labour shortage, better retention and increased sensitivity to a diverse range of needs.

It is evident that managing diversity has already made a fairly significant impact on the theory, language and practice of human resources in the Health Service. The aforementioned document underlines the fact that *'Some NHS Trusts have recently implemented managing diversity policies'.* Moreover, the driving force in this shift seems to have been the model developed by Kandola *et al.* The next question must be will it make the same impact on employment decision-making?

Fertile ground?

The training programme under development by the trust ran into some difficulties in that the management board of the partner trust was not convinced about its value or its intentions. Their main concern was health and safety rather than equalising opportunities. Initially the Training and Development Officer defended their decision by maintaining that they were at a later stage in their equal opportunities thinking. However:

> I think there also is in a sense, there's a sense in which there is some reticence within the [other trust] from some people on the steering group. I got the impression that there was concern about valuing the difference for the sake of valuing the difference. And it was not about recruiting the best people for the job it was about just the emphasis. They felt that the emphasis of the training might be that we need a diverse workforce and we'll go out and recruit as diverse a workforce as we can. And that's not the point of it. The point is to say are we recruiting the best people for the job? (R14, p.19, para.67).

He blamed an ill-informed conservative tendency for the break down in co-operation. Despite the lack of inter-trust support he had been given unilateral permission to proceed:

> [This trust was] very keen that it should be mandatory for managers, and the people we would target would be departmental managers. Those people who have the power to recruit and change policy within their areas because they would have the most impact. But they also felt that it was important for managers higher up the scale to have mandatory training as well. Although it wouldn't be a priority it would be those that have the greatest impact would be the first priority. Which is interesting in terms of what I said in terms of policy because policy is affected at the top but actually what goes on is affected much more by... the local level (R14, p.18, para.64).

It would be interesting to know whether the subsequent merger altered the agenda or whether the concerns of the partner trusts were laid to rest.

Although management boards are important the Training and Development Officer recognised that policies and programmes need to garner support from those on the ground who make the day-to-day employment decisions, as underlined by the work of Lipsky (1980). Equal opportunities, at least in its liberal form, would seem to fail to secure any substantial support from this quarter. Indeed one respondent actually stated that if goals and targets became compulsory she would ignore them unless the outcomes matched her own recruitment/promotion standards. So what hope for managing diversity?

The interview survey suggests that it may gain the popular support historically denied equal opportunities, at least nominally. For example, it requires an interpretation of identity that is fluid, with many implications for skills and the possession and use of relevant knowledge bases (Caudron 1994; Parekh 2000). Several of the interview respondents were aware of this fluidity and its implications for social interaction:

> I suppose we all represent the group that we belong to, and whether that's national origin or a profession or the colour of our hair or whatever it happens to be, and I think it just brings an awareness on every topic, that may not be there if they weren't... I mean what do I represent to you? What do I represent? There's lots of things I could represent: fathers, sons, just right across the range, and I think your identity changes as you move through structures or systems depending on what you are (R15, p.13, paras.36 & 37).

Managing diversity acknowledges the complex nature of identity and the way in which that complexity impacts upon individual and structural interactions. This is a notion readily accepted by many of the respondents both within and beyond the NHS.

Another concept, which lies at the heart of the concept, is the complex nature of discrimination. Equal opportunities focuses exclusively on discrimination on the grounds of 'race', ethnicity, gender and disability, managing diversity does not.

> Feelings of vulnerability, self-consciousness, anger, intimidation etc. can be experienced by anyone and can be caused by class, status in the organisation, language, background – even the food they eat. In short, most of us know what it feels like to be in a minority at some time or another (Kandola & Fullerton 1998: 97).

This distinction was recognised by several respondents –

> I think there's an enormous potential within this organisation, there is huge prejudice and I'm not talking about ethnic minorities. It's about medical secretaries, and MRS staff, and the medical secretaries don't do the filing, they leave it for us. So there's a huge amount of prejudice and entrenched views because people don't understand they haven't been in that role to know what the pressures are. It's like supply chains, if you know what your customer is and if you actually view people as a customer you would do things differently... You'd have an appreciation of what their pressures are, because we all constantly find ourselves moaning about another area of the organisation: why have they done this? They know it drives me mad or it makes my life hell...And it's just a lack of understanding and a lack of exposure to other people's situations. I mean I would like to have done more of that in terms of I've been an auxiliary into clinic and on the wards and it gives you a much better idea of the problems that people have to face. Even if you don't actually do the work, even if you go around with the staff for a day. But yes I think it's brilliant 'cos you really do understand it, and we started looking at a clerical training scheme where people actually have a cooks tour, so that you have an appreciation of what the pressures are. So hopefully you don't do those annoying things, or actually that improve the quality of the whole by doing your job to the best of your ability to support everyone else (R23, p.13, para.41).

> I think we're all discriminated against at times, not just ethnic groups (R16, p.13a, para.46a).

They were aware that irrational decisions are made on any number of grounds and not just those of central importance to equal opportunities policies. This suggests that managing diversity has an implicit appeal that its more conventional cousin lacks – the authors refer to this as inclusivity.

Managing diversity, by acknowledging the complex nature of discrimination, appears to have more potential because it emphasises individuality. Hussein Khatib, acting Director of Children's Services at Manchester Children's Hospital maintained that, *'Role models should be strong and should be committed to providing equal opportunities within their organisation, not just singling out particular groups such as women or ethnic minority groups'* (Stephens 2001: 23). As discussed in the previous chapter, many of the respondents from the trust emphasised the importance of treating people as individuals, of valuing individual traits and skills, rather than group-related characteristics. Employment decisions should always be taken on individual grounds

> But treating everybody as individuals, and not specifically to pick out things [ethnicity]... I treat them all as individuals, and although you think they're going to be very different, and when I came here about 10 years ago, I thought that, you know that people are going to be very different, but they're not (R13, pp.6 & 14, paras.18 & 38).

In short, despite some resistance at board level, it would seem that the ideas and the language used by Kandola *et al* may secure greater support from those making day-to-day decisions than conventional equal opportunities, even though the ability of the trust employees to treat people as individuals was highly suspect (see chapter 3 in particular). Having said that it might fall on fertile ground we need to consider whether it will work? First, we will present the empirical evidence which suggests both limited take-up and effect, before considering the possible practical and theoretical reasons for this.

The track record

The question here is two-fold. First, has managing diversity made any impact on the UK labour market, are organisations taking it on board? Second, if and when it has been taken up, what results have been forthcoming? Kandola and associates have undertaken a ten-year project to chart the course of equal opportunities in order to note any shift towards managing diversity. The original survey was designed to chart the diversity initiatives undertaken (Kandola & Fullerton 1994). The results of the second survey compiled in 1996 were similar and demonstrated that take-up has been slight and that where it has been adopted employers have largely failed to apply its precepts strategically. For example, of the 445 organisations that took part (a response rate of just 17.8%) – located in the UK and Ireland – 85% had an equal opportunities policy and only 28% reported having a managing diversity policy. Similarly, 77% regarded equal opportunities as an organisational value, compared to 23% favouring managing diversity. Most importantly perhaps, only 18% of employers claimed to have a managing diversity strategy compared to 71% with a strategy on equal opportunities (Kandola & Fullerton 1998).

Although the participants were clearly aware of the language used by Kandola *et al* in their modelling of managing diversity the most successful initiatives reported were very conventional, i.e. the formalisation of selection procedures and induction processes, the provision of carer leave etc. 60% said that having a managing diversity policy was one of the least successful initiatives. It did not feature in the list of priorities for the coming year (1997) but diversity awareness training was amongst the lowest priorities (13%). Ultimately 53% felt confident about achieving progress on equal opportunities but only 25% said the same about managing diversity.

The third survey in the series included 384 organisations in the UK, the USA and Ireland (a response rate of just 10%). They looked at implementation, success, priorities and confidence in proceeding with managing diversity. They found that although organisations in each country experienced similar problems, those in the UK and Ireland were more system and process oriented, whereas those in the USA were more individualistic, flexible and strategic. Organisations in the United States had made more progress and showed greater confidence (Dholakia 1999). Although the authors were slightly disappointed with the results they argued that for a relatively new concept the progress was surprisingly good and that the United States has benefited from its head start.

Kandola and Fullerton (1998) argue that legislation from Europe and the progress of globalisation will lend a more strategic edge to UK and Irish policies in time. However, a survey involving 389 human resource and personnel professionals across the country by the Industrial Society apparently confirmed that only 45% of firms have a diversity strategy even though 67% felt that it was a high priority and that 77% expected that priority to grow (EOR No.96, 2001). Ultimately it is fair to say that managing diversity programmes though progressing have yet to make a significant impact upon the British labour market. Where it has been embraced however we need to consider its efficacy, what have the results been like?

In many ways it is difficult to judge the success of managing diversity because it is hard to know what it is trying to achieve. For example, Kandola *et al* (1995: 34) argue that programme objectives *'need not be numerical targets, in fact...we would warn practitioners against using numerical targets'*. Although they argue that forecasts and projections ought to be part of an action plan detailing timetables and stages it would be difficult to evaluate their success without some idea of what is being measured. The idea that diversity *should* increase over time (Kandola & Fullerton 1998: 141) is not convincing. Moreover the individualistic emphasis as discussed below may be antithetical to the achievement of diversity, particularly in relation to characteristics such as gender and ethnicity. Without looking specifically at identifiable groups and prioritising their recruitment, retention and promotion (HO 1999) it would be impossible to gauge any change at all, let alone measure its success.

Research conducted by the Experimental Psychology Department at Oxford University in 1999 set out to test the progress achieved by 'managing diversity firms'. It targeted 200 FT 500 firms, though only 65 actually participated (perhaps illustrating the level of interest in the concept). Ultimately managing diversity firms (a third of respondents) were not more diverse than those declaring for conventional equal opportunities (EOR No.87, 1998).

There were areas of improvement. For example, 95% of managing diversity firms monitored their workforce compared to just 65% of the rest (although mainly in terms of age, gender and ethnicity). They were also more likely to provide flexible working, paternity leave, careers breaks and help with childcare. Senior managers were far more committed to their policies than their equal opportunities counterparts.

However they were less likely to have formal policies on harassment and special facilities for disabled people. They were no more likely to have a designated manager or to have more access to the executive board when they did. While line managers were more responsible for policy setting and implementation they were not more likely to be appraised on this basis. Nor were there any differences between the level of training and development offered to employees. Contrary to the findings above few managing diversity firms recognised any significant difference between their policies and equal opportunities policies, suggesting perhaps (confirming the worst fears of Kandola *et al.* 1995) that managing diversity is little more than a fashionable trend in terms of equality of opportunity and its pursuit.

Ultimately, the test must be actual results and there was very little to distinguish between managing diversity firms and the rest. Whereas 86% of senior management and 54% of the workforce of the former were white and male, the comparative figures for equal opportunities organisations was 87% and 49% respectively. Therefore, despite the apparent drive into the heart of the personnel functions of the NHS, it must be said that managing diversity has not made a significant impact on the UK labour market. At this stage it has not been taken up to any great extent, nor has it made a huge difference in terms of diversification, though perhaps by its own individualistic standards it could be seen as an unmitigated success. Now we must consider possible reasons for this state of affairs, doing so in both practical and theoretical terms.

Practical problems

One major problem with managing diversity, from a working relations perspective, is that it is not a popular alternative to equal opportunities policies. Trade Union activists in particular have expressed serious concerns about it. In 1997 the Trades Union Congress Black Workers Conference saw a motion passed against the development of managing diversity. Beyond that: *'Interviews with trade union officials responsible for equality issues revealed dominant attitudes ranging from scepticism to outright hostility, with diversity management being described as 'a cover-up', 'window dressing' and a 'softer term' which detracted from the equality agenda'* (Wrench 2005: 74). While it is possible to explain this as an artefact of ignorance and suspicion, a large scale shift to managing diversity still has the potential to disturb relations in an organisational context.

Ironically a different practical problem relates to the inability of managing diversity to distinguish itself from equal opportunities policies. The model set out by Kandola *et al* certainly experiences problems in this respect. We saw above that in terms of implementation it is in many ways reflective of conventional equal opportunities, albeit emphasising positive aspects of diversification, rather than the (legal) consequences of discrimination, and focusing on the importance of cultural renewal. Their task will be more difficult in the current climate, where diversity and equal opportunities are already used more or less interchangeably, both in lingual and policy terms (NHSME 1993). We need only refer to the policy framework established by 'model' equal opportunities employers such as Littlewoods (EOR No.81, 1998), Asda, Lloyds TSB and Manchester City Council (EOR No.85, 1999) to see this process in operation.

The representative of the NHSE outlined the direction the Department of Health (DoH) was taking in this respect:

> Yes...there's recently been an issue by the department called *Valuing Diversity* and it was a weighty document. Too weighty really 'cos it took a lot to plough through, which put a lot of people off. But we were asked to do a few things as

part of this. And the action plan was, at the end of it we had to come up with a 3 year action plan, which was to start January this year, and had to be simple, achievable and relevant. And to help us audit we were asked to run a few sort of focus groups with volunteers from the workforce. About a third of the workforce were encouraged to attend – and did attend. We got male/female divides and seniority divides as well, and they were asked a set of questions about their views on equal opps, and then there was a Department of Health survey came around, finding out what people's views were about equal opps, and what they understood about it. And we were sent the results back from that and we were asked to draw up an action plan, which we did. And we drew up 12 specific actions as a result of that, and the very first action was to give everybody a copy of the equal opps policy, because not everybody even knew we had one. The second was equal opps training for everyone involved in recruitment, and so it went on (R9, p.13, para.39).

Although the language has moved beyond equal opportunities towards achieving diversity, the means with which to do it are virtually identical. More than this the distinct identity created for managing diversity by writers like Kandola *et al* is in danger of being lost altogether as diversity and equal opportunities are conflated by advocates in the field.

Even those well versed in the language and precepts are placing its distinctiveness at risk. As we have seen already so-called managing diversity employers failed to take a strategic approach in implementing their policies, and the fact that managing diversity demands a cultural commitment would seem to be a stumbling block for those on the ground in the context of the NHS. As Dickens (1994) has identified, organisations prefer to adopt only the parts of the strategy that appeal to them.

In spite of the obvious support articulated by the majority of the respondents from human resources backgrounds, most had only experienced managing diversity in the context of a training programme. This is apparently all too common (Agocs & Burr 1996) and would suggest that NHS employers have focused on the skills part of the MOSAIC, *'skilled workforce: aware and fair'* (Kandola *et al* 1995: 35), rather than cultural regeneration. This would place responsibility for diversity issues onto the shoulders of managers and personnel professionals.

Indeed in-house efforts for the trust were confined to organising management training:

> So training is a 2-day programme which will concentrate on some of the issues which are important in terms of the political agenda. So race, gender, disability, we'll look at sexual orientation because that was highlighted recently as particular issue within the NHS. Age, but I think the main bulk of the training is about we're all different. What's it like to be discriminated against in some way? We have all been discriminated against, how does it feel? And let's look at it in its broadest sense. Let's look at it in terms of personalities and work styles, for example, and then the idea being that managers go away and change practices. So there will be some kind of assignment for them to do. That may be reflective in terms of their own attitudes and in a change of attitudes. But it may be in terms of actual practice in their workplace. It may be about family friendly policies, thinking of those who work shifts. It may be a self-rostering system. So it may be those kinds of things (R14, pp.3 & 18, paras.9 & 65).

Although diversity awareness training has been carried out, particularly in the United States (Caudron 1994; The Economist 1995a), and cascade training[2] has been used to combat a range of equal opportunities issues (Wilkinson 1991), very few models of managing diversity would accept this confinement to training, and this is totally alien to the model developed by Kandola *et al*. Whereas managing diversity was heralded as a pervasive cultural influence it seems to have taken on the form of a generalised anti-discriminatory training programme.

The central difference would be that it would be counselling anti-discrimination across a range of characteristics rather than simply 'race', ethnicity, gender and disability. Although the document produced by the Training and Development Officer stressed the need to change the attitudes of middle and departmental management and develop *'organisational practices which value all staff and improve the quality of patient care'*, there are no recommendations as to how the latter is to be achieved. Therefore, it seems a realistic prospect that managing diversity will never move far beyond an elaborate training programme.

---

[2] Cascade training generally involves training a small number of select employees, often though not necessarily managers, to train other members of staff, and for that training to trickle down through the organisation.

This would not satisfy the criteria for success set out by Kandola *et al*. In their view persuasion must be supplemented by enforcement and it is not entirely certain that the procedural requirements will be met, especially to the degree the authors view as necessary. The Training and Development Officer argued that changing attitudes via diversity training would enable the trust to meet any goals and timetables established by the government:

> I think it's important: 1) in terms of government strategies and achieving targets, and the new human resources strategy for the NHS (R14, p.4, para.13).

He seemed to view managing diversity and positive action working together:

> It presupposes that you do have the ethnic minorities applying for the jobs, but they're not actually getting the job at the end of the day. I suspect probably that although that might be happening to some extent, the ethnic minorities are not even applying for the job in the first place. So it's more a case of targeting those minority groups to some into nurse education or whatever, and then we get to a point at which we can decide whether or not we're truly giving people jobs on merit... The only way I can see that happening realistically is as a society giving all those people the same access to further education and developing themselves. Because one of the problems I think we have is, we as an organisation, in terms of our percentages of ethnic minorities do well as reflected in the local community. But as I say in terms of the higher echelons of the organisation we don't do particularly well. But then, if you look at the number of ethnic minorities going into nurse training, the numbers drop considerably. So therefore we have a great difficulty trying to move those people up the organisation because they're not there. So one has to target them much earlier on, in terms of getting them into university, into nurse education, and then helping them up the organisation (R14, pp.10 & 14, paras.39 & 54).

The best means of achieving ethnic diversity for this respondent would be to use positive action measures to ensure adequate levels of education amongst certain ethnic groups, and to introduce wide ranging anti-discriminatory programmes (i.e. managing diversity training programmes), so that centralised goals and targets will not run aground on prejudicial attitudes. This can be done (Agocs & Burr 1996) and would fit very neatly with a formulation such as that outlined by the IPD (1996) and Jain and Verma (1996), but bearing in mind the opinions of

Kandola *et al* about the use of positive action measures, it would amount to a chronic misuse of their model.

In practical terms then, managing diversity is in real danger of losing its integrity, either because of a lack of awareness, or, through the desire of those who understand it to manipulate it in order to gain support and/or acceptance. Even if these problems could be ironed out feminist critics in particular have argued that managing diversity has little hope of achieving significant change because it operates within the managerial culture it is trying to reform (Teicher & Spearitt 1996). In other words it has no immediate implications for radical change, and is guilty of the same failing that hampers most reform, i.e. that those with something to lose are expected to bring about their own decline (Thompson 1998). The inclusivity emphasised in the Kandolian model does not appear to entirely address this issue and indeed offers its own justifications for failure (again how to measure the achievement of individual diversity?). This leads us neatly into the area of theoretical difficulties.

Theoretical issues

The first major theoretical point bridges theory and practice, which of course illustrates the clumsy but necessary distinction we have made here. It is that the whole edifice relies on the business case for diversity. There is growing evidence of a link as the work of Schneider and Ross (2002) indicates, but there are also areas in which diversity may have very little to offer (Wrench 2005). Furthermore, the market is inherently unstable and things change rapidly:

> The problem is that fighting racism and discrimination will now only be seen as important if there is a recognisable business reason for it. Under a diversity management approach, racism is indeed argued to be unacceptable, but only when the outcome of such racism is recognised as leading to inefficiency in the utilisation of human resources. If a change in market conditions means that racism and discrimination do not lead to inefficiency, then there will no longer be any imperative to combat them (Wrench 2005: 78).

Therefore, it is vital that the moral case for equality and social justice is maintained otherwise they are likely to disappear in altogether in certain areas and at particular times.

But managing diversity also appears to have its own intrinsic theoretical difficulties. Whereas in practical terms managing diversity is in danger of disappearing, in theoretical terms, the problem appears to be that it can go too far in eclipsing the aims of group-based policies (i.e. equal opportunities). One of the potential problems with managing diversity is sold as one of its strengths. It focuses on individuals and therefore '...*jeopardizes the focus on strategies to advance the position of women and minority groups at a time when the achievements remain limited*' (Teicher & Spearitt 1996: 132; Agocs & Burr 1996; Wrench 2005).

Unfortunately, judging by research findings to which this study lends weight, society is not yet ready to see individuals and celebrate their diversity, because certain groups are still subject to prejudice and discrimination (Mason 2000; Parekh 2000). Although the ultimate aim must be to recognise individual uniqueness, managing diversity, it would seem, tries to put the cart before the horse.

One respondent argued that she would like to be seen as an individual first and foremost, but that white people prevent this:

> I mean even in here I mean people say things to me and I think, God they never learn, and I'm never rude to them or anything, Oh God your hair is so nice. And it may be nice, and I'll say well thank you very much. Oh God I just love the way you people do your hair...and it would be nice if someone said your hair looks really nice today and leave it at that 'cos I don't wake up in the morning thinking I'm black, or I'm a woman or whatever. I'm just a person... I mean it's situations like that that make me realise, or make me aware that I am black you know (R6, pp.28 & 30, paras.93, 95, 104 & 105).

Therefore, although many of the white respondents argued that they try to see the individual and not an individual's ethnicity etc. it appears that in practice minority ethnic people are often defined by their group identity.

Racism is still a part of the everyday interaction between the ethnic majority and minorities (Torkington 1991; EOR No.97, 2001). There was evidence of this from within the Health Service, and the same respondent argued that it was a major part of society also, drawing upon bitter personal experience:

> I tell you, when I was walking to do some shopping once and this old lady was walking towards me. It was really raining and very windy and she had her umbrella, sort of protecting herself from the wind and the rain, and at one point she lifted it up, and she saw me and she just freaked. She grabbed her handbag, she got hold of it really tightly and I stood there looking at her, and I said Why did you do that? Why did you behave in that way? Oh don't take my money. And I said Why do you think that I'm going to take your money and your handbag? Oh you all mug people. And I said have you ever been mugged by anybody? Well it's always on the news. These images and I just think flipping heck (R6, p.30, para.102).

Jay (1992) collected similar stories during his pilot study into racism in the south west. Despite the declarations of the trust employees and other white respondents that they view people first and foremost as individuals, there is ample evidence to suggest that they continue to define people in group-based terms.

Perhaps the biggest danger of the Kandolian model of managing diversity is that far from achieving greater diversity it might actually work in reverse and undermine efforts in that direction. Jones (1992) has argued that *'...if this continues, diversity could become the basis to eliminate corporate racial progress'* (cited in Kandola & Fullerton 1998: 12). One of the key elements to this is the possible use of individual diversity to obscure group-based issues. As mentioned above, Kandola *et al* choose to compare discrimination faced by individuals with that experienced by individuals from certain groups. In further underlining the influence of Kandola *et al*, the Training and Development Officer said:

> Diversity I see in it's broadest sense and that is we talk very much about race, gender, disability, sexual orientation and those sorts of things, but I think it's much broader than that and it spreads into things like differences in personalities and work styles. So one person may be very tidy and organised in their

workstyle, another person may be completely chaotic and a mess. But can they both do the job effectively? And how do you learn to value each other and value those differences? So that's how I see it (R14, p.2, para.6).

In effect characteristics like work style and personality are as important as ethnicity and gender where discrimination is concerned, according to advocates of managing diversity (Wrench 2005).

This is highly problematic. First, specifically with regards to tidiness, at interview those making the decisions will not be aware of the work practices of the interviewees, unless they are already employed by the organisation. If the interview is a selection/recruitment interview an interviewer will not be able to gauge tidiness where they will probably be able to ascertain ethnicity. Second, personality may be connected with ethnicity, in the way people speak or behave, and therefore act as a shield for unfair discrimination. Previously we saw that 'fitting in' was felt to be important, for example, the different sense of humour attributed to the Palestinian nurse in chapter 3 which was seen to be a cultural difference.

Third, both tidiness and personality may be relevant in a wider range of activities than ethnicity. Even the Training and Development Officer acknowledged this:

> I think it's about people questioning not about the fact that somebody, if we're looking at the example of being untidy, it's not about looking at somebody because, just saying they can't do the job because they're untidy but can they do the job effectively? And it's saying yeah, then that should be the criteria by which you judge them. If their untidiness affects their ability to do the job then it's a different matter (R14, p.2, para.8).

Several respondents were adamant that presentation and personality were important factors in selection processes because they were relevant. How a person would fit into an existing work setting had a bearing on job and team performance:

> But I just feel that if I've got somebody with motivation, who wants to do the job, is flexible, is loyal, has a good sense of humour then that's fine. But I think that would be the same in all my wards, I think that people think that if people are prepared to work, I think they don't mind, we don't have the antagonism around colour etc. that we used to have (R13, p.11, para.32).

Consequently the discrimination experienced by the 'unlikeable' or the untidy is unlikely to be as irrational or as damaging as that suffered by minority ethnic individuals. The very inclusivity, or individual emphasis of managing diversity, which explains its appeal may also be instrumental in its failure to secure greater ethnic diversity.

The reason for this is that group-based characteristics are being concealed by individualism (Agocs & Burr 1996). Managing diversity may experience difficulty in achieving ethnic diversity because ethnicity becomes lost in theoretical ambiguity and this may explain its appeal to the interview respondents. Many were keen to rehearse the breadth of definition that can be accommodated by the term 'diversity':

> But it's in everything, it's not just in culture, it's like becoming a parent, becoming a carer, any of those things in life that make you think about others differently, becoming a car driver when you were always a pedestrian. Those different perspectives (R23, p.12, para.38).

A typical example from the mail survey read:

> Different ways of approaching a problem, a wide variety of options or alternatives. Wide ranging differences in people, animals, objects etc.

Similarly, a respondent from the HSJ survey discussed in the previous chapter, said, *'Diversity issues are part of our staff charter. I'm even trying to avoid using the word "race". Diversity is about everybody'* (Agnew 2000: 13). So discrimination on the basis of ethnicity becomes no more or less important than that suffered by car drivers or the untidy. The desire to extend discrimination beyond ethnicity surely explains the unwitting support for managing diversity expressed by several of the respondents.

The potential for obscuring discrimination on the basis of ethnicity is untimely, because research demonstrates the continuing impact of racism and xenophobia in Britain and its institutions. It may lead to the displacement of majority complaints about equality measures, for example,

> It is not yet clear what valuing individual difference and diversity practically means as far as selection and recruitment are concerned, and nor has a convincing case yet been built up to demonstrate that employees will react more positively to diversity criteria of appointment than to affirmative action criteria. 'X can't do the job, she was only appointed because she's different!' might become as much of a slur as 'X was only appointed because she's a woman/from a minority group etc.' (Blakemore & Drake 1996: 200-201).

Worse still, it might lead to complete inertia in the pursuit of (ethnic) diversity. After all, what better way to justify discrimination for the white majority and against minority ethnic groups, than to argue that the white, middle-class, able-bodied male was employed because of their individual characteristics? To quote Agocs & Burr (1996: 40), *'In most instances they [managing diversity programmes] do not seriously address issues of inequality in the organisation arising from the distribution of power and opportunity; white male privilege remains intact'*. In a sense this means that redefining merit as the proponents of managing diversity seek to do, can be subverted in the way that conventional merit has arguably been subverted in the past, recall the discussion in the previous chapter, whereby merit has been set aside when convenient. For example, virtual quotas for boys taking the 11-plus, because it was thought that a predominance of females would be socially and economically detrimental (Deem 1996).

In fairness, the proponents of managing diversity do have a fall back position to retain group-based factors in their formulation. This involves defining ethnicity as one facet of an individual's characteristics that can be exploited by a firm or organisation to increase sales for example, or, perhaps, to increase the sensitivity of a service such as that provided by the Health Service (Blakemore & Drake 1996; IPD 1996: 2). They attempt to re-define merit as discussed previously. So we now need to consider the possibility that the advocates of managing diversity can have their cake and eat it – can they stress the predominance of individuality *and* retain group-based characteristics?

Needs-led diversity revisited

In earlier chapters we talked about redefining merit in an attempt to illustrate the value of ethnic diversity in the workforce, in trying to justify its achievement. Yet the problem with doing so was that it seemed to lead to general needs-led diversity, minority ethnic groups dealing with 'their' own problems and issues. Managing diversity has the same difficulty, because although it emphasises individuality it is prepared to use group-based factors to illustrate its efficacy, as discussed in the first section of this chapter.

Included under the heading of the debatable benefits attributed to managing diversity are improving customer service and increasing sales to members of minority culture groups. The suggestion here is that ethnicity as one individual characteristic can be relevant in a much broader range of activities than is currently recognised. An extended quote may help to illustrate this:

> The diverse workforce is also thought to impact on the understanding of customer needs. A report published by the Ethnic Minority Business Development Initiative in 1991 indicated that financial institutions were missing out to competitors because they failed to address the needs of black customers. Indeed, creating a workforce which reflects the customer market is likely to facilitate an understanding of customer needs through the associated diversity of perspectives (Kandola *et al* 1995: 33).

Although they are sceptical about the evidence to support the gains attached to debatable and indirect benefits of diversity and keen to point out the dangers of reinforcing stereotypical ideas about group members, the conjecture appears to be common to various models emphasising diversity and arguably the wider business case. For example, *'managing diversity'* – *that is, to ensure that organizations benefit from the particular contributions of women and black staff'* (Newman 1994: 184). Fine (1995) adds flesh to the bones erected by Newman thus:

> For example, if a manufacturing firm seeks to increase its market share by developing a new market among Hispanic consumers, it will need employees working in new product development and marketing who are knowledgeable about Hispanic culture... I am not suggesting that certain positions be reserved for members of particular cultural groups, or that, in this example, a non-Hispanic would be incapable of doing the work. I am suggesting, rather, that knowledge of Hispanic culture is necessary to accomplish the work. All things being equal, an Hispanic applicant may be more qualified for the position than a non-Hispanic (Fine 1995: 178-179; see also Parekh 2000).

The qualification set out here, and the later attempts by Kandola and Fullerton (1998) to question the indirect and debatable benefits attached to managing diversity, and to counsel against the notion of team-based diversity (see footnote 4, chapter 8), may have come too late (even if they are sincere). It seems that those working with managing diversity on the ground may see this kind of group-based specialisation (inherent in the concept of general needs-led diversity) as central to the practical operation of managing diversity. The Training and Development Officer was indicative of this, he argued that managing diversity would improve services in all the ways outlined in chapter 7, simply by virtue of diversification. However, in practice it would work like this:

> Well most of the reading I've done is around commercial organisations and how they've targeted their advertisements etc., much better, and have then been able to have a workforce that represents the community much better. Therefore, they in terms of marketing their goods have been able to target their goods much better to those ethnic minority groups etc. So I haven't seen it in practice though there have been pockets of things that I've seen and people I've known within the Health Service. A particular example is one Asian woman who works with an Asian community there and develops their services etc. so I assume that kind of thing goes on but I haven't seen it at firsthand at all (R14, p.7, para.29).

So in spite of the twin facets of individualism and cultural regeneration that make managing diversity an assumed improvement on conventional equal opportunities, it is possible that the principal effect will be to allow minority ethnic people to take on the responsibility of providing services to 'their' own communities. Ultimately it would seem that whenever diversity is related to outcomes, whenever it is operationalised, the result is general needs-led diversity.

In this respect the notion is apparently no different to any of the measures discussed in Section 3, and retains the emphasis underlined throughout. Minority ethnic communities should be identified (when convenient to white society) first and foremost as group members and held responsible for dealing with the problems 'they' themselves create (Baxter 1997). Perhaps worst of all it is dangerous in that it may serve in the long term to weaken the legislative equal opportunities deterrent that while questionable (Lester 1998; Thompson 1998; Parekh 2000) should nevertheless be defended. This is apparent when looking at the evidence from New Zealand in particular where diversity management was embraced openly as a strategy to head off tougher affirmative action measures (Wrench 2005).

Conclusion

Managing diversity, as defined by Kandola *et al*, is different in many ways to conventional equal opportunities. In essence the differences are theoretical, and it may be its individualistic aspects that appeal to both personnel professionals and those making employment decisions on a day-to-day basis. It is certain that the Kandolian model has already made an impact within the Health Service, and that this may have been prompted by the government's growing concern with ethnic diversity (certainly in the trust involved in the interview survey). Only with more research can the progress of each be determined. Furthermore, it would seem that the ideas and language of managing diversity may appeal to a wider range of people than equal opportunities ever has, and as Wrench (2005) argues, with a more radical emphasis and placed within an equality framework it might be that managing diversity can be crafted to become a useful tool..

However, there are both practical and theoretical problems that may impact upon the ultimate success of managing diversity as defined by Kandola *et al*. In practical terms the distinctiveness of managing diversity is under threat because those who are not aware of its existence are using diversity and equal opportunities interchangeably. Even those well versed in its language and precepts seem unable or unprepared to implement it as the authors intended, because there will be very little support for the cultural approach they recommend. Managing diversity may be the weapon that personnel professionals have grasped to counter their marginalisation in the New Public Management revolution. Positive action may be too late on the scene, but this does not mean that managing diversity will not also find itself on the periphery, the preserve of human resources and personnel departments. It remains outside the core business after all. Perhaps aware of the range of options at his disposal the Training and Development Officer appears to favour the use of managing diversity as a training programme in support of proposed goals and timetables.

On a more theoretical note, the problem is not that it may lose itself, but that it might go too far. The very individualism that makes it so appealing may well lead to its use as a means of obscuring group-based identities. The evidence seems to suggest that diversity as a phrase is already becoming fairly meaningless in terms of equality theory – it can relate as easily to plants, animals and car drivers as to matters of ethnicity or gender.

In order to retain the relevance of ethnicity the authors have tried to make it just one aspect of individuality and to show its usefulness in these terms, but all that really happens is that we end up with general needs-led diversity, minority ethnic individuals taking responsibility for 'their' communities. In essence managing diversity has not really solved the question of how to make ethnicity another individualistic characteristic. Individualisation *may* even lead to the justification of illegal discrimination.

Ultimately, diversity has the potential to be misused by everyone, assuming the best of intentions. On the part of those who seek to shift the language and theory of equal opportunities towards diversity, there is a certain amount of self-justification. Writers like Kandola *et al* have secured themselves a distinct place in the equalities industry, although *they* accuse writers such as Jones (1992 cited in Kandola & Fullerton 1998; for a discussion of the rise of 'experts' around 'race' issues in the United States see Lasch-Quinn 2001) of self-interest in trying to underline group-based differences. Similarly, those who aim to translate their ideas into practice appear to have gained more influence than before, particularly at a time when ethnic diversity has become such a major issue. For those who seek to improve the prospects of minority ethnic groups, they have been lured into using economic and work-based arguments rather than morality, even though their crusade is really a moral one.

The danger though is that all of these factions risk selling individuals into ethnically specific roles they will not be able to escape from – perpetual ethnic specialists, as has happened reputedly to Section 11 workers in social services and education. In this possibility lies the greatest danger for ethnic minority communities, because at a time when the government is trying to increase the numbers of minority ethnic people in public services, perhaps it is time to ask why? Maybe it is simply a well-intentioned response to the aftermath of the MacPherson Report. This seems a plausible suggestion. Yet there are other possibilities. For one thing it might be a simple device to buy off discontent by co-opting the more vociferous and dangerous elements into the middle-classes as has happened in the United States., this is commonly referred to as decapitation (Cockburn 1995).

Another possibility is that as ethnic diversity tends towards the general needs-led, the government may simply be abdicating responsibility onto communities themselves. The best case scenario would be that services suddenly improve because the individuals manage to successfully define the needs of their communities, ensure access and appropriate services. This enables white professionals and the government to do what they have always done.

The worst case scenario might be that it does not make any difference. Services continue to be inaccessible, inappropriate and ultimately ineffective. In this case the government can argue that these individuals were drafted in to improve things, they were best placed to do so, and if they have failed then that is a problem for the communities themselves. Should this happen, as seems likely, the Health Service and the government will be able to wash their hands of the issues and let minority ethnic communities continue to take the strain.

CHAPTER 10:

Conclusion

Key questions

A number of key questions provided the main framework for this project. The most important revolved around the notion of pursuing ethnic diversity in the workforce and particularly within the NHS. What does it mean? How will it work in practice? In order to evaluate these questions a number of others first had to be addressed. For instance, does the NHS provide a sensitive service for minority ethnic communities? If not, why not? What has been done or is being planned both nationally and in the research area? Has this potential, has it been realised? In order to draw the material together here we will summarise briefly the three sections as they appear in the text.

Failings and consequences

An enormous amount of literature, reviewed in chapters 2 and 3, underline the ways in which minority ethnic communities have been failed to some extent by the Health Service. The consultation exercise carried out in the area shortly before the interview survey took place underlined the inadequacy of local service provision in three main areas:

- Language provision.

- Cultural misunderstandings.
- The inappropriateness of service provision.

The primary focus of the interview material was communication, i.e. a combination of lingual and cultural barriers. Although commentators such as Bhopal & White (1993) have argued that this deflects attention away from more important matters, its importance should not be underestimated, because it remains a significant problem for many people (whatever the underlying cause). The primary problem that policy-makers may face in the region will be the massive discrepancies in the views of those who provide and those who use services.

The majority of the employees were happy with the level of service they provide, despite the problems their accounts often contained. It was apparent that the majority felt that where problems occur they are due to the cultural deviancy of minority ethnic communities, and that those communities ought to bend to fit the shape of the service provided, it should not be the responsibility of the service to meet diverse (therefore by definition illegitimate) needs.

One of the recurring themes of literature in this area relates to the impact discrimination has on the quality of service provision to minority ethnic communities. Yet the consultation document did not reflect that. When confronted with this the HA representative argued that discrimination is only a problem identified by activists and is not a major issue for communities *per se*. She did not consider the possibility, identified by the unofficial user representatives, that minority ethnic individuals might be intimidated into silence. As this occurs, according to Bagilhole and Stephens (1999), where individuals are working in a professional environment, how much more difficult might it be for relatively powerless individuals to speak out about institutional racism? The employees of the trust shared the view that discrimination was not a major issue. Where it did occur it was mainly the preserve of white 'elderly' patients suffering the after-effects of two World Wars or too set in their ways to accept their diverse new reality. Ultimately the MacPherson Report was blamed for creating divisions and tensions open to the exploitation of opportunists.

The evidence, as stated above, does not support these arguments and the majority of the unofficial user representatives argued that discrimination was the foundation stone of service failure. Although these same respondents did not interpret the MacPherson Report in relation to discrimination directly, it was clear from their opinions that the definition of institutional discrimination/racism provided was too weak. They consequently devised an alternative model that could be termed direct institutional discrimination, and reflected the complex interacting 'racisms' discussed by Patel (1993), whereby institutions and individuals are informed by an inner colonialism. The inadequacies of the institution, according to the unofficial user representatives, are the result of a conscious aggregation of racist attitudes and actions informed by this inner colonial dialogue.

Although this model might not satisfy the exacting criteria required in the sociology of 'race' to establish the existence of institutional discrimination (see Mason 2000, for example), there was some evidence to support their claims in fact if not extent. The 'non-attendance' policy is used to replace minority ethnic nurses where white racists demand it, but the same option is not open to minority ethnic communities even when there are good reasons to support their claims. According to Mavunga (1992) such differential treatment can only be explained with reference to racism. Ultimately a difficult road lies ahead for policy-makers eager to overcome problems of racism and institutionalised discrimination.

Plans and policies

The area of policy development in a national context is a vast area and has been ably summarised by Smaje (1995). This same author raised a number of possibilities which might have a bearing on the quality of service provided to minority ethnic communities in the near future. These, with the exception of ethnic monitoring, for reasons outlined in the introduction, were all explored through the perceptions of the interview respondents, but most particularly the innovation of the internal market. As set out in detail in chapter 4, aside from the general benefits that the market discipline was predicted to have, there were also potential benefits for minority ethnic communities.

The interview respondents felt that the experiment embodied in the form of the internal market had been a failure on both counts, in relation to the needs of the general population and to those specific to minority ethnic communities. The trust employees generally felt that there had been no discernible improvement (largely because the service was already adequate). Only a small minority were prepared to credit it with any impact at all. Their main concern was that the Patient's Charter (PC) had created an enormous amount of expectation that could not be satisfied and a compensation culture to rival that of the United States. As minority ethnic individuals were viewed by the majority of the trust employees as opportunists, it may be surmised that they have misused the PC to the greatest extent.

The user representatives were generally more concerned about the role of the HA. The head of the CHC argued that the rate of reform had prevented it from successfully defining its role, but more than this, that it would not have been able to apply the pressure on providers anyway. It was operating within the context of severe resource constraints (as were providers) and removing contracts would have destabilised local services.

The unofficial user representatives were much more cynical, and one in particular, who had direct experience of dealing with the HA, argued that it had not carried out its function as a purchaser as had been hoped (by commentators such as Hopkins & Bahl 1993) because it did not want to create 'a fuss'. It wanted a quiet life and wanted to provide trusts with the same. In fact, the representative of the HA confirmed this to some extent by virtually dismissing the promises that had been made, and in emphasising the value of user participation revealed a disturbing ulterior motive. It seems that where users have been involved in the policy-making process it has largely been an exercise in buying off discontent, to generate sympathy for the plight of providers. (This reflects the ulterior motives which may have influenced the adoption of managing diversity policies as outlined in chapter 9; i.e. that trusts can either avoid diversification by emphasising the individualistic aspects or place the main responsibility for improving service provision with minority ethnic communities themselves by emphasising the group-based aspects of the concept.) Consequently, it was apparent that the reforms, just as many have argued, did not deliver on their promise. Furthermore, on the limited evidence provided there was little confidence that the development of PCGs would lead to meaningful reform.

In terms of the policy promises demanded by the local community, as just stated, there seemed little hope that language provision and the cultural awareness of white staff in the region would improve significantly in the near future. Trust employees were satisfied with their current procedures, which appear to revolve around, in many cases, allowing the friends, relatives and professional acquaintances to provide informal interpreting services. Where this fails minority ethnic members of staff are called in to fill the breach. Similarly, the prospect of establishing universal CAT to reduce the level of cultural misunderstandings, flawed though it undoubtedly is, would appear to be small. Even then minority ethnic members of staff have been encouraged to take on the task without adequate support, and on a day-to-day basis they are expected to act as counsellors for their white colleagues. As Baxter (1988) maintained well over a decade ago, the attention of minority ethnic staff is directed to the needs of minority ethnic communities when it suits the white majority.

One respondent even suggested that this reliance on minority ethnic health workers ought to be formalised into a supportive network for white colleagues. No doubt this would not alter the unrecognised and unrewarded nature of the activity (Baxter 1988; Bagilhole & Stephens 1997). The persistent message appeared to be – it's 'their problem let 'them' deal with it, while 'we' (white health workers, managers and administrators) continue to concentrate on the core business.

Ethnic diversity: its shape and implications

Having said all this, the policy framework for dealing with minority ethnic health needs sketched out in the HAs report and action plan could be viewed as an example of best available practice. For instance, Greenwood (1997) set out the initiatives taken by Birmingham Health Authority in this light, which included:

- Cultural awareness training for all staff in the area.
- Quarterly meetings with providers.
- Links with the local university to establish the best means of recruiting more minority ethnic students onto health-based programmes.
- The development of 'community mums', a broadly based link working service.

There were slight differences between the policy frameworks. For example, in Birmingham there were quarterly meetings with providers, which may have been part of the local HAs plans, but if so I was not made aware of them. Furthermore, although the 'community mums' initiative was largely a link working service, it also provided link workers with future opportunities to train as health professionals, an innovation that was not recognised by the local HA.

Other than this there were few differences between the two policy frameworks, and so it is possible to conclude, taking Greenwood's recommendation for granted that the HA is an exemplar. Yet despite the promises that had been made there was very little commitment to their delivery. The HA representative continually stressed the obstacles as she saw them – resource constraints and small numbers. This would appear to underline the claim that '...race-related policies which are not put into meaningful practice serve as a protective cover allowing the institution to sit back and make no real change'

(Torkington 1991: 26). The effects of New Public Management, as identified by Carter (2000), appear to have enabled NHS managers to dismiss equality issues and avoid change.

Even if proposed policies were put into place there must be some doubts about their transformative potential. There is no recognition of the part that discrimination and/or racism play in the failure of the Health Service to provide a sensitive and appropriate service to a diverse society (Ahmad 1993a; Fernando 1993; Batsleer et al 2003). The answer seems to be to challenge the false, though well meaning, assumptions of white health workers, and to give the bulk of responsibility over to minority ethnic groups and individuals wherever possible.

As set out in the third section, this brings into sharp relief the role of minority ethnic health workers and the practical implications of greater ethnic diversity. Stubbs (1993) has questioned the traditional focus on interpreting and cultural awareness and the implications for minority ethnic workers. He suggests that it is vital that their role should be clearly articulated, and where that requires (ethnically) specific activities then that ought to be recognised and adequately rewarded (see also Baxter 1988, 1997; Anionwu 1996). One of the key issues for the local communities as set out in the report and action plan of the HA was the achievement of greater ethnic diversity in the local workforce. This reflects the recommendations of several major reports recently, for example, Alexander (1999), MacPherson (1999), Parekh (2000) and is consequently a policy priority for the Labour government (Straw 1999; DoH 2000; HO 1999; DoH 2003a).

The value of ethnic diversity was first expressed, it seems, in the context of the higher education system of the United States and the commercial sector quickly moved to embrace diversity in a much broader sense (Ross & Schneider 1992). This became the business case for equal opportunities and despite much scepticism (Rubenstein 1986; Hancock 1992; Blakemore & Drake 1996) was adapted by the CRE to form a quality case for the public sector.

The benefits of greater ethnic diversity are thought to include, as discussed in chapter 4, increased social harmony, the engagement of the full range of available talent, but most importantly, the ability to provide more sensitive services to a diverse community. The evidence is not altogether convincing on any of these points and the shape of ethnic diversity has only really been hinted at. The primary objective of the third section was to explore this issue through the perceptions of the mail and interview respondents. Although the trust employees were not happy with the whole notion of 'representation' particularly in a numerical sense, they were able to identify a number of benefits, many of which feature in the relevant literature. Indeed there was something of a consensus throughout that greater ethnic diversity would improve the standard of health care in the UK.

There was a certain amount of agreement among the interview respondents at least about the shape that diversity ought to take. It was interesting to note that the alternatives proposed by Iganski and Johns (1998) were not exhaustive, see Table 4.

Table 4: Models of ethnic diversity

Diversity model	Profile of each model
Proportional diversity	Here the objective is to achieve a workforce that reflects society, using either a local or national benchmark
Structural diversity	Although structural diversity can be operationalised in proportional terms, the central difference between the models is the policy emphasis. The latter prioritises diversity in executive and managerial positions. It is possible to achieve proportional diversity without affecting the upper echelons of an organisation (Law 1996)

Needs-led diversity	This notion attempts to tailor diversity directly to the needs of patients and users. It comes in various shapes i.e. segregational, specific and general. It requires that minority ethnic individuals take responsibility for the needs of 'their' communities

The interview respondents were asked to describe what ethnic diversity would look like and how it would work in practice. Generally, their interpretations altered as the interviews progressed. Invariably they began from a position of proportionality, until it became clear that this could be contained by ensuring that those recruited remain at the lower and lowest levels of an organisation. The overwhelming majority then drifted through the structural model – prioritising diversity at the higher and highest levels (NAHA 1988; NHSE 1993) – with a view to getting minority ethnic individuals throughout the organisation to work to actively improve the service provided to 'their' communities.

Essentially the respondents favoured what Iganski and Johns (1998) referred to as needs-led diversity, a form of diversity that is shaped by the needs of minority ethnic communities. This works on the basis of representation. At the more extreme end of the continuum (which emerged out of the interview data) lies segregational needs-led diversity, where minority ethnic communities have their own separate service(s). The Chinese community in the research area had asked for their own clinic but this would not be provided due to resource constraints (as they had been informed) but also because of the danger of enhancing societal tensions (which they had not). A compromise was proposed, what we have called specific needs-led diversity, this would very much reflect the legal notion of genuine occupational qualifications, although there is a great deal of confusion around this whole area. This would require that minority ethnic health workers should be available wherever necessary to deal with specific issues.

However, it soon became clear that the way in which the majority of the interview respondents viewed diversity was general needs-led diversity, expanding the areas in which ethnicity is seen to be relevant. Minority ethnic individuals are expected to work together, throughout the organisation, to actively improve the service to 'their' communities. In other words they would become community representatives. Whether or not this was what the local communities wanted when they demanded greater ethnic diversity is impossible to determine, and the debate about the willingness or ability of individuals to act as representatives has been going on for some time. The essential danger of ethnic diversity as a means of improving services to minority ethnic communities is that they will be charged with making the improvements, and where they are not able to do so, due to marginalisation (i.e. section 11 posts, Penketh & Ali 1997), the alleged deviant nature of minority ethnic communities will be underlined. Even minority ethnic communities cannot solve the problems that 'they' create.

Despite the fact that ethnic diversity, appears to tend inevitably towards the general needs-led and the problems this creates the government have made the pursuit of ethnic diversity a key policy priority for the public sector. Their strategy involves the renewed centralisation of equal opportunities after the perceived failure of managerial devolution (Carter 2000) and an attempt to mainstream 'race' equality issues (see chapter 8). Throughout the relevant literature calls for more radical, though legal, measures have been sounded. Many commentators favour the adoption of strong positive action measures (Parekh 2000; Iganski *et al* 2001) but there may be difficulties with implementation even though policy appears to be moving in this direction to some extent (DoH 2000; DoH 2003a).

Repeated survey evidence, to which this research lends weight, shows that equal opportunities has been slow to develop within the NHS, and there has been great resistance to the use of positive action, particularly the establishment of goals and targets (Cameron 1993: Blakemore & Drake 1996). Although there are areas of good practice they remain all too uncommon, and are located in the more diverse areas, which is not sufficient due to geographical and demographic change (Straw 1999).

The interview survey provides an insight into the processes at work, and the principal issue for those making day-to-day employment decisions it would seem is individualism. They want to treat people as individuals in spite of the fact that all the evidence points to the contrary. There was very little support at all for goals and targets, even from the unofficial user representatives, as many feared they would inevitably lead to quotas. It may be as Hurstfield (1998) suggested that NHS boards need to be convinced about the value of equal opportunities in general and positive action in particular, but it is similarly important to persuade those at grassroots level (Lipsky 1980). The irony is that in many ways the respondents were more radical than the government, and even went beyond the use of positive discrimination, by effectively redefining the merit principle to give a much larger role to ethnicity. In short, that people could and perhaps should be employed taking their ethnicity into account, because ethnicity has implications for the performance of occupations in a service setting (as maintained by the CRE 1995b, for example).

All this really demonstrates, however, is that the rhetoric that has grown up around the issue of the business case for equal opportunities and the practical worth of ethnic diversity has been widely disseminated. When these implications were reflected back at the respondents (as per the active interviewing method outlined by Holstein and Gubrium 1997), where they recognised the paradox which was relatively rare, they quickly retreated to the safety of the status quo – i.e. that ethnicity is largely irrelevant and equal treatment is paramount.

Carter (2000) speculated that policy-makers committed to more radical, centralised equal opportunities measures might be able to rely on the human resources and personnel professionals in the NHS. The argument was that as they had been effectively undermined by the decentralisation of management, they would be natural allies. Yet it soon became clear from the mail and the interview surveys that they may have already found a means of justifying their existence and possibly greater influence – namely managing diversity. This is a fairly new addition to equalities theory and practice, and is essentially individualistic. The mail survey indicated that the model devised by Kandola *et al.* (1994, 1995, 1998) has begun to make an impact on the personnel function of the NHS, and this was supported by the interview data – the trust were in the process of organising an managing diversity training programme. The cultural implications for managing diversity are not being heeded it seems, as it is turned into a more comprehensive version of anti-discriminatory training. It could be that this is due to the theoretical blurring that has occurred between matters of equal opportunities and diversity, or, in good management theory style, it could be that an exercise in self-justification has been adapted even further to that end.

Even if managing diversity was employed in exactly the manner that Kandola *et al.* (1995) advise it has the potential to be extremely dangerous (Wrench 2005). On the one hand it encourages diversity to be stretched beyond meaningful bounds, so that personality and workstyle are viewed as equally important (in terms of evaluating discrimination) as group-based identities such as ethnicity, gender and disability. At times, as both sets of respondents showed, this can extend to ridiculous proportions, to take into account bio-diversity (that diversity can include everything including plants and flowers as one mail respondent suggested) for instance. The risk is that this could provide employers with an ideal opportunity to discriminate against minority groups and perhaps get away with it. For example it would be perfectly reasonable – theoretically at least – to recruit middle-class, able-bodied, heterosexual white males almost exclusively and argue that each was selected, promoted etc. on the basis of their unique individual characteristics, and not because they happen to be white and male. Kandola and Fullerton (1998: 20) criticise the defensive legalistic emphasis of conventional equal opportunities, but go on to say, *'...it is important to recognise that anti-discrimination legislation covers different subjects in different countries. By adopting a diversity-oriented approach organisations can prepare themselves for any eventuality'*. They redefine equal opportunities in individualistic terms with potentially discriminatory results.

On the other hand, managing diversity provides employers with the option of redefining merit by emphasising group-based characteristics in harmony with the business case for equal opportunities. It tries to square the circle by using group-based identities where they will help employers, and even if we are to take a charitable view of this and point to the lengths the authors later go to question such notions (Kandola & Fullerton 1998), the idea has certainly influenced those who intend to implement their ideas. (See for example the example of managing diversity working in practice offered by the Training and Development Officer in chapter 9). If a gap in the market exists in relation to the Chinese community, for example, then it would be advisable to employ Chinese people to exploit it. They are the surest route into that community. In the same way it might be possible to apply the same argument to the operation of the Health Service echoing the quality case for diversity (CRE 1995b).

The problem is that whichever method is used to achieve diversity, and however diversity is operationalised, it unerringly ends up in theoretical terms (and probably in practice, judging by the history of ethnic diversity in the NHS) as general needs-led diversity. The result of this is that we end up with the same segregation; minority ethnic communities dealing with 'their' own issues and problems while the mainstream service remains largely untouched. This it seems is one of the primary recurring features of ethnic relations in the NHS.

Summary

The Health Service fails to provide an adequate service to minority ethnic communities, certainly in the research area and according to the relevant literature. However, there does not appear to be any real intention to solve the problem. The central contention appears to be that diverse needs are not part of the core business of the NHS and that if minority ethnic communities are not satisfied with the existing provision, then it is their responsibility to change things. One way in which this might be done is to pursue greater ethnic diversity in the workforce, and particularly at the higher and highest levels. This has been a long-term demand in the literature (Baxter 1988, 1997; Bagilhole 1997; Mason 2000; Parekh 2000; Iganski *et al* 2001), has been a central thrust of official reports (NAHA 1988; Alexander 1999; MacPherson 1999; Parekh 2000) and featured strongly in the demands of the local communities.

Diversity is going to be difficult to achieve, however, because even if the government are successful in reclaiming centralised control over the personnel function of the NHS there promises to be firm opposition to anything that resembles differential treatment. Furthermore, it appears that the natural allies of the government in this enterprise, namely personnel directors and human resources professionals, have already launched their bid for greater influence under a competing flag, that of managing diversity. Even if ethnic diversity were to be achieved throughout the Health Service, there is a very real danger that it will lead to greater marginalisation and isolation for minority ethnic individuals, and may offer nothing in terms of improved services. For when the skin is peeled away from ethnic diversity needs-led diversity invariably emerges. The implicit message seems to be if they improve things then that is a bonus; but if they do not or cannot then no more can be done. Until the service recognises that it must provide a sensitive service to everyone, and that *that* is its core business the failure, taking into account some regional and marginal improvements, will continue.

APPENDICES

APPENDIX 1: GLOSSARY OF TERMS

Black – Generally used to denote political organisation amongst minority ethnic communities (Sivanandan 1984). For example, the participating Chinese organisation identified its members as Black.

Culture – *'Cultural norms provide guidelines for understanding and action, guidelines which are flexible and changing, open to different interpretations across people and across time, structured by gender, class, caste and other contexts, and which are modulated by previous experience, relations, resources and priorities'* (Ahmad 1996: 190).

Discrimination – Under the relevant legislation (the Race Relations Act 1976) discrimination comes in different forms. Direct discrimination simply means less favourable treatment on the basis of one's 'race', ethnicity, ethnic or national origins etc. although it is possible to be guilty of direct discrimination simply by responding to the discrimination of others – i.e. by employing a white shop assistant to assuage white customers. Indirect discrimination refers to policies or procedures that although applied equally to everyone have the effect of disproportionately disadvantaging one section of the community to their detriment, and which have no bearing on the job in question. The MacPherson Report thrust institutional discrimination (racism) onto the agenda, but was too weak for some (McLaughlin & Murji 1999) and too strong for others (the police service and the right wing media). Here we also talk about direct institutional discrimination – the tendency for majority individuals to consciously create structures which reflect their own interests and respond to their needs.

Ethnicity – *'Shared origins or social background; shared culture and traditions that are distinctive, maintained between generations, & lead to a sense of identity and group; and a common language or religious tradition'* (Senior & Bhopal 1994: 330). Ethnicity can be internally or externally ascribed, or both (Kelleher

1996). I have tried to acknowledge the contextual nature of ethnicity and explore its relationship to health provision (Ahmad 1995; Nazroo 1997).

Ethnocentric – A tendency to normalise one's own culture or belief system and to marginalise or exclude that of others. In terms of health care this would simply mean that provision is geared to the needs of one community (in this case the white majority) preventing sensitive provision to other communities. Health problems and underutilisation are generally explained with reference to cultural deficiency rather than structural factors (Senior & Bhopal 1994).

Minority ethnic groups/communities – There has been a great deal of controversy about culture and ethnicity in the literature (Sheldon & Parker 1992; Smaje 1995; Law 1996; Hillier & Kelleher 1996), here however minority ethnic communities stand for 'visible' minorities, that is, visible by virtue of skin colour or cultural symbolism. This is justifiable in that the purpose of the research was to explore the appropriateness of services, rather than to explore relative health status or outcomes, and because this allowed the respondents room to articulate their own notions of ethnic diversity. As Senior and Bhopal (1994: 330) suggest *'definitions of ethnicity may need to be devised to suit the needs of a particular research project'*. However, national, religious or ethnic identities are differentiated where necessary, particularly in terms of respondent definitions and the presentation of other research findings. This is not to negate the experiences of white minorities (i.e. the Irish, Hickman & Walter 1997, the Polish or the majority of travellers) merely to parallel the recent priorities of government which have been to improve the position of 'black' and 'Asian' groups (NHSME 1993).

Needs-led diversity – This is a form of ethnic diversity that is pursued in order to meet the specific needs of minority ethnic communities. This is legitimate under the provisions of the RRA 1976 in a limited number of areas however there are various types of needs-led diversity as illustrated in chapter 7.

New Commonwealth – An official label attached to minority ethnic people from Commonwealth countries, including Pakistan only until 1972 (Australasia and Canada, the Old Commonwealth). *'It is often viewed as a euphemism for 'black'* (Baxter 1988: 2).

Proportional diversity – Unlike needs-led diversity, proportional diversity is simply about numbers, attempting to reflect the local or national population in the workforce. It is organically related to the notion of positive action (in particular goals and targets)

Structural diversity – Although structural diversity can be subsumed under proportional diversity it need not be. Structural diversity essentially reflects a policy priority to diversify the higher and highest areas of the labour market, to get more minority ethnic people into positions of influence.

'Race' – Wherever this term appears – unless as part of a quote – it will be enclosed by inverted commas, to denote the pseudo-scientific nature of the term. In reality scientists have continually shown 'race' to be a social construct not a genuine biological category (Miles 1989; Bradby 1995).

Racism – Despite the scientific evidence to support the non-existence of 'race', it has been argued in some circles that racism ought to be retained as a concept because of the popular perception that it exists and to provide a rallying point for resistance (Miles 1989; Bradby 1995; Mason 2000). Although it is widely recognised that racism comes in many guises and that 'racisms' is more appropriate, this is not the way that racism will be understood here. For the purposes of this research, as we are talking about the relationship between white health workers their colleagues and patients, racism refers to *'the structural* *manifestation of power inequalities'* (Thorogood 1989: 320). This means fewer life chances, greater disadvantage and more ill-health (Kelleher 1996).

APPENDIX 2: ABBREVIATIONS

AMBC – Asian Mother and Baby Campaign

CAT – Cultural Awareness Training

CRE – Commission for Racial Equality

DoH – Department of Health

DHSS – Department of Health and Social Security

ENB - English National Board for Nursing, Midwifery and Health Visiting.

EOC – Equal Opportunities Commission

EOR – Equal Opportunities Review

GOQ – Genuine occupational qualification

HA – Health Authority

MD – Managing Diversity

NAHA – National Association of Health Authorities

NAHAT – National Association of Health Authorities and Trusts (superseded NAHA)

OPCS – Office of Population Censuses and Surveys

PA – Positive action

PCGs – Primary Care Groups

PD – Positive discrimination

REC – Racial Equality Council

SEN – State Enrolled Nursing

SRN – State Registered Nursing

UKCC – United Kingdom Central Council

APPENDIX 3: QUESTIONNAIRE

DIVERSITY IN THE NHS: A SURVEY

Please tick or circle the appropriate answer and give details where necessary   [   ]

DIVERSITY

In recent times much policy exhortation has focused on the issue of achieving an ethnically diverse workforce, in order to increase the sensitivity of health provision.

1. Below is a list of statements detailing the way in which diversity has been interpreted, please rank them in order of priority, annotating 1 as the highest priority, and 6 as the lowest:

Diversity means allowing health care to be delivered in the context of a free market.   _

Diversity means designing services in accordance with the expressed needs of users.   _

Diversity means increasing the number of health Professionals from minority ethnic groups.   _

Diversity means increasing the number of people from Minority ethnic groups in managerial positions.   _

Diversity means ethnically matching professionals and Patients to deal with specific cultural needs.   _

Diversity means changing the culture of important Institutions such as the health service.   _

2. Below are a number of statements relating to diversity in the workforce, please indicate your agreement, disagreement or neutrality by circling the appropriate number, where: 1 = strongly agree; 2 = agree; 3 = neutral; 4 = disagree; and 5 = strongly disagree:

Services ought to be designed according to the expressed needs of users.   1   2   3   4   5

Resources are too scarce to permit a user-led service.   1   2   3   4   5

Users are not necessarily the best placed to judge their own health needs.   1   2   3   4   5

Services would improve by increasing the number of minority ethnic health workers.   1   2   3   4   5

A workforce which reflects the community would be better equipped to meet its needs.   1   2   3   4   5

The proportion of ethnic minority health workers should correspond with that in the local area.   1   2   3   4   5

Minority ethnic workers should act as representatives for their respective groups.	1	2	3	4	5
Services have improved where the workforces is diverse.	1	2	3	4	5
Minority ethnic groups should be represented at all levels in the health service.	1	2	3	4	5
Minority ethnic communities need more role models in the context of employment.	1	2	3	4	5
A diverse workforce would cultivate trust between providers and communities.	1	2	3	4	5
Diversity is a matter of social justice.	1	2	3	4	5
Diversity would maximise the talent in society.	1	2	3	4	5
Diversity makes good business sense.	1	2	3	4	5
Some needs can only be met by workers from the same ethnic backgrounds as users.	1	2	3	4	5
Ethnicity is more important than qualifications.	1	2	3	4	5
Diversity is important in terms of one-to-one provision.	1	2	3	4	5
Patients prefer workers from their own ethnic group.	1	2	3	4	5
Diversity would lead to professional segregation.	1	2	3	4	5
Ethnic matching might be used to excuse racism.	1	2	3	4	5
A diverse workforce would reduce discrimination.	1	2	3	4	5
For diversity to be valued the culture of the Health service would have to change.	1	2	3	4	5
There are no barriers to minority ethnic Recruitment and promotion.	1	2	3	4	5
The practical value of diversity is unclear.	1	2	3	4	5
Diversity is a divisive concept.	1	2	3	4	5
Diversity is racist because group identity is	1	2	3	4	5

340

held to be more important than individuality.

Diversifying the workforce would ease social tensions.	1	2	3	4	5

EQUAL OPPORTUNITIES POLICY

	Yes	No
3. Does your trust/unit have a written equal opportunities policy?		☐
☐		
4. Does the policy cover ethnicity?	☐	☐
5. Does your trust/unit have a draft equal opportunities policy?	☐	☐

6. If there is a draft equal opportunities policy, when is it likely to be formally approved?...
....

ACTION PLANS

In 1992 the Employment Department issued a 10-point plan for employers, encouraging them to meet the goals set out under the Opportunity 2000 campaign. Action plans detailing action taken or planned were to be submitted to the NHSME.

	Yes	No
7. Does your trust/unit have an action plan?	☐	☐
8. Does the action plan cover ethnicity?	☐	☐
9. Is the plan oriented to service provision or employment?		
10. Is your trust/unit currently formulating an action plan?	☐	☐

RECRUITMENT AND SELECTION

	Yes	No
11. Are recruitment and selection processes for employment regularly reviewed?	☐	☐
12. Are person specifications always drawn up for all employment vacancies?	☐	☐
13. Are records always kept of the reasons for short listing or non-short listing of job applicants	☐	☐

14. Are records always kept of the reasons for appointment   □   □
or non-appointment of job applicants?

15. Are records regularly analyzed for equal opportunities   □   □
purposes?

16. Are the selection processes for training regularly reviewed?   □   □

17. Is your trust/unit having any recruitment/retention problems   □   □
for some groups of staff? *(If yes, please give details)*
....
....
....
....

HARASSMENT

                                                   Yes   **No**

18. Is racial harassment included in the staff discipline and   □   □
grievance procedures?

19. Does your trust/unit have an established procedure which   □   □
concerns racial abuse and harassment of staff by patients and visitors?

20. To whom would staff make complaints of harassment in the first instance?
....
....
....

21. Is there a counselling or support facility available for staff who have   □   □
suffered harassment? *(If yes, please provide details)*
....
....
....
....

EQUALITY AUDIT AND ETHNIC MONITORING

An audit involves a regular appraisal of the workforce to establish what human resources are available and to identify where they are within the organisation. It also involves an evaluation of employment practices to prevent legal challenges.

                                                   Yes   **No**

22. Has your trust/unit conducted an equality audit?   □   □

23. When was it last carried out?
....
....
....

24. Has a report been produced as a result of the audit? ☐ ☐

25. Has any action been taken? ☐ ☐
   (If yes, please specify)
   ....
   ....
   ....
   ....

26. Is an audit being planned? ☐ ☐

27. Bearing in mind the demographic profile of the area in which your trust/unit recruits how do you feel 'Black' and 'Asian' minority ethnic groups (as defined in the 1991 Census) are represented in the following areas?

	Underrepresented		Overrepresented		Well represented	
	'Black' groups	'Asian' groups	'Black' groups	'Asian' groups	'Black' groups	'Asian' groups
Medical and dental	☐	☐	☐	☐	☐	☐
Nursing and midwifery	☐	☐	☐	☐	☐	☐
Student nurses	☐	☐	☐	☐	☐	☐
All other nursing	☐	☐	☐	☐	☐	☐
Professional and technical	☐	☐	☐	☐	☐	☐
Scientific and professional	☐	☐	☐	☐	☐	☐
P.A.M.S.	☐	☐	☐	☐	☐	☐
Admin and clerical	☐	☐	☐	☐	☐	☐
Works/maintenance	☐	☐	☐	☐	☐	☐
Ancillary	☐	☐	☐	☐	☐	☐
Ambulance	☐	☐	☐	☐	☐	☐
Other/miscellaneous	☐	☐	☐	☐	☐	☐

	Yes	No
28. Is information collected on the ethnicity of job applicants?	☐	☐
29. Is this information analysed regularly?	☐	☐

TRAINING

	Yes	No
30. Does your trust/unit provide training on equal opportunities issues?	☐	☐

31. Is an equal opportunities component included in:

Induction training?	☐	☐
Management training?	☐	☐

32. Is attendance on a recruitment and selection course mandatory for:

All staff involved in the selection of new employees?	☐	☐
All staff involved in the selection of existing employees for training courses provided or funded by your trust/unit?	☐	☐

POSITIVE ACTION

33. Have any of the following positive action measures (permissible under the Race Relations Act 1976) been undertaken by your trust/unit?

	Yes	**No**
Additional training for minority ethnic groups?	☐	☐
The setting of goals and/or timetables for minority ethnic employment?	☐	☐
Out-reach recruitment efforts (to schools, colleges etc.)?	☐	☐
Advertising in minority ethnic publications or media?	☐	☐

Other *(please specify)*

....
....
....

POSITIVE DISCRIMINATION

In the United States calls for positive discrimination have been justified in the pursuit of diversity. here positive discrimination, which is not permissible under the Race Relations Act 1976 can be taken to imply the adoption of preferential selection policies designed to improve the employment position of minority ethnic groups.

34. A list of statements about positive discrimination (hereafter PD) is presented below, please indicate your agreement, disagreement or neutrality by circling one of the accompanying numbers, where 1 = strongly agree and 5 = strongly disagree, as above.

PD is required to compensate minority ethnic groups for past disadvantage.	1	2	3	4	5
PD is needed to overcome present disadvantages.	1	2	3	4	5
PD is necessary to avoid civil unrest.	1	2	3	4	5
PD would enhance social tensions.	1	2	3	4	5

344

PD deprives better qualified applicants.	1	2	3	4	5
PD undermines service quality.	1	2	3	4	5
Qualifications do not always predict ability.	1	2	3	4	5
Deprived areas need PD more than ethnic minorities.	1	2	3	4	5
Women need PD more than ethnic minorities.	1	2	3	4	5
Disabled people need PD more than ethnic minorities.	1	2	3	4	5
Appointments should only be made on the basis of merit.	1	2	3	4	5
In certain circumstances ethnicity can be classed as an element of merit.	1	2	3	4	5

	Yes	**No**
35. Do you believe that positive discrimination has occurred, or does occur, within the health service *(if yes, please explain)*	☐	☐

....
....
....
....
....
....
....

ACHIEVING DIVERSITY

36. Which of the following strategies would you favour as a means of achieving diversity *(Please tick as many boxes as you require to illustrate your preference)*:

Turning health provision over to the free market? ☐

Enforcing the existing legislation (i.e. RRA 1976)? ☐

Adopting a rigorous equal opportunities policy? ☐

Employing positive action measures? ☐

Engaging in positive discrimination? ☐

Name and designation of completing officer

....
....
....
....
....
....
....

Thank you very much for completing this questionnaire. Please return it in the pre-paid envelope to: Nick Johns, Faculty of Human Sciences, Department of Social Policy and Social Work, 20 Portland Villas, Drake Circus, Plymouth Devon PL4 8AA.

An abstract of the findings will be forwarded to your unit on the completion of the research. Thank you once again for your participation.

APPENDIX 4: INTERVIEW SCHEDULE

Interview Schedule

Provision

1) Are you aware of any problems this trust, or the NHS more widely, experiences in providing health care for minority ethnic groups?

2) Such as:

a) Language barriers
b) Cultural differences
c) Discrimination (individual/institutional)

3) How would you deal with these?

4) What about

a) language
      (i)   interpreting services
      (ii)   phrase books
      (iii)   translated literature
      (iv)   technology
      (v)   language classes

b) Culture

      (i)   printed guides
      (ii)   cultural training

c) Discrimination

      (i)   enforcing RRA 1976
      (ii)   anti-racist training

5) Any other issues?

Policy

1) Do you think any of these measures, which have been discussed as possible ways of improving the service to minority ethnic groups, will be any value:

a) NHS reforms

b) ethnic monitoring

c) link workers

Diversity

1) Do you feel that minority ethnic groups are fairly represented at all levels of the trust, or, in the NHS more widely?

2) How would you explain this?

3) Do you think that a diverse workforce would be better able to provide a sensitive service to minority ethnic communities and the community more generally?

4) How would you define diversity?

5) What would you expect diversity to achieve?

6) Barriers?

7) Seen diversity?

8) Is diversity racist?

9) Does anything for whites?

10) Any attempts at diversity?

Achieving Diversity

1) What would be the best way of achieving diversity?

APPENDIX 5: DESIGNATION OF RESPONDENTS

Respondent number	Designation and Type
R1*	Co-ordinator of the local language project (Unofficial user rep)
R2	Head of the local link working organisation (Unofficial user rep)
R3	Part-time volunteer/part-time NHS worker (Unofficial user rep)
R4	Head of the local Chinese organisation (Unofficial user rep)
R5	Case worker for the local REC (Unofficial user rep)
R6	Co-ordinator of the Sickle Cell Clinic (Unofficial user rep)
R7	Chief Executive of enterprise agency (Unofficial user rep)
R8	Mental health charity volunteer (Unofficial user rep)
R9	Personnel Manager for the regional office of the NHSE
R10	Administrative Co-ordinator (Trust employee)
R11	HA representative (Official user rep)
R12	Head of local CHC (Official user representative)
R13	Ward Manager (Trust employee)
R14	Training and Development Officer (Trust employee)
R15	Radiologist (Trust employee)
R16	Ward Sister (Trust employee)

R17	Ancillary Manager (Trust employee)
R18	Health Visitor (Trust employee)
R19	Catering Manager (Trust employee)
R20	Nurse Trainer
R21	Support Services Manager (Trust employee)
R22	Dietetic Co-ordinator (Trust employee)
R23	Record Office Manager (Trust employee)
R24	Disability Co-ordinator (Trust employee)
R25	Ward Manager (Trust employee)
R26	District Nurse (Trust employee)
R27	Administrative Officer (Trust employee)
R28	Personnel Adviser (Trust employee)
R29	Ward Sister (Trust employee)
R30	Physiotherapy Co-ordinator (Trust employee)
R31	Administrative Manager (Trust employee)
R32	Personnel Director of a local Trust (exploratory only)

REFERENCES

Aanchawan, T. (1996). 'Room at the top', *Health Service Journal*, 7/3/96, pp.26-28.

Abdussalam, M. & Käfferstein, F. (1996). 'Food beliefs and taboos', *World Health*, No.2, March/April, pp.10-11.

Abrams, F. (1997). 'Equality law could bring more female MPs', *The Independent*, 29/12/97, p.3.

Adams, G.R. & Schvaneveldt, J.D. (1991). *Understanding Research Methods (2nd ed)*, London: Longman.

Adeboale, V. (2004). 'Marginal points', *Health Service Journal*, 3/6/04, ppp.24-25.

Admani, K. (1993a). 'Black and ethnic minority doctors in the National Health Service', in Hopkins, A. & Bahl, V. (eds) *Access to health care for people from black and ethnic minorities*, London: RCP.

Admani, K. (1993b). 'Special needs of elderly Muslims', in Hopkins, A. & Bahl, V. (eds) *Access to health care for people from black and ethnic minorities*, London: RCP.

Agnew, T. (1998a). 'Minority action', *Health Service Journal*, Vol.108, No.5622, September, pp.14-15.

Agnew, T. (1998b). 'Survey finds failure in NHS equality practice', *Health Service Journal*, Vol.108, No.5621, September, p.2.

Agnew, T. (2000). 'Down equality street', *Health Service Journal*, Vol.110, No.5699, April, pp.12-13.

Agocs, C. & Burr, C. (1996). 'Employment equity, affirmative action and managing diversity: assessing the differences', *International Journal of Manpower*, Vol.17, No.4/5, pp.30-45.

Ahmad, W. (1992). 'The maligned healer: the 'Hakim' and Western medicine', *New Community*, Vol.18, No.4, pp.521-536.

Ahmad, W.I.U. (1993a). 'Introduction', in Ahmad, W.I.U. (ed) *'Race' and Health in Contemporary Britain*, Buckingham: Open University Press.

Ahmad, W.I.U. (1993b). 'Promoting equitable health and health care: A case for action', in Ahmad, W.I.U. (ed) *'Race' and Health in Contemporary Britain*, Buckingham: Open University Press.

Ahmad, W.I.U. (1993c). 'Making black sick: 'race', ideology and health research', in Ahmad, W.I.U. (ed) *Race' and Health in Contemporary Britain*, Buckingham: Open University Press.

Ahmad, W.I.U. (ed) (1993d). *Race and Health in Contemporary Britain*, Buckingham: Open University Press.

Ahmad, W.I. (1994). 'Reflections on the consanguinity and birth outcome debate', *Journal of Public Health Medicine*, Vol.16, No.4, pp.423-428.

Ahmad, W. (1995). 'Review article: 'Race' and health', *New Community*, Vol.17, No.3, pp.418-429.

Ahmad, W.I.U. (1996). 'The trouble with culture', in Kelleher, D. & Hillier, S. (eds) *Researching Cultural Differences in Health*, London: Routledge.

Ahmad, W.I.U., Baker, M. & Kernohan, E. (1991). 'General Practitioner's perceptions of Asian and non-Asian patients', *Family Practice – An International Journal*, Vol.8, No.1, pp.52-56.

Ahmad, W.I.U. & Sheldon, T. (1992). ''Race' and statistics', in Ahmad, W.I.U. (ed) *The Politics of Race and Health*, Bradford: Race Relations Unit of Bradford & Ilkley Community College.

Ainsworth, S. (1998). 'Opportunities knock', *Health Service Journal*, Vol.108, No.5628, 29/10/98, p.31.

Airy, C., Bruster, S., Calderwood, L., Erens, B., Pitson, L., Prior, G. & Richards, N. (1999). *National Surveys of NHS Patients, Coronary Heart Disease 1999. National Report. Summary of Key Findings*, London: DoH.

Alexander, Z. (1999). *Study of Black, Asian and Ethnic Minority Issues*, London: DoH.

Alibhai, Y. (1993). 'Black Nightingales', in Walmsley, J., Reynolds, J., Shakespeare, P. & Woolfe, R. (eds) *Health, Welfare and Practice*, London: Sage.

Alibhai-Brown, Y. (1998a). 'Not the right sort of Asians', *The Guardian*, 19/1/98, p.15.

Alibhai-Brown, Y. (1998b). 'Black nurses' blues', *The Guardian*, 18/3/98, p.22.

Alibhai-Brown, Y. (1998c). 'The media and race relations', in Blackstone, T., Parekh, B. & Sanders, P. (eds) *Race Relations in Britain: a developing agenda*, London: Routledge.

Alibhai-Brown, Y. (1999). 'The case of the racist kidneys reveals a sickness in the NHS', *The Independent*, 8/7/99, p.4.

Alibhai-Brown, Y. (2005a). 'Never mind those six pledges – here are six reasons why you shouldn't vote Labour', *The Independent*, 14/2/05.

Alibhai-Brown, Y. (2005b). 'The reality of modern men (and women)', *The Independent*, 18/4/05, p.31.

Alibhai-Brown, Y. (2005c). 'People matter more than holy books', *The Independent*, 23/5/05, p.31.

Ananthanarayanan, T.S. (1989). 'Cultural Factors in the Organisation of a Pyschogeriatric Service for Elderly Asians in North Staffordshire', in Cox, J.L. & Bostock, S. (eds) *Racial Discrimination in the Health Service*, Staffordshire: Penrhos.

Anderson, J.M., Blue, C. & Lau, A. (1991). 'Women's perspectives on chronic illness: ethnicity, ideology and restructuring of life', *Social Science and Medicine*, Vol.33, No.2, pp.101-113.

Andrews, A. & Jewson, N. (1993). 'Ethnicity and infant deaths: the implications of recent statistical evidence for materialist explanations', *Sociology of Health and Illness*, Vol.15, No.2, pp.137-153.

Anionwu. E.N. (1993). 'Sickle cell and thalassaemia: community experiences and official responses', in Ahmad, W.I.U. (ed) *'Race' and Health in Contemporary Britain*, Buckingham: Open University Press.

Anionwu, E.N. (1996). 'Ethnic origin of sickle and thalassaemia counsellors: does it matter?', in Kelleher, D. & Hillier, S. (eds) *Researching Cultural Differences in Health*, London: Routledge.

Anwar, M. (1990). 'Ethnic classifications, ethnic monitoring and the 1991 Census', *New Community*, Vol.16, No.4, July, pp.607-615.

Anwar, M. & Ali, A. (1987). *Overseas Doctors: Experience and Expectations: A Research Study*, London: CRE.

Anwar, M., Roach, P. & Sondhi, R. (eds) (2000). *From Legislation to Integration? Race Relations in Britain*, London: Macmillan.

Association of American Colleges and Universities (AACU). (1998). 'Establishing diversity as an educational and civic priority', *http://www.aacu-edu.org/Initiatives/Priority 4.html*.

Atkin, K., Cameron, E., Badger, F. & Evers, H. (1989). 'Asian elders' knowledge and future use of community social and health services', *New Community*, Vol.15, No.3, pp.439-445.

Atkin, K., Lunt, N., Parker, G. & Hirst, M. (1994). 'Ethnic Origin and Practice Nursing: The Effect of a Possibly Controversial Question on a Postal Survey', *Sociology*, Vol.28, No.1, pp.163-169.

Au, S. (1990). 'Bridging the cultural gap', *OPENMIND*, No.46, Aug/Sept 1990, p.4.

Austin, H. (1996) 'Sickle cell treatment holds hope for young', *The Observer*, 11/8/96, p.13.

Bagilhole, B. (1993). 'Managing to be fair: implementing equal opportunities in a local authority', *Local Government Studies*, Vol.19, No.2, pp.163-175.

Bagilhole, B. (1997). *Equal Opportunities and Social Policy*, London: Longman.

Bagilhole, B. & Stephens, M. (1997). 'Women Speak Out: Equal opportunities in employment for ethnic minority women workers in a National Health Service Trust Hospital', *Social Services Research*, No.1, pp.11-25.

Bagilhole, B. & Stephens, M. (1998). 'Equal Opportunities in an NHS Hospital: Perspectives from Ethnic Minority Female Employees and Management', *The Journal of Contemporary Health*, Issue 7, Autumn; pp.83-6.

Bagilhole, B. & Stephens, M. (1999). 'Management responses to equal opportunities for ethnic minority women within an NHS Trust', *Journal of Social Policy*, Vol.28, No.2, pp.235-248.

Bhopal, R. & White, M. (1993). 'Health promotion for ethnic minorities: past, present and future', in Ahmad, W.I.U. (ed) *Race and Health in Contemporary Britain*, Buckingham: Open University Press.

Bhui, K. (2002). *Racism and Mental Health: prejudice and suffering*, Philadelphia P.A.: Jessica Kingsley.

Black, J. (1985).'The difficulties of living in Britain', *British Medical Journal*, Vol.290, pp.615-617.

Black, J. (1985). 'Contact with the health services', *British Medical Journal*, Vol.290, pp.689-692.

Blackstock, C. (1999). 'Straw to set job targets for minorities', *The Guardian*, 5/7/99, p.6.

Blackstone, T. (1998). 'Towards a learning society', in Blackstone, T., Parekh, B. & Sanders, P. (eds) *Race Relations in Britain: a developing agenda*, London: Routledge.

Blackstone, T., Parekh, B. & Sanders, P. (eds) (1998). *Race Relations in Britain: a developing agenda*, London: Routledge.

Blakemore, K. and Drake, R. (1996). *Understanding Equal Opportunity Policies*, London: Prentice Hall/Harverster Wheatsheaf.

Bodi, F. (2000). 'Don't label me please', http://www.guardian.co.uk/Archive/Article/0,4273,4069013,00.html

Bolton, J. (1979). *People Skills*, London: Touchstone.

Booth, T. (1988). *Developing Policy Research*, Aldershot: Avebury.

Boseley, S. (1998). 'Merit awards overhaul for top doctors', *The Guardian*, 10/8/98, p.4.

Bothamey, R. (1996). 'Issues of race', *Journal of Community Nursing*, Vol.10, No.10, October, pp.22-24.

Bourne, J. (1980). 'Cheerleaders and ombudsmen: the sociology of race relations in Britain', *Race and Class*, Vol.21, No.4, pp.331-352.

Bowers, H. (1993). 'Seeing health in black and white', *Practice Nurse*, 15-31 October, pp.612-622.

Bowers, J. & Franks, S. (1980). *Race and Affirmative Action*, Fabian tract 471, Civic Press Limited.

Bowler, I. (1993). 'They're not the same as us': midwives' stereotypes of South Asian descent maternity patients', *Sociology of Health and Illness*, Vol.15, No.2, pp.157-177.

Brach, C. & Fraser, I. (2000). 'Can cultural competency reduce racial and ethnic health disparities?'. *Medical Care Research and Review*, Vol.57, No.1, pp. 181–217.

Bradby, H. (1995). 'Ethnicity: not a black and white issue', *New Community*, Vol.17, No.3, June, pp.405-417.

Brah, A. (1992). 'Difference, diversity and differentiation', in Donald, J. & Rattansi, A. (eds) *'Race', Culture and Difference*, London: Sage/OUP.

Brah, A. (1994). 'Time place and others: discourses of race, nation and ethnicity', *Sociology*, Vol.28, No.3, pp.805-813.

Branigan, T. (2001a). 'Race relations high on list of UK concerns', *The Guardian*, 22/6/01, p.5.

Branigan, T. (2001b). 'Sisters in arms', *The Guardian (G2)*, 12/2/01, pp.8-9.

Brasher, S. (1996). 'Labour women have last laugh', *New Statesman & Society*, 12 January, p.7.

Brass, E. & Koziell, S.P. (1997). 'This green and revolting land', *The Big Issue (South West)*, No.240, July 7-13, pp.20-1.

Brent Community Health Council. (1981). *Black People and the Health Service*, London: Brent CHC.

Brindle, D. (1996a). 'Family care 'lacking for elderly blacks and Asians'', *The Guardian*, 7/8/96, p.7.

Brindle, D. (1996b). 'Worry grows over nurses', *The Guardian*, 5/9/96, p.9.

Brindle, D. (1997a). 'NHS's ethnic nurse numbers decline', *The Guardian*, 21/4/97, p.6.

Brindle, D. (1997b). 'NHS trusts hiring no minorities', *The Guardian*, 24/7/97, p.8.

Brindle, D. (1997c). 'Finding proof positive', *The Guardian (Society)*, 13/8/97, p.13.

Brindle, D. (1998). 'Psychiatric needs of blacks 'ignored'', *The Guardian*, 27/9/98, p.7.

Brindle, D. (1999). 'NHS looks abroad for midwives', *The Guardian*, 31/7/99, p.2.

British Medical Journal. (1992). 'Are doctors from ethnic minorities discriminated against?', Vol.304, p.1513.

Brown, G. (1996). 'In the real world', *The Guardian*, 2/8/96, p.13.

Brown, J. (2005). 'Britons struggle more than others to get ahead', *The Independent*, 25/4/05, p.6.

Brown, C. & Morris, N. (2005). 'Tories join Blair to condemn party's immigration strategy', *The Independent*, 23'4'05, p.8.

Browne, A. (2001). 'Nurses desert NHS for good life', *The Observer*, 19/8/01, p.5.

Bryan, B,. Dadzie. S. & Scafe, S. (1985). *Heart of the Race: Black Women's Lives in Britain*, London: Virago.

Bryman, A. (1984). 'The debate about quantitative and qualitative research: a question of method or epistemology?', *British Journal of Sociology*, Vol.35, No.1, pp.75-92.

Bryman, A. (1988). *Quantity and Quality in Social Research*, London: Routledge.

Bryman, A. & Cramer, D. (1997). *Quantitative Data Analysis: with SPSS for Windows*, London: Routledge.

Buchan, J. (2000). 'Happy landings', *Health Service Journal*, Vol.110, No.5719, pp.24-25.

Burden, A. (1993). 'Diabetes: impact upon black and minority ethnic people', in Hopkins, A. & Bahl, V. (eds) *Access to health care for people from black and ethnic minorities*, London: RCP.

362

Burnard, P. (1995). 'Unspoken meanings: qualitative research and multi-media analysis', *Nurse Researcher*, Vol.3, No.1, September, pp.55-65.

Butcher, T. (1998). 'Managing the Welfare State', in Jones, H. & MacGregor, S. (eds) *Social Issues and Party Politics*, London: Routledge.

Butler, P. (1999). 'My way', *Health Service Journal*, Vol.109, No.5636, 7 January, p.10.

Butler, A. & Landells, M. (1994). *Telling Tales out of School: Research into sexual harassment of women academics*, Equality Research Group Working Papers No.1, University of Plymouth.

Butt, J. (1994). 'Exploring and Using the Black Resource in Research', *Research Policy & Planning*, Vol.12, No.2, pp.9-12.

Calman. K. (1992). 'Health of black and ethnic minorities', reprinted from *On the State of Public Health for the year 1991*, London: DoH.

Calvillo, E.R. & Flaskerud, J.H. (1993). 'Evaluation of the Pain Response by Mexican American and Anglo American Women and their Nurses', *Journal of Advanced Nursing*, Vol.18, pp.451-459.

Cameron, I. (1993). 'Formulating an equal opportunities policy', *EOR*, No.47, January/February, pp.16-20.

Campbell, T. (1998). 'Downsizing and mentoring at Digital', *EOR*, No.78, March/April, p.24.

Campbell, D. (1999). 'Met race policy goes all the way to the top', *The Guardian*, 16/3/99, p.6.

Carlisle, D. (2004). 'Overseas recruitment: planet poaching or doing a world of good?', *Health Service Journal*, 15/7/04, pp.8-9.

Carlisle, D. (2005). 'Needed by the NHS but denigrated by the politicians', *Health Service Journal*, 5/5/05, pp.12-13.

Carmichael, C. (1996) 'Inner-city blues', *Health Service Journal*, Vol.106, No.5529, 14 November, pp.30-31.

Carr-Hill, R. & Rudat, K. (1995). 'Unsound Barriers', *Health Service Journal*, 9 February, pp.28-29.

Carter, J. (2000). 'New public management and equal opportunities in the NHS', *Critical Social Policy*, Vol.20, No.1, pp.61-83.

Cartice, J. & Heath, A. (2001). 'Is the English Lion About to Roar', *British Social Attitudes Survey: Focusing on Diversity 2000/01*, No.17, London: BSA.

Carvel, J. (2001). 'Search for staff to fulfil health pledges', *The Guardian*, 23/5/01, p.17.

Caudron, S. (1994). 'Diversity ignites effective work teams', *Personnel Journal*, Vol.73, No.9, pp.54-8.

Chaudhary, V. (1998). 'Students allege race bias in exam marking', *The Guardian*, 11/3/98, p.11.

Chevannes, M. (1991). 'Access to health care for black people', *Health Visitor*, Vol.64, p.1.

Chowdery, S. (2005). 'Do we really need these patronising awards', *The Independent*, 28/5/05, p.35.

Cicourel, A.V. (1964). *Method and Measurement in Sociology*, London: Collier-MacMillan.

Clarke, L. (1994). *Discrimination*, London: Institute of Personnel Management.

Clarke, M. & Clayton, D.G. (1983). 'Quality of obstetric care provided for Asian immigrants in Leicestershire', *British Medical Journal*, Vol.286, pp.621-623.

Clements, P. & Spinks, A. (2000). *The Equal Opportunities Guide (2nd edition)*, London: Kogan Page.

Cochrane, R. & Stopes-Roe, M. (1980). 'The mental health of immigrants', *New Community*, Vol.23, No.1-2, pp.123-8.

Cockburn, A. (1995). 'Letterfrom: America', *New Statesman & Society*, 4 August, p.4.

Cockburn, C. (1989). 'Equal opportunities: the short and long agenda', *Industrial Relations Journal*, Vol.20, pp.213-25.

Cohen, C. (1979). 'Race and the Constitution', in Wasserstrom, R.A. (ed) *Today's Moral Problems*, London: Collier Macmillan.

Cohen, P. (1995a). 'National survey reveals worrying trends', *Health Visitor*, Vol.68, No.3, March, p.90.

Cohen, P. (1995b). 'Racism rampant within NHS', *Health Visitor*, Vol.68, No.12, December, pp.484.

Coker, N. (1997). 'High culture', *Health Service Journal*, 28 August, pp.30-1.

Cole, A. (1987). 'Limited Access', *Nursing Times*, Vol.83, No.24, 17 June, pp.29-30.

Cole, A. (1994). 'Prescription for unequal opportunities', *Health Visitor*, Vol.67, No.7, July, pp.221-222.

Cole, T. (1989). 'Researching Race and Racism', *Social Studies Review*, November, pp.62-64.

Collier, R. (1998). *Equality in Managing Service Delivery*, Buckingham: Open University Press.

Collins, H. (1992). *Equality Matters. Equal opportunities in the '90s: background and current issues*, London: Library Association Publishing.

Collins, H. (1995). *Equality in the Workplace. An Equal Opportunities Handbook for Trainers*, Oxford: Blackwell.

Collins, S. (1993). 'The African way', *OPENMIND*, No.65, Oct/Nov, pp.20-21.

Commission for Racial Equality. (CRE) (1983). *Ethnic Minority Hospital Staff*, London: CRE.

CRE. (1985). *Positive Action and Equal Opportunity in Employment*, London: CRE.

CRE. (1991). *NHS Contracts and Race Equality*, London: CRE.

CRE. (1995a). *Racial Equality Means Business. A Standard for Racial Equality for Employers*, London: CRE.

CRE. (1995b). *Racial Equality Means Quality. A Standard for Racial Equality for Local Government in England and Wales*, London: CRE.

CRE. (2000). *Race Equality and NHS Trusts*, London: CRE.

CRE. (2001). *The General Duty to Promote Racial Equality. Guidance for public authorities on their obligations under the Race Relations (Amendment) Act 2000,* London: CRE.

CRE. (2002). *Towards Racial Equality – An Evaluation of the Public Duty to Promote Race Equality and Good Race Relations in England and Wales,* London: CRE.

Cook, S.W. (1978). 'Interpersonal and attitudinal outcomes in co-operating interracial groups', *Journal of Research and Development in Education,* Vol.12, No.4, pp.23-38.

Cooper, C. (1991). 'Closed to interpretation, *OPENMIND,* No.51, June/July, p.5.

Cooper, G. (1998). 'Alarm at shortage of new nurses', *The Independent,* 5/8/98, p.7.

Cooper, R. (1994). 'Fair employment priorities', *EOR,* No.53, January/February, pp.17-18.

Cope, R. (1989), 'The compulsory detention of Afro-Caribbean's under the Mental Health Act', *New Community,* Vol.15, No.3, pp.343-356.

Cortis, J.D. (1993). 'Transcultural nursing: appropriateness for Britain', *Journal of Advances in Health and Nursing Care,* Vol.2, No.4, pp.67-77.

Cortis, J.D. & Rinomhota, A.S. (1996) 'Leading the race', *Nursing Management,* Vol.3, No.3, June, pp.8-9.

Coussey, M & Jackson, H. (1991). *Making Equal Opportunities Work,* London: Pitman/Longman.

Cox, J. (1989). 'Racial Discrimination and the Health Service', in Cox, J. & Bostock, S. (eds) *Racial Discrimination in the Health Service,* Staffordshire: Penrhos.

Cox, J. & Bostock, S. (eds) (1989). *Racial Discrimination in the Health Service,* Staffordshire: Penrhos.

Culley, L. (1996). 'A critique of multiculturalism in health care: the challenge for nurse education', *Journal of Advanced Nursing,* Vol.23, No.3, March, pp.564-571.

Cunningham, J. (2000). 'The hearing aide', *The Guardian (Society),* 1/11/00, p.6.

Cunningham, S. (1992). 'The Development of Equal Opportunities Theory and Practice in the European Community', *Policy and Politics,* Vol.20, No.3, pp.177-189.

Czaja, R. & Blair, J. (1996). *Designing Surveys: A Guide to Decisions and Procedures,* London: Pine Forge Press.

Daly, M. (1998). 'Doctor challenged to take his own ECT', *The Big Issue,* No.283, 11-17 May, p.4.

Davies, J. (2001). 'Waste not, want not', *Health Service Journal,* Vol.111, No.5757, 31 May, pp.24-27.

Davies, S., Modell, B. & Wonke, B. (1993). 'The haemoglobinopathies: impact upon black and ethnic minority people', in Hopkins, A. & Bahl, V. (eds) *Access to health care for people from black and ethnic minorities,* London: RCP.

Deem, R. (1996). 'Women and educational reform', in Hallett, C. (ed) *Women and Social Policy: An Introduction*, London: Prentice Hall/Harvester Wheatsheaf.
Department of Health and Social Security (DHSS). (1987). *Asian Mother and Baby Campaign: A Report by the Director Miss Veena Bahl*, London: DHSS.
DHSS. (1988). *Ethnic Minority Health (A report of a management seminar)*, London: DHSS.
Department of Health (DoH). (1990).*The National Health Service and Community Care Act, 1990*, London: HMSO.
DoH. (1991). *The Patient's Charter*, London: HMSO.
DoH. (1992). *Health of the Nation –a strategy for health in England*, London: HMSO.
DoH. (1997). *The New NHS: Modern and Dependable*, London: HMSO.
DoH. (2000). *The Race Equality Agenda of the Department of Health*, London: DoH.

DoH. (2001). *Equal opportunities goals and objectives*, http://www.dh.gov.uk/PolicyAndGuidance/HumanResourcesAndTraining/Model Employer/EqualityAndDiversity/EADGoalsObjectives/fs/en?CONTENT_ID=405 1986&chk=XyiYkI.

DoH. (2003a). *Equalities and Diversity Strategy & Delivery Plan to Support the NHS*, London: HRD.

DoH. (2003b). *Equalities and Diversity in the NHS: Progress and Priorities*, London: HRD.

DoH. (2004a). *New equality champion for the NHS 13/10/04*, http://www.dh.gov.uk/PublicationsAndStatistics/PressReleases/PressReleasesNoti ces/fs/en?CONTENT_ID=4091141&chk=nHKml/.

DoH. (2004b). *About the Positively Diverse programme*, http://www.nhsemployers.org/EmployerExcellence/positively_diverse_programm e.asp.
DoH. (2004c). *Race Equality Plan*, London: DoH.

DoH. (2005). *Race Equality Scheme 2005-2008*, London: DoH.

De Vaus, D.A. (1990). *Surveys in Social Research (2nd ed)*, London: Unwin Hyman.
Dholakia, B. (1999). 'Managing diversity – and international perspective', *EOR*, No.86, July/August, pp.33-36.
Dickens, L. (1994). 'The business case for women's equality: is the carrot better than the stick?', *Employee Relations*, Vol.16, No.8, pp.5-18.
Dickinson, R. & Bhatt, A. (1994). 'Ethnicity, health and control: results from an exploratory study of ethnic minority communities' attitudes to health', *Health Education Journal*, Vol.53, pp.421-9.
Dillner, L. (1995) 'Manchester tackles failure rate of Asian Students', *British Medical Journal*, Vol.310, p.209.

366

Dobson, F. MP, Secretary of State for Health, (1999). *All staff must have a voice in the new NHS*, http://www.dh.gov.uk/PublicationsAndStatistics/PressReleases/PressReleasesNotices/fs/en?CONTENT_ID=4025675&chk=vnB9Qn.

Dodd, V. (1997). 'Race for life', *The Guardian (Society)*, 25/11/97, p.16.

Dodd, V. (2004). 'Met plan to fast track black recruits', *The Guardian*, 17/4/04.

Dominelli, L. (1988). *Anti-Racist Social Work*, London: MacMillan.

Donaldson, L.J. (1986). 'Health and social status of elderly Asians: a community survey', *British Medical Journal*, Vol.293, pp.1079-1082.

Donovan, J.L. (1984). 'Ethnicity and Health: A Research Review', *Social Science and Medicine*, Vol.19, No.7, pp.663-670.

Donovan, J.L. (1986a). *We Don't Buy Sickness, It Just Comes*, Aldershot: Gower.

Donovan, J.L. (1986b). 'Black people's Health: A Different Approach?', in Rathwell, T. & Phillips, D. (eds) *Health Race & Ethnicity*, London: Croon Helm.

Douglas, J. (1996). 'Developing with Black and minority ethnic communities, health promotion strategies which address social inequalities', in Bywaters, P. & McLeod, E. (eds) *Working for Equality in Health*, London: Routledge.

Douki, S. & Tabbane, K. (1996). 'Culture and depression', *World Health*, No.2, March-April, pp.22-23.

Doyal, L. & Gough, I. (1991). *A Theory of Human Needs*, London: Macmillan.

Doyal, L., Hunt, G. & Mellor, J. (1981). 'Your Life in Their Hands: Migrant Workers in the National Health Service', *Critical Social Policy*, Vol.1, No.2, Autumn, pp.54-73.

Dreachslin, J.L., Weech-Maldonado, R., Kathryn, K.H. & Dansky, H. (2004).'Racial and ethnic diversity and organizational behavior: a focused research agenda for health services management', *Social Science and Medicine*, Vol.59, No.5, September, pp.961-971.

Dunn, J. & Fahy, T.A. (1990). 'Police Admissions to a Psychiatric Hospital: Demographic and Clinical Differences between Ethnic Groups', *British Journal of Psychiatry*, Vol.156, pp.373-78.

Dworkin, R. (1981). 'Reverse Discrimination', in Braham, P., Rhodes, E. & Pearn, M. (eds) *Discrimination and Disadvantage in Employment*, London: Harper Row.

Eaton, L. (1997). 'Race against time', *Health Service Journal*, Vol.107, No.5544, 13 March, p.18.

Eboh, W. (1996). 'Sickle cell disease', *Practice Nursing*, Vol.7, No.1, pp.25-30.

Edmonds, D. (1994). 'Race against positive discrimination', *New Statesman & Society*, 15 April, pp.22-23.

Edwards, A. & Talbot, R. (1994). *The Hard-pressed Researcher*, Harlow: Longman.

Edwards, J. & Batley, R. (1978). *The Politics of Positive Discrimination*, London: Tavistock.

Edwards, J. (1988). 'Facing up to positive discrimination', *New Community*, Vol.14, No.3, Spring, pp.405-411.

Edwards, J. (1994). 'Group Rights v. Individual Rights: The Case of Race-Conscious Policies', *Journal of Social Policy*, Vol.23, No.1, pp.55-70

Edwards, J. (1995). *When Race Counts*, London: Routledge.

Einterz, E.M. (1996). 'Who are we to say?', *World Health*, No.2, March-April, pp.20-21.

Elliott, P. (1998). 'Hidden talents', *Health Service Journal*, Vol.108, No.5622, 7 September, p.28.

Ellis, C. & Sollenfeld, J.A. (1994). 'Diverse approaches to managing diversity', *Human Resources Management*, Vol.33, No.1, pp.79-109.

Equal Opportunities Commission (EOC). (1991). *Equality Management. Women's Employment in the NHS*, Manchester: EOC.

Equal Opportunities Review (EOR). (1989). 'Equal opportunity at the Ford Motor Company', No.24, March/April, pp.9-12.

EOR. (1989). 'Equal opportunities in the Civil Service', No.26, July/August, pp.26-32.

EOR. (1990). 'Equal opportunities at Littlewoods', No.33, September/October, pp.11-19.

EOR. (1993). 'Action for race equality: an EOR survey of employer initiatives', No.48, March/April, pp.14-20.

EOR. (1994). 'Equal opportunities in the health service: a survey of NHS trusts', No.53, January/February, pp.24-31.

EOR. (1995). 'Impact of positive action measures limited', says study', No.59, January/February, p.8.

EOR. (1997). 'Employers lack strategy on diversity' No.73, May/June, pp.4-5.

EOR. (1998). 'Partnership to tackle racism in NHS', No.76, November/December, pp.7-8.

EOR. (1998). 'Limited positive discrimination allowed', No.77, January/February, pp.38-41.

EOR. (1998). 'Ethnic minority goals set for armed forces', No.78, March/April, p.7.

EOR. (1998). 'Workplace diversity - new challenges, new opportunities', No.78, March/April, pp.18-24.

EOR. (1998). 'Inequality in pay and promotion in the NHS', No.79, May/June, pp.7-8.

EOR. (1998). 'Littlewoods: increasing diversity, increasing profits', No.81, September/October, pp.20-8.

EOR. (1998). 'Sex bias in nursing', No.85, September/October, p.7.

EOR. (1998). 'Managing diversity firms not more diverse', No.87, September/October, pp.5-6.

EOR. (1999). 'Action to tackle racial harassment in the NHS', No.84, March/April, p.11.

EOR. (2000). 'Job prospects worse for ethnic minorities', No.89, January/February, pp.9-10.

EOR. (2000). 'Ethnic minority police up – but progress slow', No.93, September/October, p.7.

EOR. (2001). 'Mixed progress for Home Office race equality targets', No.95, January/February, p.2.

EOR. (2001). 'Most employers lack a diversity strategy', No.96, March/April, p.3.

EOR. (2001). 'NHS fails on race equality action', No.96, March/April, p.8.

EOR. (2001). 'A third of Blacks and Asians experience workplace racism', No.97, May/June, pp.5-6.

EOR. (2001). 'Step closer for sexual harassment ban', No.98, July/August, pp.7-8.

Esmail, A. (1997.) 'Tackling racism in the NHS', *British Medical Journal*, Vol.314, pp.618-619.

Esmail, A. & Everington, S. (1993). 'Racial discrimination against doctors from ethnic minorities', *British Medical Journal*, Vol.306, pp.691-2.

Esmail, A. & Everington, S. (1994). 'Complaints may reflect racism', *British Medical Journal*, Vol.308, p.1374.

Esmail, A., Nelson, P., Primarolo, D. & Toma, T. (1995). 'Acceptance into medical school and racial discrimination', *British Medical Journal*, Vol.310, pp.501-2.

Etzioni, A. (1997). 'Community Watch', *The Guardian*, 28/6/97, p.21.

Evans-Pritchard, A. (1994). 'Race to disaster', *The Sunday Telegraph*, 20/11/94.

Ezard, J. (1998). 'Merit is our only test for entry, Cambridge tells state pupils', *The Guardian*, 2/7/98, p.6.

Fairhall, D. (1998). 'General vows that his 'crusade' against racism will change the guard at Buckingham Palace', *The Guardian*, 6/3/98, p.9.

Farooqi, A. (1993). 'How can family practice improve access to health care for black and ethnic minority patients', in Hopkins, A. & Bahl, V. (eds) *Access to health care for people from black and ethnic minorities*, London: RCP.

Fenton, J. (1995) 'A backlash running ahead of schedule', *The Independent*, 25/9/95.

Fenton, S. (1989). 'Racism is Harmful to your Health', in Cox, J. & Bostock, S. (eds) *Racial Discrimination in the Health Service*, Staffordshire: Penrhos.

Fenton, S. & Sadiq-Sangster, A. (1996). 'Culture, relativism and the expression of mental distress: South Asian Women in Britain', *Sociology of Health and Illness*, Vol.18, No.1, pp.66-85.

Fernando, S. (1989). 'Racist Psychiatry', in Cox, J. & Bostock, S. (eds) *Racial Discrimination in the Health Service*, Staffordshire: Penrhos.

Fernando, S. (1992). 'Black Europeans', *OpenMind*, No.54, Dec 1991/Jan 1992, p.15.

Fernando, S. (1993). 'Combating racism in mental health services', *OpenMind*, No.61, Feb/Mar 1993, pp.18-19.

Fernando, S. (1994). 'Race and Europe', *OpenMind*, No.66, Dec 1993/Jan 1994, p.6.

Fernando, S. (1998). *The Guardian (letters page)*, 31/7/98: 19.

Fine, M.G. (1995). *Building Successful Multicultural Organizations: Challenges and Opportunities*, London: Quorum Books.

Fink, A. & Litwin, M. (1995). *The Survey Kit: How to measure survey reliability and validity*, Thousand Oaks, California: Sage.

Fisk, R. (2005). 'I may not be sure about God or the Devil, but I still believe in the United Nations', *The Independent*, 23/4/05, p.35.

Fletcher, M. (1997). 'Equal health services for all', *Journal of Community Nursing*, Vol.11, No.7, pp.20-25.

Flew, A. (1981). *The Politics of Procrustes*, London: Temple Smith.

Flew, A. (1986). 'Three Concepts of Racism', *The Salisbury Review*, October 1986, pp.2-6.

Foolchand, M. (2000). 'Behind closed doors', *Health Service Journal*, 13 April, p.30.

Forbes, I. (1991). 'Equal opportunity: radical, liberal and conservative critiques', in Meehan, E. & Sevenhuijsen, S. (eds) *Equality, Politics and Gender*, CLA: Sage.

Foster, J.J. (2001). *Data Analysis: Using SPSS for Windows. New edition: Versions 8-10*, London: Sage.

Foster, L. & James, S. (2001). 'Getting even', *Health Service Journal*, Vol.111, No.5743, pp.28-29.

France-Dawson, M. (1990). 'Sickle cell conditions and health knowledge', *Nursing Standard*, Vol.4, No.35, 23 May, pp.30-4.

Francis, E. (1993). 'Psychiatric Racism and Social Police: Black People and the Psychiatric Services', in James, W. & Harris, C. (eds) *Inside Babylon: The Caribbean Diaspora in Britain*, London: Verso.

Francis, E. (1996). 'Community care, danger and black people', *OPENMIND*, Apr/May, pp.4-5.

Franklin, A. (1994). 'Anti-Racist Research Guidelines', *Research Policy & Planning*, Vol.12, No.2, pp.18-19.

Frey, J.H. & Oishi, S.M. (1995). *How to Conduct Interviews by Telephone and in Person*, London: Sage

Friedman, M. (1962). *Capitalism and Freedom*, Chicago: University of Chicago Press.

Friedman, M. (1980). 'The Power of the State', *The Listener*, 21/2/80, pp.229-30.

Friedman, M. & Friedman, R.D. (1980). *Free to Choose*, Avon: New York.

Gates Jnr, H.L. (1997). 'Black flash', *The Guardian (The Week)*, 19/7/97, pp.1-2.

George, M. (1994) 'Racism in nursing', *Nursing Standard*, Vol.8, No.18, pp.20-21.

Gerrish, K., Husband, C. & Mackenzie, J. (1996). *Nursing for a Multi-Ethnic Society*, Buckingham: Open University Press.

Giggs, J. (1986). 'Ethnic Status and Mental Illness in Urban Areas', in Rathwell, T. & Phillips, D. (eds) *Health Race & Ethnicity*, London: Croon Helm.

370

Gillam, S.J., Jarman, B., White, P. & Law, R. (1989). 'Ethnic differences in consultation rates in urban general practice', *British Medical Journal*, Volume 299, pp.953-957.

Gillespie, R. (1993). 'Multi-Cultural Health Provision', *Health Services Management*, March 1993, pp.24-25.

Gilroy, P. (1987). *There Ain't No Black in the Union Jack*, London: Hutchinson.

Gilroy, P. (1990). 'The end of anti-racism', *New Community*, Vol.17, No.1, October, pp.71-83.

Glaser, B.G. (1965). 'The Constant Comparative Method of Qualitative Analysis', *Social Problems*, Vol.12, pp.436-445.

Glazer, N. (1983). *Ethnic Dilemmas 1964-1982*, London: Harvard University Press.

Glazer, N. (1998). *'In defence of preference'*, *The New Republic*, Vol.4, 6 April, p.342.

Godlee, F. (1996). 'The GMC, racism, and the complaints against doctors', *British Medical Journal*, Volume 312, pp.1314-1315.

Goldman, A.H. (1979). *Justice and Reverse Discrimination*, Princeton, NJ: Princeton University Press.

Gordon, P. & Klug, F. (1986). *New Right New Racism*, Nottingham: Searchlight.

Griffith, J., Wilson, P. & Tedeschi, P. (1986). 'Does Race Affect Hospital Use?', in Rathwell, T. & Phillips, D. (eds) *Health Race & Ethnicity*, London: Croon Helm.

Greenwood, L. (1996). 'Black and right', *NHS Magazine*, Spring, p.13.

Greenwood, L. (1997). 'All things being equal', *NHS Magazine*, Winter, p.7.

Grimsley, M. & Bhat, A. (1988). 'Health', in Bhat, A., Carr-Hill, R. & Ohri, S. (eds) *Britain's Black Population (2nd ed)*, London: Radical Statistics Race Group.

Gunaratnam, Y. (1993). *A Starting Point for Managers on Improving Services for Black Populations*, London: King's Fund Centre.

Gunaratnam, Y. (2001). 'Eating into multiculturalism: hospice staff and service users talk food, 'race', ethnicity, culture and identity', *Critical Social Policy*, Aug, Vol.21, No.3, pp.287-310.

Hakim, C. (1987). *Research Design*, London: Unwin Hyman.

Hancock, C. (1992). 'Managing equal opportunities in the public sector', *Senior Nurse*, Vol.12, No.1, pp.6-9.

Harding, L. (2005). 'NHS bodies clock up 108 race warnings', *Health Service Journal*, 5/5/05, p.7.

Harding, M. (2003). 'Diverse harmony', *Health Service Journal*, 6/11/03, pp.38-39.

Hari, J. (2005). 'If only we did have a compensation culture', *The Independent*, 1/6/05, p.31.

Harker, J. (2001). 'The usual suspects', *The Guardian (G2)*, 24/4/01, p.4.

Harvey, L. (1990). *Critical Social Research*, London: Unwin Hyman.

Haskey, J. (1997) 'Population review (8): The ethnic minority and overseas-born populations of Great Britain', *Population Trends*, No.88, Summer, pp.13-30.

371

Haslam, J. (1997). 'A change of culture', *The Guardian (Education)*, 4/11/97, p.6.
Hattersley, R. (1997). 'How to give a break to black Britons', *The Guardian*, 15/10/97, p.19.
Hattersley, R. (1998). 'A vision thing', *The Guardian*, 14/9/98, p.17.
Health Education Authority (HEA). (1994). *Health-Related Resources for Black Minority Ethnic Groups*, London: HEA.
Healey, P. (1998). 'Milburn sets out five-year staff strategy', *Health Service Journal*, 24 September, p.5.
Health Service Journal (HSJ). (1998). 'Joined-up thinking on Human Resources Strategy', 24/9/98, p.19.
HSJ. (2004). 'Mountains to climb (racial diversity special report)', 30/9/04,pp.39-43.
Helms, J.E. (ed) (1990). *Black and White Racial Identity: Theory, Research, and Practice*, Westport, Connecticut: Praeger.
Henley, A. (1982). *Asian Patient's in Hospital and at Home*, Oxford: Oxford University Press.
Henley, A. (1986). 'Nursing Care in a Multi-Racial Society', *Senior Nurse*, Vol.4. No.2, February, pp.18-20.
Henley, A. (1991). *Asians in Britain. Caring for Hindus and their Families: religious aspects of care*, London: HEC/DHSS/King Edward's Hospital Fund for London.
Hennings, J., Williams, J. & Haque, B.N. (1996). 'Exploring the health needs of Bangladeshi women: a case study in using qualitative research methods', *Health Education Journal*, Vol.55, pp.11-26.
Her Majesty's Stationery Office (HMSO). (1999). Modernising Government, London: HMSO. http://www.cabinet-office.gov.uk/moderngov/whtpaper/index.htm.
Hillier, S. & Rahman, S. (1996) 'Childhood development and behavioural and emotional problems as perceived by Bangladeshi parents in East London', in Kelleher, D. & Hillier, S. (eds) *Researching Cultural Differences in Health*, London: Routledge.
Hiscock, D. (2004). 'Show the way', *Health Service Journal*, 15/4/04, pp.32-33.
Hoare, T., Thomas, C., Biggs, A., Booth, M., Bradley, S. & Friedman, E. (1994). 'Can uptake of breast screening by Asian women be increased? A randomized controlled trial of a linkworker intervention', *Journal of Public Health Medicine*, Vol.16, No.2, pp.179-185.
Holstein, J.A. & Gubrium, J.F. (1997) 'Active Interviewing', in Silverman, D. (ed) *Qualitative Research: Theory, Method and Practice*, London: Sage.
Home Office (HO). (1999). *Race Equality – The Home Secretary's Employment Targets*, London: HO.
HO. (2000). *Towards Diversity. Promoting Cultural Change*, Home Office Communication Directorate.
Hopkins, A. (1993) 'Envo', in Hopkins, A. & Bahl, V. (eds) *Access to health care for people from black and ethnic minorities*, London: RCP.

Hopkins, A. & Bahl, V. (eds) (1993). *Access to health care for people from black and ethnic minorities*, London: RCP.

Humphreys, J. & Rubery, J. (1995). *The Economics of Equal Opportunities*, Manchester: EOC.

Hurstfield, J. (1999). *Equal opportunities and monitoring in NHS trusts: a survey of 420 NHS trusts in England and 25 case studies of good practice in equal opportunities*, London: IRSR.

Huston, P. (1990). 'Invisible agents for change', *World Health*, April-May 1990, p.13.

Hutton, J. MP, Minister of State for Health, (2003). *Speech: Leadership - Breaking Through, 15 October 2003*, http://www.dh.gov.uk/NewsHome/Speeches/SpeechesList/SpeechesArticle/fs/en?CONTENT_ID=4071806&chk=gU6KaF.

Hutton, W. (2000). *New Life for Health*, London: Vintage.

Iganski, P. (1995). 'Re-thinking positive discrimination', *Public Policy Review*, Vol.3, No.1, pp.42-44.

Iganski, P. & Payne, G. (1996). 'Declining racial disadvantage in the British labour market', *Ethnic and Racial Studies*, Vol.19, No.1, 1 January 1996, pp.113-131.

Iganski, P. & Payne, G. (1999). 'Socio-economic re-structuring and employment', *The British Journal of Sociology*, Vol.50, No.2, pp.195-215.

Iganski, P. & Johns, N.R. (1998). 'The problem of 'diversity' and health care provision for minority ethnic communities', *Journal of Contemporary Health*, Issue 7, Autumn, pp.87-89.

Iganski, P., Spong, A., Mason, D., Humphreys, A. & Watkins, M. (1998). *Recruiting minority ethnic groups into nursing midwifery and health visiting*, London: ENB.

Iganski, P., Mason, D., Humphreys, A. & Watkins, M. (2001). 'Equal opportunities and positive action in the British National Health Service; some lessons from the recruitment of minority ethnic groups to nursing and midwifery', *Ethnic and Racial Studies*, Vol.24, No.2, March 2001, pp.294-317.

Ineichen, B. (1986). 'Compulsory admission to psychiatric hospital under the 1959 Mental Health Act: the experience of ethnic minorities', *New Community*, Vol.13, No.1, Spring-Summer, pp.86-93.

Ineichen, B. (1987). 'The mental health of Asians in Britain: a research note', *New Community*, Vol.14, No.1/2, Autumn, pp.136-141.

Ineichen, B. (1989). 'Afro-Caribbeans and the incidence of schizophrenia: a review', *New Community*, Vol.15, No.3, April, pp.335-341.

Institute of Personnel Development (IPD). (1996). *Managing Diversity. An IPD position paper*, London: IPD.

IRS. (1999). 'Equal opportunities in the NHS: the state of play', *IRS Employment Trends*, No.671, January, p.3.

IRS. (2001). 'From the margins to the mainstream: race equality at the Home Office', *IRS Employment Trends*, No.728, May, pp.11-16.

Irsahd, S. (1994). 'The Islamic path to inner health', *OPENMIND*, No.69, June/July, pp.13-14.

Jackson, S.E. And Associates. (1992). *Diversity in the Workplace*, London: The Guildford Press.

Jahoda, M. (1960). *Race Relations and Mental Health*, UNESCO.

Jain, H.C. & Verma, A. (1996). 'Managing workforce diversity for competitiveness: The Canadian experience', *International Journal of Manpower*, Vol.17, No.4/5, pp.14-29.

Jamdagni, L. (1996). 'Race against time', *Health Service Journal*, 7 March, pp.30-31.

James, D. & Willitts, M. (2000). 'House of unrepresentatives', *Health Service Journal*, Vol.110, No.5372, 23 November, pp.32-33.

Jay, E. (1992). *'Keep Them in Birmingham'. Challenging Racism in south-west England*, London: CRE.

Jayaratnam, R. (1993). 'The need for cultural awareness', in Hopkins, A. & Bahl, V. (eds) *Access to health care for people from black and ethnic minorities*, London: RCP.

Jewson, N. & Mason, D. (1986). 'The theory and practice of equal opportunities policies: liberal and radical approaches', *Sociological Review*, Vol.34, No.2, pp.307-334.

Jewson, N. & Mason, D. (1993). *Equal Employment Opportunities in the 1990s: A Policy Principle come of Age. University of Leicester Discussion Papers in Sociology*, University of Leicester.

Jewson, N., Mason, D., Waters, S. & Harvey, J. (1990). *Ethnic Minorities and Employment Practice*, London: Employment Department Research Paper No.76.

Johns, N.R. (1999). 'The Lawrence report: an old present newly wrapped?', *Crime Prevention and Community Safety: An International Journal*, Vol.1, No.2, pp.47-50.

Johnson, B. (2000). 'Am I guilty of racial prejudice? We all are', http://www.guardian.co.uk/Archive/Article/0,4273,3965660,00.html.

Johnson, M.R.D. (1986). 'Inner City Residents, Ethnic Minorities and Primary Care in the West Midlands', in Rathwell, T. & Phillips, D. (eds) *Health Race & Ethnicity*, London: Croon Helm.

Johnson, M.R.D. (1987). 'Towards racial equality in health and welfare', *New Community*, Vol.14, No.1/2, Autumn, pp128-135.

Johnson, M.R.D. (1992). 'Health and social services', *New Community*, Vol.18, No.4, pp.611-618.

Johnson, M.R.D. (1993). 'Equal opportunities in service delivery: responses to a changing population?', in Ahmad, W.I.U. (ed) *Race and Health in Contemporary Britain*, Buckingham: Open University Press.

Johnson, M. MP. (2004). *Speech given at the Mary Seacole Awards, 27th October 2004,*

374

http://www.dh.gov.uk/NewsHome/Speeches/SpeechesList/SpeechesArticle/fs/en?
CONTENT_ID=4093015&chk=yfMVI8.

Jones, H. (1994). *Health and Society in Twentieth-Century Britain*, London: Longman.

Joppke, C. (2004). 'Ethnic diversity and the state', *British Journal of Sociology*, Sep, Vol.55, No.3, pp.451-463.

Jordan, B. & Düvell, F. (2003). *Irregular Migration: the dilemmas of transnational mobility*, Cheltenham : Edward Elgar.

Joyce, E. (1997). 'The crisis ahead', *The Guardian*, 6/8/97, p.15.

Joyram, P. (1994) 'Bringing about change for the Asian community', *OPENMIND*, No.70, Aug/Sept, p.8.

Judge, K. & Solomon, M. (1993). 'Public Opinion and the National Health Service: Patterns and Perspectives in Consumer Satisfaction', *Journal of Social Policy*, Vol.22, No.3, pp.299-327.

Kandola, R. & Fullerton, J. (1994). *Managing the Mosaic. Diversity in Action*, London: IPD.

Kandola, R. & Fullerton, J. (1998). *Diversity in Action. Managing the Mosaic (2ⁿᵈ ed)*, London: IPD.

Kandola, R., Fullerton, J. & Ahmed, Y. (1995). 'Managing diversity: succeeding where equal opportunities has failed', *EOR*, No. 59, January/February, pp.31-6.

Karmi, G. (1993). 'Management structures for recognising and meeting the health needs of black and ethnic minority people', in Hopkins, A. & Bahl, V. (eds) *Access to health care for people from black and ethnic minorities*, London: RCP.

Kavanagh, K.H. & Kennedy, P.H. (1992). *Promoting Cultural Diversity*, London: Sage.

Kelleher, D. (1996) 'A defence of the use of the terms 'ethnicity' and 'culture', in Kelleher, D. & Hillier, S. (eds) *Researching Cultural Differences in Health*, London: Routledge.

Kelleher, D. & Hillier, S. (eds) (1996). *Researching Cultural Differences in Health*, London: Routledge.

Kershaw, A. (2005). 'Africans not included', *The Independent*, 4/6/05, pp.12-13.

Kingman, S. (1992). 'Black Students still underrepresented at UK medical schools', *British Medical Journal*, Vol.304, p.66.

King's Fund Equal Opportunities Task Force. (1987). *A Model policy for Equal Opportunities in Employment in the NHS*, London: King Edward's Hospital Fund for London.

King's Fund. (1990).*The Work of the Equal Opportunities Task Force 1986-1990. A Final Report*, King Edward's Hospital Fund for London.

King's Fund. (1990). *Racial equality: the nursing profession. Equal Opportunities Task Force Occasional Paper No.6*, London: King's Fund Centre.

King's Fund. (2001). 'King's Fund calls for urgent action to eradicate racism from medicine', (News), http://www.kingsfund.org.uk/pr010619.html

Kirkpatrick, J. (1999). 'Rage against ageism', *The Guardian*, 31/3/99, p.16.

Kirton, G, & Greene, A.M. (2002). 'The dynamics of positive action in UK trade unions: the case of women and black members', *Industrial Relations Journal*, Jun, Vol.33, No.2, pp.157-172.

Kossek, E.E. & Lobel, S.A. (1996). *Managing Diversity: Human resource strategies for transforming the workplace*, Oxford: Blackwell.

Krause, I.B. (1991) 'Culture trap', *OPENMIND*, No.51, June/July, pp.12-13.

Kundnani, H. (1999). 'Loss of nerve', *The Guardian (Society)*, 8/12/99, pp.6-7

Kurtz, Z. (1993). 'Better health for black and ethnic minority children and young people', in Hopkins, A. & Bahl, V. (eds) *Access to health care for people from black and ethnic minorities*, London: RCP.

Kushnick, L. (1988). 'Racism, the National Health Service, and the Health of Black People', *The International Journal of Health Services*, Vol.18, No.3, pp.457-470.

Lambert, H. & Sevak, L. (1996). 'Is 'cultural difference' a useful concept?: Perceptions of health and the sources of ill health among Londoners of South Asian origin', in Kelleher, D. & Hillier, S. (eds) *Researching Cultural Differences in Health*, London: Routledge.

Larbie, J. (ed) (1988). *The Training Needs of Health Workers in a Multiracial Society*, London: National Extension College.

Lasch-Quinn, E. (2001). Race Experts, London: W.W. Norton & Company.

Laurance, J. (2005). 'Medical staff quit for the West, leaving health service in crisis', *The Independent*, 27/5/05, p.2.

Law, I. (1996). *Racism, Ethnicity and Social Policy*, London: Harvester Wheatsheaf.

Le Grand, J. (1982). *The Strategy of Equality*, London: Allen & Unwin.

Leibel, D.J. (1997). 'NHS must show its true colours', *The Guardian (Letters)*, 10/9/97, p.16.

Leininger, M.M. (ed) (1991). *Culture Care Diversity and Universality: A Theory of Nursing*, New York: National League for Nursing Press.

Leiston, R. & Richardson, J. (1996). 'The ethnicity question', *Journal of Community Nursing*, Vol.10, No.4, April, pp.28-29.

Lester, A. (1996) 'The Politics of the Race Relations Act 1976', *The Runnymede Bulletin*, No.297, 1 September, pp.6-7.

Lester, A. (1998). 'From legislation to integration: twenty years of the Race Relations Act', in Blackstone, T., Parekh, B. & Sanders, P. (eds) *Race Relations in Britain: a developing agenda* London: Longman.

Lethbridge, J. (1993). 'Health promotion and education for black and ethnic minority groups', in Hopkins, A. & Bahl, V. (eds) *Access to health care for people from black and ethnic minorities*, London: RCP.

Lewin, A.E. & Rice, B. (1994). *Balancing the Scales of Opportunity: Ensuring Racial and Ethnic Diversity in the Health Professions*, Washington: National Academy Press.

Lewis, A. (1997). 'Tragedy of 'white' universities', *The Guardian*, 27/5/97, p.17.

Liff, S. (1989). 'Assessing equal opportunities policies', *Personnel Review*, Vol.18, No.1, pp.27-34.

Liff, S. (1996). 'Managing Diversity: New Opportunities For Women', *Warwick Papers in Industrial Relations*, University of Warwick: Coventry.

Linton, M. (1995). 'Poll shows opposition to women-only shortlists', *The Guardian*, 30/9/95, p9.

Lipsedge, M. (1993). 'Mental health: access to care for black and ethnic minority people', in Hopkins, A. & Bahl, V. (eds) *Access to health care for people from black and ethnic minorities*, London: RCP.

Lipsey, D. (1987). 'Big 'no' to positive discrimination', *New Society*, Vol.79, No.1254, 9 January, p.5.

Lipsky, M. (1980). *Street-Level Bureaucracy*, New York: Russell Sage Foundation.

Littlewood, R. (1992). 'Psychiatric diagnosis and racial bias: empirical and interpretative approaches', *Social Science and Medicine*, Vol.34, No.2, pp.141-9.

Littlewood, R. & Lipsedge, M. (1988). 'Psychiatric illness among British Afro-Caribbeans', *British Medical Journal*, Vol.296, pp.950-951.

Lucas, J. (1994). 'Race and culture in Europe', *OpenMind*, No.69, June/July, p/18.

McCormick, A., Charlton, J. & Fleming, D. (1995). 'Who sees their general practitioner and for what reason?', *Health Trends*, Vol.27, No.2, pp.34-35.

MacEwen, M. (1994). 'Anti-Discrimination law in Great Britain', *New Community*, Vol.20, No.3, pp.353-370.

McFarland, E., Dalton, M. & Walsh, D. (1989). 'Ethnic minority needs and service delivery: the barriers to access in a Glasgow inner-city area', *New Community*, Vol.15, No.3, pp.405-415.

McGauran, A. (2000). 'Race lost on points', *Health Service Journal*, Vol.110, No.5710, 22 June, pp.16-17.

McGauran, A. (2001). 'Handle with care', *Health Service Journal*, Vol.111, No.5738, 18 January, pp.16-17.

McGrath, M. (1997). 'For life, liberty and the pursuit of money', *The Guardian (Weekend)*, 2/8/97, pp.15-23.

McIver, S. (1994). *Obtaining the Views of Black Users of Health Services*, London: King's Fund Centre.

McKeigue, P.M., Richards, J.D.M. & Richards, P. (1990). 'Effects of discrimination by sex and race on early careers of British medical graduates during 1981-7', *British Medical Journal*, Vol.301, pp.961-964.

McLaughlin, E. & Murji, K. (1999). 'After the Stephen Lawrence Report', *Critical Social Policy*, Vol.19, No.3, August, pp.371-385.

McManus, I.C. (1998). 'Factors affecting the likelihood of applicants being offered a place in medical schools in the UK in 1996 and 1997: retrospective study', *British Medical Journal*, Vol.317, pp.1111-1117.

McManus, I.C. & Richards, P. (1984). 'Audit of admission to medical school: I - Acceptances and rejects', *British Medical Journal*, Vol.289, pp.1201-4.

McManus, I.C., Richards, P. & Maitlis, S.L. (1989). 'Prospective study of the disadvantage of people from ethnic minority groups applying to medical schools in the United Kingdom', *British Medical Journal*, Vol.298, pp.723-6.

McManus, I.C., Richards, P., Winder, B.C., Sproston, K.A. & Styles, V. (1995). 'Medical school applicants from ethnic minority groups: identifying if and when they are disadvantaged', *British Medical Journal*, Vol.310, pp.496-500.

McNaught, A. (1987). *Health Action and Ethnic Minorities*, London: Bedford Square Press.

McNaught, A. (1988). *Race and Health Policy*, London: Croon Helm.

MacPherson, W. R., Rt Hon the Lord (1999). *The Stephen Lawrence Inquiry*. London: HMSO, http://www.official-documents.co.uk/document/cm42/4262/sli-00.htm.

Madden, M.S. (1994). 'Nursing in the years to come', *World Health*, No.5, September-October, pp.34-35.

Major, L.E. (1998). 'Emergency wealth check', *The Guardian (Higher)*, 1/9/98, p.vi.

Malek, B. (1997). 'Not Such Tolerant Times', *Soundings*, Issue 6, pp.140-152.

Malone, A. & Byrne, C. (1998). 'Constituencies defy Blair on women MPs', *The Mail on Sunday*, 12/2/98 p.10.

Marable, M. (1995). *Beyond Black and White*, London: Verso.

Markham, G. (1996). 'Gender in leadership', *Nursing Times*, Vol.3, No.1, April, pp.18-19.

Mason, D. (1990). 'A rose by any other name...? Categorisation, identity and social science', *New Community*, Vol.17, No.1, October, pp.123-133.

Mason, D. (1990). 'Competing Conceptions of 'Fairness' and the Formulation and Implementing of Equal Opportunity Policies, in Ball, W. & Solomos, J. (eds) *Race and Local Politics*, London: Macmillan.

Mason, D. (2000). *Race and Ethnicity in Modern Britain (2nd ed)*, Oxford: Oxford University Press.

Matheson, K., Echenburg, A., Taylor, D.M., Rivers, D. & Chow, I. (1994). 'Women's Attitudes Towards Affirmative Action: Putting Actions in Context', *Journal of Applied Social Psychology*, Vol.24, No.23, pp.2075-2096.

Mavunga, P. (1992). 'Probation: A Basically Racist Service', in Gelsthorpe, L. (ed) *Minority Ethnic Groups in the Criminal Justice System: papers presented to the 21st Cropwood Roundtable Conference, 1992*, Cambridge: University of Cambridge.

May, T. (1993). *Social Research: Issues, Methods and Processes*, Buckingham: Open University Press.

Mehta, G. (1993). 'The ethnic elderly', *Journal of Community Nursing*, March, pp.16-20.

Meikle, J. (1997a). 'Civil unrest warning', *The Guardian*, 5/3/97, p.9.

Meikle, J. (1997b). 'Time for 'home truths'', *The Guardian (Society)*, 26/11/97, pp.2-3.

378

Meikle, J. (2001). 'Milburn to pledge big rise in NHS staff', *The Guardian*, 15/2/01, p.5.

Mensah, J. (1996). 'Everybody's problem', *Nursing Times*, Vol.92, No.22, May 29, pp.26-27.

Merrill, J. (1989). 'Attempted Suicide by Deliberate Self-Poisoning Amongst Asians', in Cox, J.L. & Bostock, S. (eds) *Racial Discrimination in the Health Service*, Staffordshire: Penrhos.

Miles, R. (1989). *Racism*, London: Routledge.

Millar, B. (1997). 'Cell out', *Health Service Journal*, Vol.107, No.5540, 13th February 1997, p.12.

Millar, B. (1997). 'Rocky road to equal rights', *Health Service Journal*, Vol.106, No.5542, p.14.

Miller, B. & Crail, M. (1998). 'The human touch', *Health Service Journal*, Vol.109, No.5624, 1 October, pp.11-12.

Miller, B. & Crail, M. (1998). 'New strategy gets warm welcome, but doubts remain', *Health Service Journal*, Vol.109, No.5624, 1 October, pp.12-13.

Miller, J. & Glassner, B. (1997). 'The 'Inside' and the 'Outside': Finding Realities in Interviews', in Silverman, D. (ed) *Qualitative Research: Theory, Method and Practice*, London: Sage.

Mind. (1994). *Directory of Mental Health Services 1994*, London: Longman.

Mitchell, S. (2000). 'Local police force unwittingly proves that racism is not taken seriously', *The Big Issue* (South West), No.333, 3-4 May, pp.4-5.

Modood, T. (1988). 'Black', racial equality and Asian identity', *New Community*, Vol.14, No.3, pp.397-404.

Modood, T. (1997). 'Employment', in Modood, T. & Berthoud, R. (eds) *Ethnic Minorities in Britain*, London: PSI.

Modood, T. (1998). 'Ethnic diversity and racial disadvantage in employment', in Blackstone, T., Parekh, B. & Sanders, P. (eds) *Race Relations in Britain: a developing agenda*, London: Longman.

Modood, T. & Berthoud, R. (eds) (1997). *Ethnic Minorities in Britain*, London: PSI.

Moore, A. (2003). 'A gender for change', *Health Service Journal*, 13/11/03, p.15.

Moore, W. (1996). 'Like speaking unto like?', *Health Service Journal*, 3 October, pp.24-27.

Moore, W. (1998). 'Self service', *The Guardian (G2)*, 25/3/98, pp.2-3.

Morgan, D.L. & Kreuger, R.A. (1993). 'When to Use Focus Groups and Why', in Morgan, D.L. (ed) *Successful Focus Groups. Advancing the State of the Art*, London: Sage.

Morris, N. (2005). 'Research shows immigration boosts economy', The Independent, 14/5/05, p18.

Mwasamdube, P. & Mullen, C. (1998). *Survey of Ethnically Sensitive Services in the NHS Executive South & West Region*, Portsmouth NHS Trust.

National Association of Health Authorities (NAHA). (1988). *Action not Words*, Birmingham: NAHA.

National Association of Health Authorities and Trusts. (NAHAT). (1996/7). *NHS Handbook 1996/7*, London: HMSO.

NAHAT & King's Fund Centre. (1993). *Equality Across the Board*, London: King's Fund Centre.

National Health Service Confederation (2004). *Briefing*, Issue 107, September, London: NHS Confederation.

National Health Service Executive (NHSE). (1994*). Collection of ethnic group data for admitted patients*, EL(94) 77, London: HMSO.

NHSE. (1998). *Working Together: Securing a quality workforce for the NHS*, London: HMSO.

NHSE. (1999). *The NHS Performance Assessment Framework*, London: HMSO.

National Health Service Management Executive (NHSME). (1991a). *Assessing health care needs*, London: DoH.

NHSME. (1991b). *Moving forward – needs, services and contracts*, EL(91)(40), London: DoH.

NHSME. (1992a). *Health Service guidelines – meeting the spiritual needs of patients and staff*, HSG(92)2, London: NHSME.

NHSME. (1992b). *Local voices – the views of local people in purchasing for health*, London: NHSME.

NHSME. (1993). *Ethnic Minority Staff in the NHS. A Programme for Action*, London: NHSME.

National Health Service Training Authority (NHSTA). (1989). *Equal Opportunities. A Management Guide to the Implementation of a Strategy*, Bristol: NHSTA.

Nakajima, H. (1996). 'Editorial: Culture and health', *World Health*, No.2, March-April, p.3.

National Association of Care and Resettlement of Offenders (NACRO). (1992). *Race Policies into Action. The Implementation of equal Opportunities Policies in the Criminal Justice Agencies*, London: NACRO.

Nazroo, J.Y. (1997). *The Health of Britain's Ethnic Minorities*, London: PSI.

Nelson, P. (1990). 'Equal opportunities: dilemmas, contradictions, white men and class', *Critical Social Policy*, Issue 28, Summer, pp.25-42.

Neuberger, J. (1987). *Caring for Dying People of Different Faiths*, London: Austen Cornish.

Newman, J. (1994). 'The Limits of Management: Gender and the Politics of Change', in Clarke, J., Cochrane, A. & McLaughlin, E. (eds). *Managing Social Policy*, London: Sage.

Nguyen-Van-Tam, J., Simpson, J., Madeley, R. & Davies, L. (1995). 'Health care experiences of Vietnamese families in Nottingham', *Health Trends*, Vol.27, No.4, pp.106-110.

Nickel, J.W. (1979). 'Preferential Policies in Hiring and Admissions: A Jurisprudential Approach', in Wasserstrom, R.A. (ed) *Today's Moral Problems*, London: Collier Macmillan.

380

Nickel, J.W. (1990). 'Strong Affirmative Action', *New Community*, Vol.17, No.4, October, pp.49-58.

Noon, M. & Ogbonna, E. (eds) (2001). *Equality, Diversity and Disadvantage in Employment*, Basingstoke: Palgrave.

Norton-Taylor, R. (1998). 'Military 'must wage war' on racism', *The Guardian*, 11/11/98, p.8.

Nursing Times. (1995). 'School bridges ethnic divide', Vol.91, No.39, p.6.

Oakley, A. (1981). 'Interviewing women: a contradiction in terms', in Roberts, H. (ed) *Doing Feminist Research*, London: Routledge.

Office of National Statistics (ONS). (1999). *Britain 1999. The Official Yearbook of the United Kingdom*, London: HMSO.

Office of Population and Census Studies (OPCS). (1993). *Ethnic Group of Residents*, London: OPCS.

O'Donnell, M. (1992). Your Good Health?' *Sociology Review*, September, pp.22-25.

OpenMind. (1993). 'Bid to tackle raw deal for minority ethnic communities', No.63, June/July, p.7.

OpenMind. (1994). 'The Islamic path to inner health', No.69, June/July, pp.13-14.

OpenMind. (1995). 'Black People in Mind', No.78, December 1995/January 1996, p.21.

OpenMind. (1997) 'Launch of African/Caribbean Users Forum', No.83 January/February, p.4.

Osler, A. (1997). 'Any career prospects?', *The Guardian (Education)*, 4/11/97, p.6.

Ouseley, H. (1995). 'Talent spotting', *The Guardian (Careers)*, 25/2/95, pp.2-3.

Owen, D. (1994). *Ethnic Minority Women and the Labour Market: Analysis of the 1991 Census*, Manchester: EOC.

Pandya, N. (1997). 'Why equal opportunities initiatives are sideshow to the main event', *The Guardian (Jobs)*, 23/3/97, pp.26-27.

Pandya, N. (1999). 'Public sector recruitment targets extended', *The Guardian (Jobs)*, 31/7/99, p.17.

Pandya, N. (1999). 'Drive to get ethnic minorities in the boardroom', *The Guardian (G2)*, 11/9/99, p.3.

Parekh, B. (1986). 'The 'New Right' and the Politics of Nationhood', in *The New Right: image and reality*, London: The Runnymede Trust.

Parekh, B. (1992).'The case for positive discrimination', in Hepple, B. & Szyszczak, E.M. (eds.) *Discrimination: the Limits of the Law*, London: Mansell Publishing.

Parekh, B. (1998). 'Integrating minorities', in Blackstone, T., Parekh, B. & Sanders, P. (eds) *Race Relations in Britain: a developing agenda*, London: Longman.

Parekh, B. (2000). *The Future of Multi-Ethnic Britain*, London: Profile Books.

Parsons, L., McFarlane, A. & Golding, J. (1993). 'Pregnancy, birth and maternity care', in Ahmad, W.I.U. (ed) *Race and Health in Contemporary Britain*, Buckingham: Open University Press.

Patel, N. (1993). 'Healthy margins: Black elders' care. Models, policies and prospects', in Ahmad, W.I.U. (ed) *'Race' and Health in Contemporary Britain*, Buckingham: Open University Press.

Patton, L. (1997). 'Widespread bias against Asians in civil service', *The Guardian*, 13/10/97, p.11.

Payne, D. (1995). 'Racism widespread in wards and jobs', *Nursing Times*, Vol.91, No.45, pp.8-9.

Pearson, M. (1986). 'The politics of ethnic minority health studies', in Rathwell, T. & Phillips, D. (eds) *Health Race & Ethnicity*, London: Croon Helm.

Pearson, M. (1987). 'Racism: The Great Divide', *Nursing Times*, Vol.17, No.24, 17 June, pp.25-26.

Penketh, L. & Ali, Y. (1997). 'Racism and Social Welfare', in Lavalette, m. & Pratt, A. (eds), *Social Policy. A Conceptual and Theoretical Introduction*, London: Sage.

Pennicott, E. (1997). 'Reading Identity: Young Black British Men', *Soundings*, Issue 6, pp.153-162.

Peterson, R.S. (1994). 'The Role of Values in Predicting Fairness Judgements and Support of Affirmative Action', *Journal of Social Issues*, Vol.50, No.4, pp.95-115.

Phillips, M. & Phillips, T. (1998). 'Black and British', *The Guardian (Weekend)*, 16/5/99, pp.38-46.

Phillips, E.M. & Pugh, D.S. (1994). *How To Get a PhD: A handbook for students and their supervisors (2nd ed)*, Buckingham: Open University Press.

Phillips, D. & Rathwell, T. (1986). 'Ethnicity and Health: Introduction and Definitions', in Rathwell, T. & Phillips, D. (eds) *Health Race & Ethnicity*, London: Croon Helm.

Phillips, A. (1999). *Which Equalities Matter?*, Cambridge: Polity Press.

Phillips, T. (1997). 'Let culture collide with culture', *The Guardian (Media)*, 13/10/97, pp.6-7.

Phillips, T. (1999). 'Rooting out racism', *The Guardian*, 8/12/99, p.22.

Phillips, T. (2004). 'Diversity no charity case', *Health Service Journal*, 30/9/04, p.26.

Potrykus, C. (1994). 'Government tackles NHS race barriers', *Health Visitor*, Vol.67, No.2, February, p.45.

Potrykus, C. (1994). 'Victimisation challenge', *Health Visitor*, Vol.67, No.2, February, p.45.

Practice Nurse. (1997). 'Training programme to expand smear uptake', Vol.8, No.15, 23 September, p.10.

Pressley, S.A. (1997). 'Ruling makes minorities feel unwanted on campus', *The Guardian*, 2/9/97, p.15.

Proctor, E.K. & Davis, L.E. (1994). 'The Challenge of Racial Difference: Skills for clinical Practice', *Social Work*, Vol.39, No.3, pp.314-323.

Rae, D. (1981). *Equalities*, Cambridge, MA: Harvard University Press.

Ragin, C. (1994). *Constructing Social Research*, London: Pine Forge Press.

Rao, J. & Ramaiah, S. (2000). 'Lip service', *Health Service Journal*, 6 April, p.30.

Rathwell, T. & Phillips, D. (1986). 'Ethnicity and Health: An Agenda for Progressive Action!', in Rathwell, T. & Phillips, D. (eds) *Health Race & Ethnicity*, London: Croon Helm.

Rauyajin, O. & Yoddumnern-Attig, B. (1993). 'Social cost of maternal deaths', *World Health*, No.3, May-June 1993, pp.18-19.

Rawaf, S. (1993) 'Purchasing for the health of black and ethnic minority people: some practical considerations', in Hopkins, A. & Bahl, V. (eds) *Access to health care for people from black and ethnic minorities*, London: RCP.

Rawaf, S. & Bahl, V. (1998) (eds). *Assessing the Health Needs of People from Minority Ethnic Groups*, London: RCN.

Rayner, C. (1998). 'Instead of a truly national charter for patient's rights, all we have is yet another dose of garbage-can management', *The Observer*, 13/12/98, p.31.

Reed, C. (1995). 'University scraps affirmative action', *The Guardian*, 22/7/1995, p.2.

Reed, C. (1996). 'University discriminated in favour of rich students', *The Guardian*, 22/3/96, p.12.

Reesal-Hussain, N. (1989). 'In a Critical Condition ‐ A Diagnosis of the National Health Service Equal Opportunities Policies', in Cox, J. & Bostock, S. (eds) *Racial Discrimination in the Health Service*, Staffordshire: Penrhos.

Rehman, H. & Walker, E. (1995). 'Researching black and minority ethnic groups', *Health Education Journal*, Vol.54, pp.489-500.

Renn, M. (1987). 'One Step Forward...?', *Nursing Times*, Vol.83, No.24, 17 June, pp.30-31.

Rentoul, J. (1995). 'Pressure grows on Labour over all-women lists', *The Observer*, 24/9/95, p.2.

Rex, J. (1968). 'The Race Relations Catastrophe', in *Matters of principle. Labour's last chance*, London: Penguin.

Richards, J.R. (1994). *The Sceptical Feminist (2nd ed)*, London: Routledge & Kegan Paul.

Robbins, D. (1982). 'Affirmative action in the USA: A lost opportunity?', *New Community*, Vol.8, No.3, Winter 1981/Spring 1982, pp.399-406.

Robinson, M.R.D. (1987). 'Towards racial equality in health and welfare: what progress?', *New Community*, Vol.14, No.1/2, Autumn, pp.128-136.

Robinson, R.K.,McClure, G. & Terpstra, G. (1994). 'Diversity in the '90s: avoid conflict with EEO laws', *Human Resources Focus*, Vol.71, No.1, January, p.9.

Robson, C. (1993). *Real World Research*, Oxford: Blackwell.

Rocheron, Y. (1988). 'The Asian Mother and Baby Campaign', *Critical Social Policy*, Vol.22, pp.4-23.

Rose, D. (1997). 'A black mark for justice', *The Observer*, 20/4/97, p.31.

Rosewell, R. (1996). 'The Liberals happy to see blacks suffer', *The Mail on Sunday*, 11/8/96, p.33.

Ross, R. & Schneider, R. (1992). *From Equality to Diversity*, London: Pitman.

Rowden, R. (1990). 'Colouring Attitudes', *Nursing Times*, Vol.86, No.24, 13 June, pp.47-48.

Rowe, A. (1995). 'Two way stretch', *The Guardian*, 30/10/95, p.12.

Rubenstein, M. (1986). 'Positive action and positive discrimination', *EOR*, No.10, November/December, p.40.

Rudat, K. (1994). *Black and Minority Ethnic Groups in England: Health and Lifestyles*, London: HEA.

Runnymede Bulletin. (1996). 'Reviewing the 1976 Act', No.297, 1 September, p.5.

Russell, M. (2001). 'Quotas are good for democracy', *The Guardian*, 5/7/01, p.19.

Saggar, S. (1993). 'The politics of race policy in Britain', *Critical Social Policy*, Vol.37, pp.32-51.

Sagovsky, R. (1989). 'Career Survey of Overseas Psychiatrists', in Cox, J. & Bostock, S. (eds) *Racial Discrimination in the Health Service*, Staffordshire: Penrhos.

Sanders, P. (1998). 'Tackling racial discrimination', in Blackstone, T., Parekh, B. & Sanders, P. (eds) *Race Relations in Britain: a developing agenda*, London: Longman.

Sashidhran, S.P. (1997). 'NHS must show its true colours', *The Guardian (Letters page)*, 10/9/97, p.16.

Sardar, Z. (1999). '...and nor is demonising the Met', *New Statesman*, 5 March, p.21.

Sashidharan, S.P. & Francis, E. (1993). 'Epidemiology, ethnicity and schizophrenia', in Ahmad, W.I.U. (ed) *Race and Health in Contemporary Britain*, Buckingham: Open University Press.

Sassoon, M. (1993). 'A voice for black users', *OpenMind*, No.62, April/May, p.25.

Saunders, P. (1996). *Unequal But Fair? A Study of Class Barriers in Britain*, London: Institute of Economic Affairs.

Scarman, L.G. (1982). *The Scarman Report: the Brixton disorders 10-12 April 1981; report of an inquiry*, Harmondsworth: Penguin.

Schneider, R. & Ross, R. (2002). *The Business of Diversity*, London: HMSO.

Seidman, I.E. (1991). *Interviewing as Qualitative Research*, New York: Teachers College Press.

Sell, H.L. (1996). 'Ritual and culture', *World Health*, No.2, March-April, p.13.

Shannon, C. (2004). 'Equal measures', *Health Service Journal*, 29/1/04, p.16.

Sharda, A. (1993). 'Purchasing for the health of black and minority ethnic people: some theoretical considerations', in Hopkins, A. & Bahl, V. (eds) *Access to health care for people from black and ethnic minorities*, London: RCP.

Sheldon, T.A. & Parker, H. (1992). 'Race and ethnicity in health research', *Journal of Public Health Medicine*, Vol.14, pp.104-110.

Sher, G. (1979). 'Justifying Reverse Discrimination in Employment', in Rachels, J. (ed) *Moral Problems*, New York: Harper & Row.

Shipman, M.D. (1972). *The Limitations of Social Research*, London: Longman.

Silverman, D. (ed) (1997). *Qualitative Research: Theory, Method and Practice*, London: Sage.

Singh, R. (1990). 'Ethnic Minority Experience in Higher Education', *Higher Education Quarterly*, Vol.44, No.4, Autumn, pp.344-359.

Sivanandan, A. (1976). 'Race, class and the state: the Black experience in Britain', *Race and Class*, Vol.17, No.4, pp.347-368.

Sivanandan, A. (1982). *A Different Hunger*, London: Pluto Press.

Sivanadan, A. (1983). 'Challenging racism: strategies for the '80s', *Race & Class*, Vol.25, No.2, pp.3-11.

Sivanadan, A. (1995) 'La trahison des clercs', *The Newstatesman & Society*, 14 July, pp.20-22.

Skellington, R. (1996). *'Race' in Britain Today (2nd Edition)*, London: Sage.

Sly, F., Thair, T. & Risdon, A. (1999). 'Trends in the labour market participation of ethnic groups', *Labour Market Trends*, Vol.107, No.12, December, pp.631-639.

Smaje, C. (1995). *Health 'Race' and Ethnicity*, London: King's Fund Institute.

Smaje, C. (1996). 'The Ethnic Patterning of Health: New Directions for Theory and Research', *Sociology of Health and Illness*, Vol.18, No.2, pp.139-171.

Smaje, C. & Le Grand, J. (1997). 'Ethnicity, Equity and the Use of the Health Services in the British NHS', *Social Science and Medicine*, Vol.45, No.3, pp.485-496.

Smith, D.J. (1980). *Overseas Doctors in the NHS*, London: PSI.

Smith, R. (1987). 'Prejudice against doctors and students from ethnic minorities', *British Medical Journal*, Vol.294, pp.328-329.

Smith, M. (2005). 'Recruits face three-year wait to join the police...because they're white', *The Mail on Sunday*, 8/5/05, p15.

Smith, K. & Dickson, M. (1998). 'Silent majority', *Health Service Journal*, Vol.108, No.5635, 17 December, p.33

Smithers, R. (1996). 'Blair may scrap final all-women selections after ruling', *The Guardian*, 10/1/96, p.8

Smithers, R. (2001). 'Apartheid claim over Islam school', *The Guardian*, 10/2/01, p.5.

Snell, J. (1996). 'Warning: racism at work', *Nursing Times*, Vol.92, No.22, 29 May, pp.30-32.

Solomos, J. (1989). 'Equal Opportunities Policies and Racial Inequality: The Role of Public Policy', *Public Administration*, Vol.67, Spring, pp.79-93.

Solomos, J. & Back, L. (1994). 'Conceptualising Racisms: Social Theory, Politics and Research', *Sociology*, Vol.28, No.1, pp.143-161.

Sowell, T. (1994). 'Lucrative bigotry', *Forbes*, Vol.153, No.10, 9 May, p.117.

Sowell,T. (1996a). 'Vitriolic facts: blaming emotional reactions for truths', *Forbes*, Vol.158, No.12, 18 November, p.52.

Sowell, T. (1996b). 'The right to be wrong', *Forbes*, Vol.157, No.12, p.50.

Sowell, T. (1997). 'How 'affirmative action' hurts blacks. (it casts suspicions on legitimate black achievement and otherwise depicts them as incapable)', *Forbes*, Vol.160, No.7, 6 October, p.64.

Sperling, L. (1997). 'Quango's: Political Representation & Women Consumers of Public Services', *Policy and Politics*, Vol.25, No.2, April, pp.112-127.

Stephens, F. (2001). 'Positive moves to end inequality', *NHS Magazine*, July/August, pp.22-23.

Stone, M. (1981). *The Education of the Black Child in Britain*, London: Fontana.

Strauss, A. & Corbin, J. (1997). *Grounded Theory in Practice*, London: Sage.

Strauss, A. & Corbin, J. (1998). *Basics of Qualitative Research. Techniques and Procedures for Developing Grounded Theory (2nd ed)*, London: Sage.

Straw, J. (1999). 'Ethnic minority targets set for police', EOR, No.85, May/June, pp.21-24.

Streeter, M. (1997). 'Irvine calls for more black judges', The Independent, 29/11/97, p.9.

Stubbs, P. (1993). 'Ethnically sensitive' or 'anti-racist'? Models for health research and service delivery', in Ahmad, W.I.U. (ed) *'Race' and Health in Contemporary Britain*, Buckingham: Open University Press.

Tam, S.T. (1994). 'The Politics of Race Research: A Chinese Case Study', *Research Policy & Planning*, Vol.12, No.2, pp.13-17.

Tanna, K. (1990). 'Excellence, equality and educational reform: the myth of South Asian achievement levels', *New Community*, Vol.16, No.3, pp.349-368.

Tarkka, M.T. & Paunonen, M. (1996). 'Social support provided by nurses to recent mothers on a maternity ward', *Journal of Advanced Nursing*, Vol.23, No.6, June, pp.1202-1206.

Tate, C.W. (1996). 'Minority networks', *Nursing Management*, Vol.3, No.1, April, p.7.

Tate, C.W. (1996) 'Race into action', *Nursing Times*, Vol.92, No.22, May, pp.28-30.

Taylor, J. (1997). 'The racist double standard: how whites are made to feel guilty & "hateful" for loving their own people and culture', *http://www.stormfront. org.*

Taylor, L. (1999). 'Off Cuts', *The Guardian (Society)*, 28/7/99, p.6.

Taylor, M.C. (1995). 'White Backlash to Workplace Affirmative Action: Peril or Myth?', *Social Forces*, Vol.73, No.4, June, pp.1385-1414.

Taylor, P. (1992). 'Ethnic Group Data and Applications to Higher Education', *Higher Education Quarterly*, Vol.46, No.4, Autumn, pp.359-374.

386

Teicher, J. & Spearitt, K. (1996). 'From equal employment opportunity to diversity management', *International Journal of manpower*, Vol.17, No.4/5, pp.109-133.

Terkel, S. (1992). *Race*, London: Minerva.

The Economist. (1991). 'The Quota Question', 30 November, pp.51-52.

The Economist. (1995a). 'Affirmative action: why bosses like it', 11 March, p.65.

The Economist. (1995b). 'America's 30-year itch', 4 March, p.14.

The Economist. (1995c). 'In black and white', 22 July, pp.47-48.

The Economist. (1995d). 'Poisoned Chalice', 26 August, p.42.

The Economist. (1995e). 'Fighting over favouritism', 17 February, pp.51-52.

The Economist. (1997). 'The hard fact: race and education', 4 October, p.32

The Guardian. (1996). 'Applications for university down 2%', 16/2/96, p.6.

The Guardian. (1997). 'Tackling the white ceiling: where are the blacks and Asians in government?', 22/7/97, p.16.

The Guardian. (1997). 'Army's anti-racist drive', 10/10/97, p.4.

The Guardian. (1998). 'Black suicides climbing', 21/3/98, p.21.

The Guardian. (1998). 'Staff quit NHS', 4/9/98, p.10.

The Independent. (1997). 'Court helps women shatter glass ceilings', 12/11/97, p.15.

The Observer. (1998). 'Race Canard', 21/6/98, p.24.

The Independent. (1999). 'There can be no apartheid within the health service', 8/7/99, p.3.

Thompson, N. (1993). *Anti-discriminatory Practice*, London: Macmillan.

Thompson, N. (1998). *Promoting Equality*, Hampshire: PALGRAVE.

Thorogood, N. (1989). 'Afro-Caribbean women's experience of the health service', *New Community*, Vol.15, No.3, pp.319-334.

Thorogood, N. (1992). 'Private medicine: 'you pays your money and gets your treatment'', *Sociology of Health and Illness*, Vo.14, No.1, pp.23-38.

Titmuss, R. (1962). *Income Distribution and Social Change*, London: Allen & Unwin.

Torkington, P. (1987). 'Sorry, Wrong Colour', *Nursing Times*, Vol.83, No.24, 13 June, pp.27-28.

Torkington, P. (1991). *Black Health: A Political Issue*, London & Liverpool: Catholic Association for Racial Justice/Liverpool Institute of Higher Education.

Townsend, P. & Davidson, N. (1982). Inequalities in Health: The Black Report, Harmondsworth: Penguin.

Toynbee, P. (2000). 'An end to waiting – that's a promise to the health service', *The Guardian*, 31/5/00, p.22.

Tran, M. (1997). 'Affirmative action faces court test', *The Guardian*, 6/10/97, p.10.

Travis, A. (1997). 'Straw sets up race inquiry, *The Guardian*, 25/7/97, p.2.

Travis, A. (1998). 'Rainbow alliance', *The Guardian (Society)*, 4/2/98, pp.2-3.

Travis, A. (1999). 'Words of hope', *The Guardian (Society)*, 14/4/99, pp.6-7.

Tarvis, A. (1999). 'Anger at block on equality reforms', *The Guardian*, 17/11/99.

Travis, A. & Rowan, D. (1997). 'A beacon burning darkly', *The Guardian*, 12/10/97, p.17.

Tully, M. (2005).'The army history forgot', *The Independent*, 3/6/05, pp.16-17.

Urban, M. (1999). 'Which is the true face of England?', *The Guardian (2)*, 5/5/99, p.12.

Wainwright, M. (1999). 'Hidden racism triggered by hard times', *The Guardian (Jobs)*, 17/7/99, p.21.

Walby, S. & Greenwell, J. (1994). 'Managing the National Health Service', in Clarke, J., Cochrane, A. & McLaughlin, E. (eds) *Managing Social Policy*, London: Sage.

Walker, M. (1997). 'God Bless (white) America', *The Guardian*, 17/5/97, p.5.

Walker, S., Spohn, C. & DeLonc, M. (1996). *The Colour of Justice: Race, Ethnicity and Crime in America*, London: Wadsworth.

Walmsley, J., Reynolds, J., Shakespeare, P. & Woolfe, R. (eds) (1993). *Health, Welfare and Practice*, London: Sage.

Walters, N. (1997). 'They thought they could change politics. Perhaps politics has changed them...', *The Observer*, 30/11/97, p.7.

Ward, L. (1993). 'Race equality and employment in the National Health Service', in Ahmad, W.I.U. (ed) *'Race' and Health in Contemporary Britain*, Buckingham: Open University Press.

Ward, L. (1998). 'Middle-age white men fill the council chambers', *The Guardian*, 20/3/98, p.8.

Wasserstrom, R.A. (ed) (1975). *Today's Moral Problems*, London: Collier Macmillan.

Watt, N. (1998). 'Police must reach black recruit goal', *The Guardian*, 19/10/98, p.7.

Watt, N. (1999). 'New candidate for London mayor', *The Guardian*, 15/3/99, p.2.

Watt, N. (2000). 'Race row as rightwinger joins Tory home affairs team', *The Guardian*, 26/7/00, p.12.

Wavell, S. (1995). 'Wrestling for an equal share', *The Sunday Times*, 26/3/95, pp.8-10.

Weale, A. (1978). *Equality and Social Policy*, London: Routledge and Kegan Paul.

Weale, A. (1983). *Political Theory and Social Policy*, London: Macmillan.

Weale, S. (1995). 'Equal last', *The Guardian (G2)*, 20/6/95, pp.2-4.

Webb, J. & Liff, S. (1988). 'Play the white man: the social construction of fairness and competition in equal opportunity policies', *The Sociological Review*, Vol.36, August, pp.532-551.

Weir, M. (1993). 'From equal opportunity to 'the new social contract': race and the politics in the United States', in Cross. M. & Keith, M. (eds) *Racism, the City and the State*, London: Routledge.

Weissberg, R. (1993). 'The gypsy scholars', *Forbes*, Vol.151, No.10, p.138.

Weston, D. & Welsh, A. (2003). 'Chapter and Diverse', *Health Service Journal*, 1/5/03, p.30.

Westwood, S. (1994). 'Racism, Mental Illness and the Politics of Identity', in Rattansi, A. & Westwood, S. (eds) *Racism, Modernity and Identity: on the Western Front*, Cambridge: Polity.

Wilkinson, B. (1991). 'Sexual harassment: an organisational challenge', *EOR*, No.36, March/April, pp.9-13.

Williams, F. (1989). *Social Policy: A Critical Introduction*, Cambridge: Polity.

Willmott, J. (1996). 'Poor recognition, poorer services for black women', *OpenMind*, No.81, September/October, pp.8-9.

Wilson, M. (1996). 'In the Black', *Health Service Journal*, 7 March, p.29.

Winant, H. (1993) 'Difference and inequality: postmodern racial politics in the United States', in Cross. M. & Keith, M. (eds) *Racism, the City and the State*, London: Routledge.

Wintour, P. (1998). 'Straw acts to boost ranks of black police', *The Observer*, 18/10/98, p.12.

Wintour, P. (2000). 'Whitehall mandarins 'balking' black staff', *The Guardian*, 15/4/00, p.7.

Wintour, P. (2000). 'Police fail on ethnic minority targets', *The Guardian*, 3/8/00, p.13.

Woolley, S. (2005). 'No party can take black voters for granted', *The Independent*, 15/4/05, p43.

Woolf, M. (2005). 'Britain has a 'disgraceful' record on ethnic-minority candidates', *The Independent*, 28/4/05, p.22.

Workforce Directorate. (2004). *Sharing the Challenge, Sharing the benefits. Equality and Diversity in the Medical Workforce*, London: DoH.

Worsthorne, P. (1999). 'Thought control is not the answer', *New Statesman*, 5 March, p.20.

Wrench, J. (2005). 'Diversity management can be bad for you', *Race and Class*, Jan-Mar, Vol.46, No.3, pp.73-84.

Young, R. (1986). 'Affirmative Action and the Problem of Substantive Racism', in Combs, M.V. & Gruhl, J. (eds) *Affirmative Action: Theory, Analysis and Prospects*, USA: McFarland.

Younge, G. (1997). 'Heroes of my generation', *The Guardian*, 31/7/97, p.17.

Younge, G. (2000). 'Stars and bars', *The Guardian*, 9/10/00, p.19.

Younge, G. (2001). 'What was that all about?', *The Guardian*, 26/4/01, p.19.

INDEX